Progress in Epileptic Disorders
Volume 13

**Seizures and Syndromes
of onset in the
Two First Years of Life**

Progress in Epileptic Disorders series
International Advisory Board

Alexis Arzimanoglou – Lyon, France
Jean Aicardi – Paris, France
Ingmar Blümcke – Erlangen, Germany
François Dubeau – Montreal, Canada
Michael Duchowny – Miami, USA
Aristea Galanopoulou – New York, USA
Alexander Hammers – London, UK
Yushi Inoue – Shizuoka, Japan
Philippe Kahane – Grenoble, France
Michael Kerr – Cardiff, UK
Silvia Kochen – Buenos Aires, Argentina
Carla Marini – Florence, Italy
Doug Nordli – Chicago, USA
Graeme Sills – Liverpool, UK
Pierre Thomas – Nice, France
Torbjörn Thomson – Stockholm, Sweden
Sarah Wilson – Melbourne, Australia

**Progress in Epileptic Disorders
Volume 13**

Seizures and Syndromes of onset in the Two First Years of Life

*Solomon L. Moshé
J. Helen Cross
Julitta de Bellescize
Linda de Vries
Douglas Nordli
Federico Vigevano*

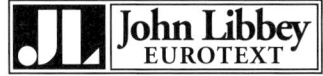

Disclosures and Acknowledgements

Proceedings of the international *Progress in Epileptic Disorders Workshop* on Seizures and Syndromes of onset in the first two years of life that took place at Grottaferrata, at the outskirts of Rome, Italy, in November 14th to 17th, 2013.

The workshop was organized by the journal *EPILEPTIC DISORDERS, Educational Journal of the ILAE*. It was supported by an unrestricted educational grant from UCB. The research association "Association ESEFNP" independently managed the grant. All participants were selected by the scientific committee on the basis of their expertise in the field and their competence in contributing to a highly interactive, collaborative and forward-looking workshop.

UCB was not involved in the content of the symposium or preparation of the proceedings; an honorarium was not provided to speakers, chairs, authors or other participating experts. All organizational issues were under the responsibility of ANT CONGRES.
The John Libbey Eurotext editions independently supported the present publication.

ANT CONGRES, the John Libbey Eurotext editions and UCB are acknowledged for their contribution to the success of the workshop and the present publication.

ISBN: 978-2-7420-1397-5
ISSN: 1777-4284
Vol. 13

Published by
Éditions John Libbey Eurotext
127, avenue de la République, 92120 Montrouge, France
Tel.: +33 (0)1 46 73 06 60
Website: www.jle.com

John Libbey Eurotext
42-46 High Street, Esther, Surrey, KT10 9KY
United Kingdom

© 2015, John Libbey Eurotext. All rights reserved.

Unauthorized duplication contravenes applicable laws.
It is prohibited to reproduce this work or any part of it without authorisation of the publisher or of the Centre Français d'Exploitation du Droit de Copie (CFC), 20, rue des Grands-Augustins, 75006 Paris.

Contents

Preface VII

Workshop participants IX

List of authors XI

SEIZURES AND SYNDROMES IN NEONATES

Foundations of neonatal epileptology: classification of seizures and epilepsies in the neonate and their etiology, electroencephalography, prognosis and pathophysiology
  Eli M. Mizrahi, Ronit M. Pressler 1

EEG monitoring in neonatal seizures: what is done, what could be done?
  Sylvie Nguyen The Tich 17

Neuro-imaging in neonatal seizures
  Lauren C. Weeke, Linda G. van Rooij, Mona C. Toet, Floris Groenendaal, Linda S. de Vries 27

Clinical and electrographical neonatal seizures: to treat or not to treat
  Lena Hellström-Westas 39

Genetics of neonatal epilepsies and the forgotten epilepsy phenotypes
  Maria Roberta Cilio, Michael S. Oldham 49

Genetic basis of epileptic encephalopathy
  Lucia Fusco, Domenico Serino, Giulia Barcia, Rima Nabbout 61

Treatment of neonatal seizures with antiepileptic drugs
  Chrysanthy Ikonomidou 71

Neonatal seizures in hypoxic-ischaemic encephalopathy:
the impact of therapeutic hypothermia
  Evonne Low, Geraldine B. Boylan 81

From conventional genetic analysis to next generation sequencing in diagnostics of epilepsies
    Johannes R. Lemke 95

Treatable newborn seizures due to inborn errors of metabolism
    Jaume Campistol, Barbara Plecko 105

Determining outcome from neonatal seizures
    Francesco Pisani, Carlotta Spagnoli 123

SEIZURES AND SYNDROMES IN INFANTS

The epidemiology of infancy onset seizures
    Christin Eltze 139

Concept of epileptic encephalopathy: is it relevant?
    Federico Vigevano, Nicola Specchio 155

The role of EEG in the management of seizures in infancy
    Thomas Bast 163

Optimizing imaging in aiding management
    William Davis Gaillard, Matthew Whitehead, Jonathan Murnick 171

"Benign" epilepsies in infants: are they always benign?
    Julitta de Bellescize, Nicola Specchio, Alexis Arzimanoglou 185

Fever-susceptibility syndromes. Predicting outcome
    Ingrid E. Scheffer, Rosemary Burgess, Christopher Reid 205

Infantile spasms semiology and pathophysiology: have we made progress?
    Douglas R. Nordli Jr 213

Trials for the treatment of infant seizures: theory, practice, ethics and potential future trends
    Andrew Lux, Finbar J. K. O'Callaghan 223

The role of ketogenic diet
    Giangennaro Coppola 235

Optimizing treatment for neonatal and infantile seizures – Do guidelines have a role in management?
    Jo M. Wilmshurst, J. Helen Cross 249

Preface

There is a very high incidence of seizures during the first two years of life. This may reflect multiple etiologies depending on the circumstances under which seizures occur; sometimes but not always seizures may lead to or herald epilepsy. In the immediate neonatal period, seizures can occur in the presence of provoked insults such as hypoxia ischemia, vascular events, traumatic injury changes in the extracellular milieu including toxic metabolic causes and drug withdrawal, as well as infections. Genetics may play an important role in the expression of acute seizures but also in the development of epilepsy later on. Genetic abnormalities may also give rise to brain dysplasias.

Within the first two years of life there is the frequent onset of difficult to control epilepsy with often devastating consequences (*i.e.* West syndrome or Dravet syndrome), although on other occasions the epileptic syndromes may have a more benign cause (*i.e.* benign familial neonatal seizures).

Ongoing efforts are to understand how seizures may occur in the developing brain, their consequences, the development of biomarkers, and effective treatments to promptly stop ongoing seizures and alter the course of epileptic encephalopathies. The simplistic view that seizures in the immature brain occur because of increased excitation and decreased inhibition is no longer pertinent as multiple age-specific (and also sex-specific) factors are intertwined, including changes in the conformation or function of channels, regional variability in the expression of various neurotransmitters and patterns of connectivity among these regions.

The topics presented in this volume address the questions raised above, and provide new insights on how it is best to approach seizures and epilepsy in the first two years of life, to systematically create a blueprint upon which diagnostic and treatment decisions can be based. The data are highly reflecting the state of the art and also individualize for the particular milieu of the patient in taking into account both nature (*i.e.* genetics), and nurture (*i.e.* events that may interfere with normal development) and result in seizures and epilepsy.

We would like to thank the authors for their keen observations, which help move forward the field.

Solomon L. Moshé and Alexis Arzimanoglou

Workshop participants

Alexis Arzimanoglou, France
Thomas Bast, Germany
Julitta de Bellescize, France
Anne Berg, USA
Geraldine B. Boylan, Ireland
Jaume Campistol, Spain
Maria Roberta Cilio, USA
Giangennaro Coppola, Italy
J. Helen Cross, UK
Paolo Curatolo, Italy
Raffallea Cusmai, Italy
Linda S. de Vries, The Netherlands
Bouchra El M'Kaddem, France
Christin Eltze, UK
Annick Fonteyne, Belgium
Lucia Fusco, Italy
William D. Gaillard, USA
Hannah Glass, USA
Giuseppe Gobbi, Italy
Pierre Gressens, France
Lena Hellström-Westas, Sweden
Hans Holthausen, Germany
Chrysanthy Ikonomidou, USA
Floor Jansen, The Netherlands
Lieven Lagae, Belgium
Marie-Dominique Lamblin, France

Johannes R. Lemke, Germany
Tobias Loddenkemper, USA
Massimo Mastrangelo, Italy
May McTague, UK
Eli M. Mizrahi, USA
Solomon L. Moshé, USA
Rima Nabbout, France
Sylvie Nguyen The Tich, France
Doug Nordli, USA
Finbar J. K. O'Callaghan, UK
Sara Olivotto, Italy
Francesco Pisani, Italy
Barbara Plecko, Switzerland
Perrine Plouin, France
Ronit M. Pressler, UK
Georgia Ramantani, Germany
Gabriel Ronen, Canada
Ingrid E. Scheffer, Australia
Nicola Specchio, Italy
Pasquale Striano, Italy
Biayna Sukhudyan, Armenia
Regina Trollmann, Germany
Federico Vigevano, Italy
Jo M. Wilmshurst, South Africa
Gabriele Wohlrab, Switzerland

Seizures and Syndromes of Onset in the Two First Years of Life
Progress in Epileptic Disorders Workshop
Grottaferrata, Italy
November 2013

Scientific Committee/Editors
Solomon L. Moshé (USA), J. Helen Cross (UK), Julitta De Bellescize (France), Linda S. de Vries (The Netherlands), Douglas Nordli (USA), Federico Vigevano (Italy)

List of authors

Alexis Arzimanoglou, Epilepsy, Sleep and Pediatric Neurophysiology Department (ESEFNP), University Hospitals of Lyon (HCL) – Lyon, France

Giulia Barcia, Reference center for Rare Epilepsies, Department of Pediatric Neurology, Necker Enfants Malades Hospital – Paris, France

Thomas Bast, Epilepsy Center Kork – Kehl, Germany

Julitta de Bellescize, Epilepsy, Sleep and Pediatric Neurophysiology Department (ESEFNP), University Hospitals of Lyon (HCL) – Lyon, France

Geraldine B. Boylan, Neonatal Brain Research Group, Irish Centre for Fetal and Neonatal Translational Research, Department of Paediatrics and Child Health, University College Cork – Cork, Ireland

Rosemary Burgess, Department of Medicine, University of Melbourne, Austin Health – Melbourne, Australia

Jaume Campistol, Neurology Department, Hospital Sant Joan de Déu, Universitat de Barcelona – Barcelona, Spain

Maria R. Cilio, Department of Neurology, Pediatric Epilepsy Center, University of California, San Francisco – San Francisco, USA

Giangennaro Coppola, Child and Adolescent Neuropsychiatry, Faculty of Medicine and Surgery, University of Salerno – Salerno, Italy

J. Helen Cross, Neurosciences Unit, UCL Institute of Child Health – London, UK

Linda S. de Vries, Department of Neonatology, Wilhelmina Children's Hospital, UMC Utrecht – Utrecht, The Netherlands

Christin Eltze, Great Ormond Street Hospital for Children, UCL Institute of Child Health – London, UK

Lucia Fusco, Neurology Division, Ospedale Pediatrico Bambino Gesù – Rome, Italy

William D. Gaillard, Center for Neuroscience and the Division of Neuroradiology, Children's National Medical Center, George Washington University School of Medicine and Health Sciences – Washington DC, USA

Floris Groenendaal, Department of Neonatology, Wilhelmina Children's Hospital, UMC Utrecht – Utrecht, The Netherlands

Lena Hellström-Westas, Department of Women's and Children's Health, Uppsala University and University Hospital – Uppsala, Sweden

Chrysanthy Ikonomidou, Department of Neurology, University of Wisconsin-Madison – Madison, USA

Johannes R. Lemke, Institute of Human Genetics, University Hospital – Leipzig, Germany

Evonne Low, Neonatal Brain Research Group, Irish Centre for Fetal and Neonatal Translational Research, Department of Paediatrics and Child Health, University College Cork – Cork, Ireland

Andrew Lux, Department of Paediatric Neurology, Bristol Royal Hospital for Children – Bristol, UK

Eli M. Mizrahi, Peter Kellaway Section of Neurophysiology, Department of Neurology, Section of Pediatric Neurology, Department of Pediatrics, Baylor College of Medicine – Houston, USA

Solomon L. Moshé, Pediatric and Clinical Neurophysiology, Einstein College of Medicine, Bronx, USA

Jonathan Murnick, Center for Neuroscience and the Division of Neuroradiology, Children's National Medical Center, George Washington University School of Medicine and Health Sciences – Washington DC, USA

Rima Nabbout, Reference center for Rare Epilepsies, Department of Pediatric Neurology, Necker Enfants Malades Hospital – Paris, France

Sylvie Nguyen The Tich, Child Neurology Unit, University Hospital of Angers. LARIS, EA7315, LUNAM University – Angers, France

Douglas R. Nordli Jr, Epilepsy Center, Ann & Robert H. Lurie Children's Hospital of Chicago – Chicago, USA

Finbar J. K. O'Callaghan, Section of Clinical Neurosciences, UCL Institute of Child Health – London, UK

Michael S. Oldham, Department of Neurology, Pediatric Epilepsy Center, University of California, San Francisco – San Francisco, USA

Francesco Pisani, Child Neuropsychiatry Unit, Neuroscience Department, University of Parma – Parma, Italy

Barbara Plecko, Division of Neurology, Children's Hospital, University of Zurich – Zurich, Switzerland

Ronit M. Pressler, Department of Clinical Neurophysiology, Great Ormond Street Hospital for Children NHS Trust – London, UK

Christopher Reid, Florey Institute of Neuroscience and Mental Health – Melbourne, Australia

Ingrid E. Scheffer, Florey Institute of Neuroscience and Mental Health, Melbourne. Department of Medicine, University of Melbourne, Austin Health. Department of Paediatrics, University of Melbourne, Royal Children's Hospital, Melbourne – Australia

Domenico Serino, Neurology Division, Ospedale Pediatrico Bambino Gesù – Rome, Italy

Carlotta Spagnoli, Child Neuropsychiatry Unit, Neuroscience Department, University of Parma – Parma, Italy

Nicola Specchio, Department of Neuroscience, Bambino Gesù Children's Hospital, IRCCS – Rome, Italy

Mona C. Toet, Department of Neonatology, Wilhelmina Children's Hospital, UMC Utrecht – Utrecht, The Netherlands

Linda G. van Rooij, Department of Neonatology, Wilhelmina Children's Hospital, UMC Utrecht – Utrecht, The Netherlands

Federico Vigevano, Department of Neuroscience, Bambino Gesù Children's Hospital, IRCCS – Rome, Italy

Lauren C. Weeke, Department of Neonatology, Wilhelmina Children's Hospital, UMC Utrecht – Utrecht, The Netherlands

Matthew Whitehead, Center for Neuroscience and the Division of Neuroradiology, Children's National Medical Center, George Washington University School of Medicine and Health Sciences – Washington DC, USA

Jo M. Wilmshurst, Department of Paediatric Neurology, Red Cross War Memorial Children's Hospital. School of Child and Adolescent Health, University of Cape Town – Cape Town, South Africa

Foundations of neonatal epileptology: classification of seizures and epilepsies in the neonate and their etiology, electroencephalography, prognosis and pathophysiology

Eli M. Mizrahi[1], Ronit M. Pressler[2]

[1] Peter Kellaway Section of Neurophysiology, Department of Neurology; Section of Pediatric Neurology, Department of Pediatrics, Baylor College of Medicine, Houston, Texas, USA
[2] Department of Clinical Neurophysiology, Great Ormond Street Hospital for Children NHS Trust, London, UK

There is a rich history of basic, translational and clinical investigations of neonatal seizures marked by important milestones which are the basis of our current understanding of these clinical and electrographic events. This discussion will consider some of the developments in semiology (classification and characterization), etiology, prognosis and pathophysiology and how they have informed our current strategies in the diagnosis and management of neonatal seizures.

■ Characterization and classification

Beginning in the 1950s there have been systematic efforts to characterize and classify clinical neonatal seizures; first recognizing and then underscoring their unique nature when compared to older children and adults. The periods of investigations have been determined both by the clinically applicable technology current to respective periods of study and data concerning the immature brain which developed concurrently with the clinical investigations themselves (Kellaway and Mizrahi, 1987).

Motor and behavioral characterization

An initial period of investigation focused upon the motor and behavioral changes considered to be neonatal seizures. The applied techniques varied: clinical observation only (Burke, 1954; Craig, 1960; Keen, 1969; McInerny and Schubert, 1969); clinical observation during recordings the neonatal electroencephalogram (EEG) (Cadilhac et al., 1959;

Harris and Tizard, 1960; Passouant and Cadilhac, 1962); and the first investigations in neonates which utilized combined EEG and cinematography (Dreyfus-Brisac and Monod, 1964). Early investigators characterized all neonatal seizures as "convulsions" or "muscular twitching" (Burke, 1954). However, there was quick recognition that these clinical events were more diverse with the identification of generalized tonic seizures and focal and multifocal clonic seizures. In addition, generalized tonic-clonic seizures were considered rare or non-existent in the neonate (Minkowski et al., 1955; Ribstein and Wather, 1958; Cadilhac et al., 1959; Dreyfus-Brisac and Monod, 1964). Early investigators also appreciated that bilateral clonic seizures of the extremities would occur simultaneously, but asynchronously on the two sides (Craig, 1960; Harris and Tizard, 1960; Passouant and Cadilhac, 1962; Dreyfus-Brisac and Monod, 1964). It was also recognized that clonic seizures could migrate both in a Jacksonian and non-Jacksonian manner (Harris and Tizard, 1960). Thus, this early period of the clinical characterization of neonatal seizures resulted in the recognition of some events which are part of current classification schemes: focal clonic, multifocal clonic and generalized tonic seizures.

This period also resulted in descriptions of more unique clinical events: apnea with cyanosis or hypotonia (Cadilhac et al., 1959); staring, pallor, hypotonia, and alternating "warding off" movements of the arms (Harris and Tizard, 1960); upward eye deviation, cyanotic apnea, slight finger contractions, sudden awakening with crying (Passouant and Cadilhac, 1962); eye opening, paroxysmal blinking, nystagmus, vasomotor changes, chewing, limb movements "resembling swimming, rowing, and pedaling" (Minkowski and Sainte-Anne-Dargassies, 1956; Dreyfus-Brisac and Monod, 1964); and abrupt changes in respiration and skin color, salivation, and alerting behavior (Schulte, 1966).

Dreyfus-Brisac and Monod (1964) summarized a 10-year period of investigations (Sainte-Anne-Dargassies et al., 1953; Minkowski et al., 1955; Dreyfus-Brisac and Monod, 1960) and emphasized the polymorphic, atypical and anarchic character of neonatal seizures compared to adults and underscored the value of combined cinematography and EEG in the analysis of clinical and EEG manfestations of neonatal seizures. Thus, during this period of investigations, the major types of clinical neonatal seizure had been identified, although there was additional work to be done to refine the classification and classification of these events.

Consolidation and confirmation of findings

This period was marked by the consolidation, confirmation and refinement of the findings mainly generated by the French investigators. Rose and Lombroso (1970) confirmed the findings of the variation seizure types described by the French group and included a group of behaviors "difficult to classify because of the peripheral phenomena were very slight" such as: changes in respiration, slight posturing of limbs, tonic eye deviation, chewing, sucking and drooling. Lombroso (1974) eventually referred to this group of events as a "minimal seizure pattern". Rose and Lombroso (1970) also recognized myoclonus as a neonatal seizure type. Freeman (1970) suggested that "the occurrence of any type of bizarre or unusual transient event" should raise the suspicion of the presence of a clinical neonatal seizure.

A seminal development in the recognition of neonatal seizures as a group of clinical events distinct from older children and adults was the 1973 publication of Volpe's discussion of neonatal seizures (Volpe, 1973). He proposed a classification system for neonatal seizures that included multifocal clonic, focal clonic, tonic and myoclonic clinical events. He also proposed that the "atypical and anarchic" seizures described primarily by the French investigators in the 1950's and 1960's and the "minimal" or "slight" seizures described by Rose and Lombroso (1970) should be classified as "subtle". Although initially behaviors such as swimming, pedaling or rowing movements were not included in Volpe's subtle seizure category, by 1977 they also became incorporated into the classification (Volpe, 1977). Volpe's subsequent work further refined his classification scheme (Volpe, 1981; 1989).

Electroclinical correlations

Another pivotal development in characterization of neonatal seizures was the work of Watanabe and colleagues (Watanabe et al., 1977) based upon the recording of neonates with seizures during EEG and polygraphic recordings and the characterization of paroxysmal behaviors which were accompanied by electrographic seizure activity. Polygraphic parameters were recorded simultaneously with EEG and clinical observation to characterize changes in respirations and heart rate. Multifocal clonic or hemiconvulsive clonic, tonic, myoclonic and four additional groups of clinical events were recorded. These four groups were: body/limb movements (swimming, rowing, pedaling, fencing); oral movements (chewing, sucking, mouthing); respiratory changes (apnea, dyspnea); and ocular changes (staring, eye opening, eye deviation, nystagmus, blinking). Thus, by this stage of clinical investigations, the full range of motor events was characterized and changes in respiration became an important focus of attention.

In the years that followed, closer attention was paid to clinical changes mediated by the autonomic nervous system. Lou and Friss-Hansen (1979) recognized increased mean arterial blood pressure during generalized and focal motor neonatal seizures. Fenichel et al. (1979) and Watanabe et al. (1982) identified changes in heart rate and respiration during apnea associated with motor seizures. Goldberg et al. (1982) studied pharmacologically paralyzed infants with EEG and noted tachycardia, systemic hypertension, and increased pO_2 during electrographic seizure activity. Perlman and Volpe (1983) demonstrated elevated cerebral blood flow velocity, systemic blood pressure, heart rate, and intracranial pressure during clinical seizures. Kellaway and Hrachovy (1983) noted that similar motor events may be accompanied both with and without autonomic changes, suggesting a more complex relationship between electrographic seizures and these clinical events.

EEG-video monitoring investigations

In the 1960s and 1970s the simultaneous recording of EEG and video was progressively applied to the characterization of various seizure types in older children and adults (Penry and Dreifuss, 1969; Penry et al., 1975; Escueta et al., 1977; Delgado-Escueta, 1979) and infantile spasms (Frost et al., 1978; Kellaway et al., 1979). In 1987, Mizrahi and Kellaway (Mizrahi and Kellaway, 1987) reported the utilization of bedside EEG-polygraphic-video monitoring of neonates experiencing seizures. This study verified the characterizations and classifications of others. They also identified clinical events which were clearly of epileptic origin and others, previously considered to be epileptic, which were of non-epileptic origin; considered the manifestation of exaggerated reflex behaviors. This latter group consisted of generalized tonic events, oral-bucal-lingual movements, some ocular signs, and movements of progression such as swimming, rowing and stepping. In addition, autonomic changes appeared to occur most often in association with motor manifestations of seizures. Subsequent applications of EEG-video monitoring in neonates have provided greater refinement of classification, formed the basis for the recognition of greater diversity of clinical manifestations of clinical events and emphasized the need for clinical training as interobserver reliability can be limited without experienced observers (Malone et al., 2009). This recording technique also allowed for the characterization of the sequence of an electroclinical seizure to treatment with antiepileptic drugs (AEDs) with initial control of the clinical seizure but persistence of the electrographic event – so-called "uncoupling" (Mizrahi and Kellaway, 1987).

ILAE classification and neonatal seizure

In the 1960s Gastaut introduced classification in the epilepsies applicable to children and adults and has since provided a framework for clinical practice (Gastaut, 1969). Historically, epilepsy classification has been largely based on clinical experience, developed by a group of eminent epileptologists with a lifetime of studying seizure disorders. Despite the fact that some of the members of the commission over the years were interested in seizures and epilepsy in infancy notably – Henri Gastaut, Warren Blume, Jean Aicardi and Perrine Plouin – neonatal seizures were not incorporated into proposals until very recently. For example, in the 1981 seizure classification, they were merely mentioned under "unclassified epileptic seizure" (Commission on Classification and Terminology of the International League Against Epilepsy, 1981). The 1989 classification of syndromes (Commission on Classification and Terminology of the International League Against Epilepsy, 1989) recognised four epilepsy syndromes plus an entity of "neonatal seizures with both generalized and focal seizures". In an attempt to classify 94 patients with neonatal seizures into the 1989 classification, Mastrangelo et al. (2005) found that > 90% of events were unclassifiable. In his special report in 2006, Engel stated that "neonatal seizures: although the components of neonatal seizures can be described in terms of the seizure types itemized above, they often display unique organizational features. Therefore, a study group will be created to more completely define and characterize the various types of neonatal seizures" (Engel, 2006). Recently the International League Against Epilepsy proposed a revised terminology for the organization of seizures and epilepsies (Berg et al., 2010) with the aim to reflect major scientific advances leading to a better understanding of epilepsy. One of the major changes are that "neonatal seizures are no longer regarded as a separate entity. Seizures in neonates can be classified within the proposed scheme". However, in the proposed scheme, the only categories of seizures which could be applicable for neonates would be "focal seizures", "unknown, subcategory, epileptic spasms" and, less frequently, "myoclonic" in the generalized category. Furthermore, electrographic seizures which may constitute up to 75% of the seizure burden in term and preterm infants would not be classifiable (Menzies et al., 2012). Based upon the data reviewed above, this proposed scheme would not be appropriate for seizures occurring in the neonatal period. This shortcoming of the 2010 proposal has been acknowledged by the ILAE and a new task force has been instituted with the aim to develop a consensus on how best to define, characterize, classify and organize neonatal seizures. A comparison of various classification schemes is presented in *Table I*.

Table I. Classifications of neonatal seizures

Reference	Type	Characterization	Ictal EEG abnormalities
Volpe (1989)	Subtle	Ocular, oral-buccal-lingual, autonomic, apnoea, limb posturing and movements	Variable
	Clonic	Repetitive jerking, distinct from jittering. Unifocal or multifocal	Common
	Myoclonic	Rapid isolated jerks Focal, multifocal or generalised	Common if generalised, uncommon if focal
	Tonic	Stiffening. Decerebrate posturing. Focal or generalised	Common if focal, uncommon if generalised
Mizrahi and Kellaway (1987; 1998)	Focal clonic	Rhythmic muscle contractions, unifocal or multifocal, synchronous or asynchronous. Not suppressed by restrain.	Epileptic
	Focal tonic	Sustained posturing of limb, trunk or neck. Also tonic eye deviation. Not provoked by external stimuli and not suppressed by restrain.	Epileptic
	Myoclonic	Random, single, rapid contractions of muscle groups. Usually not repetitive. May be generalised, focal or fragmentary. May be provoked by external stimuli.	May or may not be epileptic
	Spasms	Flexor or extensor. May occur in clusters. Not provoked by external stimuli and not suppressed by restrain.	Epileptic
	Generalised tonic	Sustained symmetric posturing; flexor, extensor or mixed; may be stimulus sensitive; may be suppressed by restrain.	Non-epileptic, no EEG correlate
	Motor automatism	Ocular, oral-buccal-lingual, progression movements of limbs May be provoked or intensified by external stimuli and suppressed by restrain.	Non-epileptic, no EEG correlate
	Electrographic	By definition none	Epileptic

Berg et al 2010*	Generalised	Tonic-clonic (in any combination)
		Absence
		  Typical
		  Atypical
		  With special features
		    Myoclonic absences
		    Eyelid myoclonia
		Myoclonic
		Myoclonic atonic
		Myoclonic tonic
		Clonic
		Tonic
		Atonic	

	Focal		
	Unknown	Epileptic spasm	

* Not specific for neonatal seizures. Only categories in bold-face are consistent with currently accepted characterizations of neonatal seizures.

Electroencephalography

The recognition of electrographic seizure discharges in neonatal EEG recordings paralleled that of the development of neonatal EEG in general. This development was pioneered predominantly by French investigators (Dreyfus-Brisac et al., 1958) as well as others who further identified neonatal EEG features (Ellingson, 1958; Kellaway, 1952; Gibbs and Gibbs, 1952). As interest in the practice of neonatal EEG increased, a period of dissemination and education ensued (Tharp, 1990; Lombroso, 1979, 1985; Kellaway, 1982; Clancy et al., 1993). Electrographic events were considered focal, multifocal and migratory. Morphology, amplitude, duration and evolution could vary (*Figure 1*). Some electrographic seizure types were considered unique to the neonatal period. Alpha seizure discharges were characterized as sustained, focal, sinusoidal discharges which were typically not associated with clinical seizures (Knauss and Carlson, 1978; Willis and Gould, 1980; Watanabe et al., 1980) (*Figure 2*). Seizure discharges of the depressed brain were characterized as focal, sustained, low voltage, monomorphic seizures which are not accompanied by clinical changes and associated with background EEG which is depressed and undifferentiated (Kellaway and Hrachovy, 1981) (*Figure 3*).

An important milestone in the application of EEG to the care of neonates with seizures was the development of cerebral function monitor (CFM) or amplitude integrated electroencephalography (aEEG) in the early 1970s (Prior et al., 1971). Over the past several years investigators have applied this technique to assess EEG background activity, to detect electrographic seizures, and to provide sustained seizure surveillance over long periods of time (Hellström-Westas, 1995; Toet et al., 2002; Mathur et al., 2008; Hellström-Westas et al., 2003). Despite some limitations related to some types and location of electrographic seizures (Rennie et al., 2004; Shellhaus et al., 2007; Clancy et al., 2011), aEEG has become an important tool in the management of neonates with seizures. However, the risk for false positive and false negative detection rate is too high for efficacy evaluation in clinical trials (Rennie et al., 2003; Glass et al., 2012).

Etiology

The earliest studies of etiology of neonatal seizures were based upon autopsy-derived data (Burke, 1954; Craig, 1960). Later studies were characterized by the increasingly sophisticated diagnostic methodology available such as lumbar puncture, biochemical assays, assays for microbiology and virology and various techniques of neuroimaging. However, in most reported series etiologies most closely associated with what is now characterized as neonatal encephalopathy have comprised almost half of the presumed causes (Burke, 1954; Craig, 1960; Harris and Tizzard, 1960; Watanabe et al., 1981; Bergman et al., 1983; Mizrahi and Kellaway, 1987; Tegkul et al., 2006). Mizrahi and Kellaway (1998) have noted the changes in relative etiologies of neonatal seizures according to the prevailing technologies and understanding of operative potential pathologies.

The recognition of the genetic basis of benign familial neonatal seizures represented an important finding in the care of newborns with seizures (Quattlebaum, 1979). The initial studies identified a genetic pedigree. Subsequent studies identified the syndrome linked to chromosome 20 (Leppert et al., 1989) and eventually the first novel potassium channel gene KCNQ2 was implicated in this inherited disorder (Singh et al., 1998). These findings have led both to improved diagnosis and the development of novel therapies such as so-called KCNQ channel openers (Raol et al., 2009).

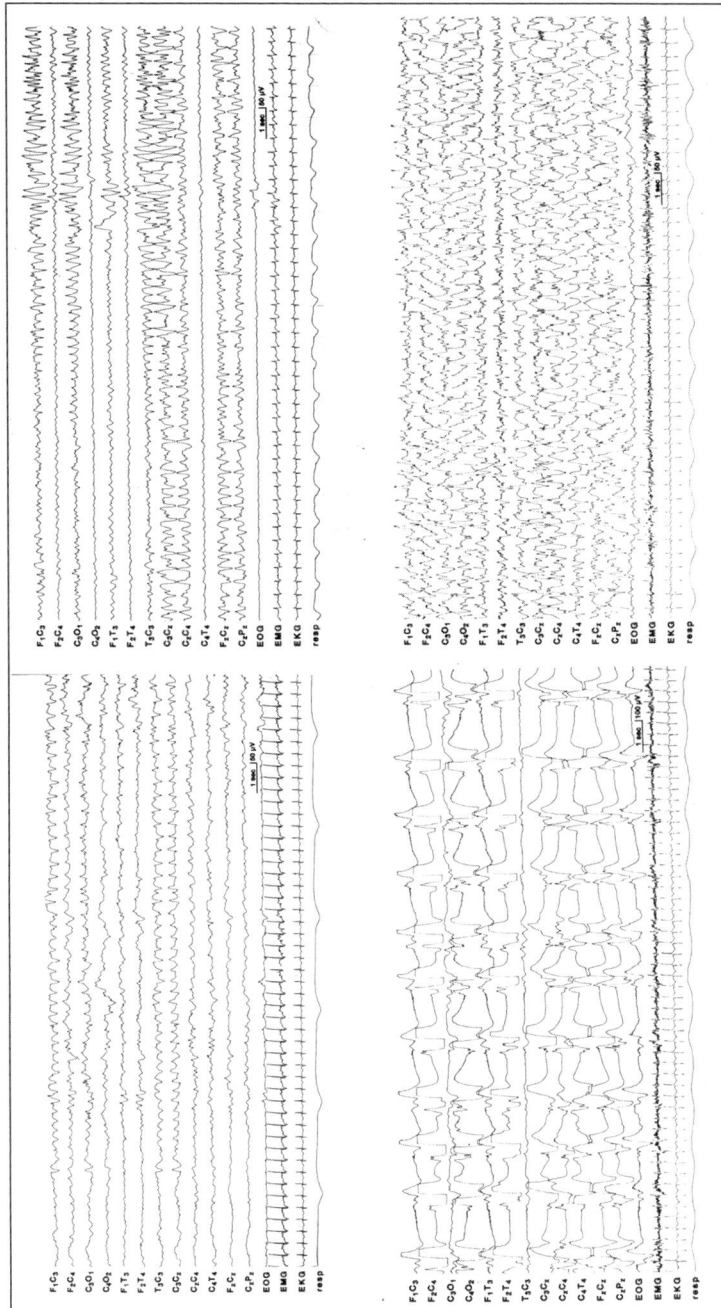

Figure 1. Electrographic seizures may be varied in morphology, frequency, duration, and location. Clockwise beginning at upper left: rhythmic discharge with initial blunted morphology which evolves to sharp waves confined to the left central region; rhythmic sharp wave discharge arising from the midline central region which migrates to the left central region; multifocal sharp wave waves appearing independently and asynchronously on the two sides; high amplitude slow rhythmic sharp and slow wave complexes over the right hemisphere with some reflection over the left.

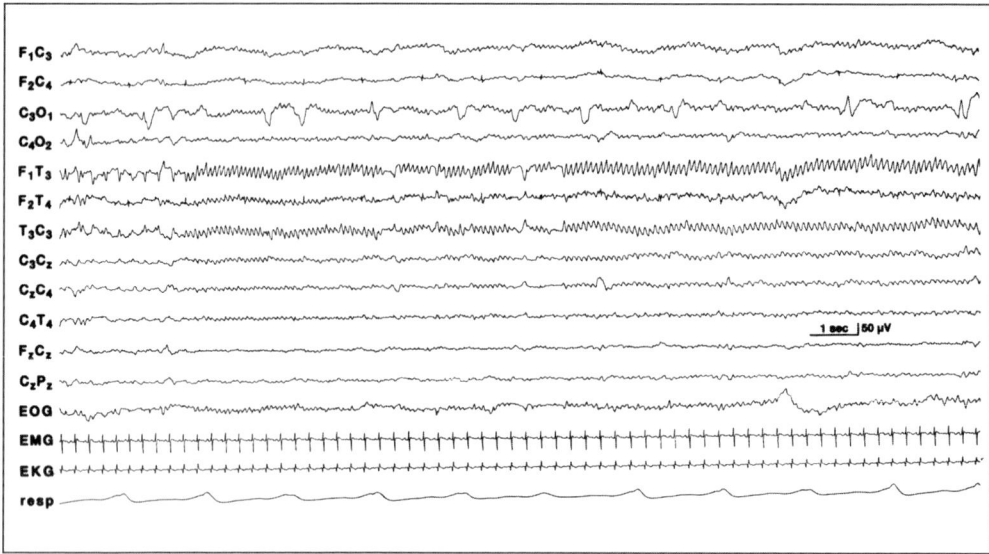

Figure 2. Alpha seizure discharge.

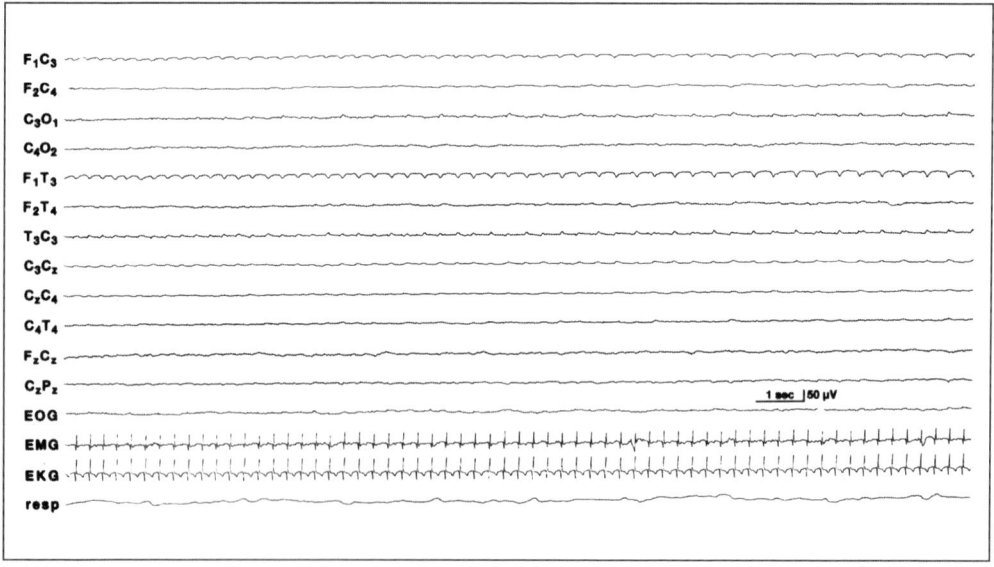

Figure 3. Seizure discharges of the depressed brain.

■ Prognosis

There have been a number of studies which have reported the outcome of neonatal seizures (*Table II*) noting significant mortality and, in survivors, neurological impairment, motor and development delay. From the earliest reports of the various outcomes of neonatal seizures discussions have focused which factor could be identified as the major determinant of prognosis: the underlying etiology and associated degree and distribution of brain injury, adverse effects of the seizures themselves, or the direct or indirect impact of AED therapy.

Recent animal data suggests that animals with electrographic seizures in the neonatal period will experience impairment in learning and behavior later in life (Holmes et al., 2009). Clinical data, however, provides conflicting data with one series suggesting impairment later in life (Glass et al., 2009) but others suggest none (Kwon et al., 2011). The potential adverse impact of AEDs on the developing brain has also been a focus of discussion, with reports of abnormal growth and development based upon specific agents. While these influences have not been discounted, their relative importance may be considered less than the overriding factor of etiology and associated degree and distribution of brain injury. Etiology has historically been considered the determinant of outcome (Cadilhac et al., 1959; Schulte, 1966; McInerny and Schubert, 1969; Brown, 1973; Volpe, 1973; Lombroso, 1975) and more recent analyses support this point of view (Lombroso, 2007).

Table II. Outcome of neonatal seizures. Neurological impairment, developmental delay and death

Study	Year	Pt Number	Deaths (%)	Abn (%)	Normal (%)
Burke	1954	46	38	17	45
Cadhilac et al.	1959	90	20	20	40
Craig	1960	374	42	3	35
Harris & Tizard	1960	41	20	27	44
Prichard	1964	56	32	36	33
Schulte	1966	57	26	45	29
Massa & Niedermeyer	1968	82	10	28	59
McInerny & Schubert	1969	95	19	25	30
Kuromori et al.	1976	130	33	24	43
Dennis	1978	50	22	36	44
Holden et al.	1982	277	35	30	35
Lombroso	1983	117	16	35	48
Clancy & Legido	1991	40	33	38	30
Ortibus et al.	1996	81	29	49	22
Bye et al.	1997	32	25	31	38
Mizrahi et al.	2001	207	28	55	45
Tekgul et al.	2006	89	NR	29	71
van der Heide et al.	2012	82	38	62	38

There has also been a greater appreciation for various risk factors which may contribute to the outcome. Notably, population studies have indicated that lower birthweight and gestation age may have adverse impacts on overall outcome (Ronen et al., 1999).

Another important milestone in the discussion of prognosis of neonatal seizures has been the recognition of the increased occurrence of post-neonatal epilepsy (Ellenberg et al., 1984). Since, there have been reports of both increased incidence of seizures following the neonatal period as well as an earlier onset compared to those without neonatal seizures. Varying series report approximately 25% of survivors have seizures after the neonatal period (Mizrahi et al., 2001).

Traditionally, outcome has been reported in terms of survival, neurological impairment, intellectual impairment, and impairment in motor skills. However, more recently, there has been an emphasis on the relationship of these outcomes which may co-exist in the same subject following neonatal seizures. While there may be distinct domains of outcome, such as developmental delay, cerebral palsy and epilepsy, they may also overlap (Garfinklle and Shevell, 2011). These findings suggest that both the understanding and reporting of prognosis may be more complex than originally described.

Pathophysiology

There is a rich scientific literature which has described epileptogenesis in the immature brain delineating enhanced excitation, an imbalance of inhibition and excitation, amplification mechanisms of seizure discharges and the role of continuing development in seizure generation. An important milestone in the understanding of epileptogenesis in the immature has been the understanding of the maturational changes in the developing brain of glutamate and GABA receptor function. It has been reported that GABA is relatively excitatory early in brain followed by eventual development of its more mature inhibitory features (Ben-Ari, 2007; Rakhade and Jensen, 2009). While some suggest this may be too simplified an observation with different evolution of transmitter function in various brain regions (Galanopoulou et al., 2011) the concept of early excitatory function of transmitters traditionally considered inhibitory has formed the basis for further understanding of enhanced risk for seizures in the neonatal period and limited efficacy of some AEDs in their treatment (Pressler and Mangum, 2013; Löscher et al., 2013).

Appropriately there has been much attention paid to the epileptic pathophysiology of neonatal seizures. Kellaway and Hrachovy (1983) and Mizrahi and Kellaway (1987) described a non-epileptic mechanism for some clinical events such as generalized tonic seizures, oral-buccal-lingual movements, some ocular signs and movements of progress including pedaling, rowing and stepping. These events occurred in infants with diffuse cerebral disturbance, altered state of consciousness and EEGs with depressed and undifferentiated background. The events could be provoked by stimulation and suppressed by restraint of the infants. It was proposed that these clinical events had features of reflex behaviors described by early physiologists (Lindley et al., 1949; Sprague and Chamber, 1954; Kreindler et al., 1958). These group of events were referred to as "brainstem release phenomena" (Kellaway and Hrachovy, 1983; Mizrahi and Kellaway, 1987).

International collaboration

The further understanding of neonatal seizures and the dissemination of information to advance the care of affected infants has been the focus of international collaboration for several years. Most recently *Guidelines on Neonatal Seizures* has been published through the joint efforts of the International League Against Epilepsy, the World Health Organization and the IRCCS Asscociazione Osasi Maria SS WHO Collaborating Center (WHO, 2011). This is an evidence-based document which provides diagnostic and management guidelines which can be used in health care settings ranging from limited to enriched.

References

- Ben-Ari Y, Gaiarsa JL, Tyzio R, Khazipov R. GABA: a pioneer transmitter that excites immature neurons and generates primitive oscillations. *Physiol Rev* 2007; 87: 1215-84.
- Berg AT, Berkovic SF, Brodie MJ, *et al*. Revised terminology and concepts for organization of seizures and epilepsies: report of the ILAE Commission on Classification and Terminology, 2005-2009. *Epilepsia* 2010; 51: 676-85.
- Bergman I, Painter MJ, Hirsch RP, Crumrine PK, David R. Outcome in neonatal with convulsions treated in an intensive care unit. *Ann Neurol* 1983: 642-7.
- Bjerre I, Quattlebaum T, Murphy JV, *et al*. A novel potassium channel gene, KCNQ2, is mutated in an inherited epilepsy of newborns. *Nat Genet* 1998; 18: 25-9.
- Brown JK. Convulsions in the newborn period. *Dev Med Child Neurol* 1973; 823-46.
- Burke JB. The prognostic significance of neonatal convulsions. *Arch Dis Child* 1954; 29: 342-5.
- Cadilhac J, Passouant P, Ribstein M. Convulsions in the newborn: EEG and clinical aspects. *Electroencephalogr Clin Neurophysiol* 1959; 11; 604.
- Clancy RR, Chung HJ, Temple JP. Neonatal electroencephalography. In: Sperling MR, Clancy RR (Eds). *Atlas of Electroencephalography*. New York: Elsevier, 1993, p. 182.
- Clancy RR, Dicker L, Cho S, *et al*. Agreement between long-term neonatal background classification by conventional and amplitude-integrated EEG. *J Clin Neurophysiol* 2011; 28: 1-9.
- Commission on Classification and Terminology of the International League Against Epilepsy. Proposal for revised clinical and electrographic classification of epileptic seizures. *Epilepsia* 1981; 22: 489-501.
- Commission on Classification and Terminology of the International League Against Epilepsy. Proposal for revised classification of epilepsies and epileptic syndromes. *Epilepsia* 1989; 30: 389-9.
- Craig WS. Convulsive movements occurring in the first 10 days of life. *Arch Dis Child* 1960; 35: 336-44.
- Delgado-Escueta AV, Nashold B, Freedman M, *et al*. Videotaping epileptic attacks during stereoelectroencephalography. *Neurology* 1979; 29: 473-89.
- Dennis J. Neonatal convulsions: aetiology, late neonatal status and long-term outcome. *Dev Med Child Neurol* 1978; 20: 143-58.
- Dreyfus-Brisac C, Monod N. Electroclinical studies of status epilepticus and convulsions in the newborn: In: Kellaway P, Petersen I (eds). *Neurological and Electroencephalographic Correlative Studies in Infancy*. New York: Grune and Statton, 1964, pp. 250-72.
- Dreyfus-Brisac C, Monod N. *Bases biologiques de la maturation. Aspect évolutif de l'électrogenèse cérébrale chez l'enfant*. Premier congrès européen de pédopsychiatrie. Paris: SPEI ed, 1960, pp. 39-51.
- Ellenberg JH, Hirtz DG, Nelson KB. Age at onset of seizures in young children. *Ann Neurol* 1984; 15(2): 127-34.
- Ellingson RJ. Electroencephalograms of normal full-term newborns immediately after birth with observations on arousal and visual evoked responses. *Electroencephalogr Clin Neurophysiol* 1958; 10: 31-50.
- Engel J Jr. Report of the ILAE classification core group. *Epilepsia* 2006; 47: 2007-18.
- Escueta AV, Kunze U, Waddell G, Boxley J, Nadel A. Lapse of consciousness and automatisms in temporal lobe epilepsy: a videotape analysis. *Neurology* 1977; 27: 144-55.
- Fenichel GM, Olson BJ, Fitzpatrick JE. Heart rate changes in convulsive and nonconvulsive apnea. *Ann Neurol* 1979: 577-82.
- Freeman JM. Neonatal seizures–diagnosis and management. *J Pediatr* 1970; 77: 701-8.
- Frost JD Jr, Hrachovy RA, Kellaway P, Zion T. Quantitative analysis and characterization of infantile spasms. *Epilepsia* 1978; 19: 273-82.

- Galanopoulou AS, Moshé SL. In search of epilepsy biomarkers in the immature brain: goals, challenges and strategies. *Biomark Med* 2011; 5: 615-28.
- Garfinkle J, Shevell MI. Cerebral palsy, developmental delay, and epilepsy after neonatal seizures. *Pediatr Neurol* 2011; 44: 88-96.
- Gastaut H. Classification of the epilepsies: proposal for an international classification. *Epilepsia* 1969a; 10: S14-S21.
- Gastaut H. Clinical and electroencephalographical classification of epileptic seizures. *Epilepsia* 1969; 10 (suppl): 2-13.
- Gibbs FA, Gibbs EL. *Atlas of Electroencephalography*, vol 2. Reading: Addison-Wesley, 1952.
- Giraud P, Bernard R, Gastaut H. [Convulsions in infancy; etiological, clinical, electroencephalographic and therapeutic study]. *Arch Fr Pediatr* 1953; 10: 667-8.
- Glass HC, Glidden D, Jeremy RJ, Barkovich AJ, Ferriero DM, Miller SP. Clinical neonatal seizures are independently associated with outcome in infants at risk for hypoxic-ischemic brain injury. *J Pediatr* 2009; 155: 318-23.
- Glass HC, Kan J, Bonifacio SL, Ferriero DM. Neonatal seizures: treatment practices among term and preterm infants. *Pediatr Neurol* 2012; 46: 111-5.
- Goldberg RN, Goldman SL, Ramsay RE, Feller R. Detection of seizure activity in the paralyzed neonate using continuous monitoring. *Pediatrics* 1982; 69: 583-6.
- Harris R, Tizard JP. The electroencephalogram in neonatal convulsions. *J Pediatr* 1960; 57: 501-20.
- Hellstrom-Westas L, de Vries LS, Rosen I. *Atlas of Amplitude-Integrated EEGs in the Newborn*. New York: Pantheon Publishing Group, 2003, p. 150.
- Hellström-Westas L, Rosén I, Svenningsen NW. Predictive value of early continuous amplitude integrated EEG recordings on outcome after severe birth asphyxia in full term infants. *Arch Dis Child Fetal Neonatal Ed* 1995; 72: F34-8.
- Holden KR, Mellitus ED, Freeman JM. Neonatal seizures. I. Correlation of prenatal and perinatal events with outcome. *Pediatrics* 1982: 165-76.
- Holmes GL. The long-term effects of neonatal seizures. *Clin Perinatol* 2009; 36: 901-14.
- Keen JH. Significance of hypocalcaemia in neonatal convulsions. *Arch Dis Child* 1969; 44: 356-61.
- Kellaway P. The development of sleep spindles and of arousal patterns in infants and their characteristics in normal and certain abnormal states. *Electroencephogr Clin Neurophyiol* 1952: 369.
- Kellaway P, Hrachovy RA. Electroencephalography. In: KF Swaiman and FS Wright (eds). *The Practice of Pediatric Neurology*, Vol. 1, 2nd ed. St. Louis: CV Mosby, 1982, pp. 96-114.
- Kellaway P, Hrachovy RA. Status epilepticus in newborns: a perspective on neonatal seizures. *Adv Neurol* 1983; 34: 93-9.
- Kellaway P, Hrachovy RA, Frost JD Jr, Zion T. Precise characterization and quantification of infantile spasms. *Ann Neurol* 1979; 6: 214-8.
- Kellaway P, Mizrahi EM. Neonatal seizures. In: Lüders H, Lesser RP (eds). *Epilepsy: Electroclinical Syndromes*. Berlin: Springer-Verlag, 1987, pp. 13-47.
- Kreindler A, Zuckerman E, Steriade M, Chimion D. Electroclinical features of convulsions induced by stimulation of brain stem. *J Neurophysiol* 1958; 21: 430-6.
- Kwon JM, Guillet R, Shankaran S, Laptook AR, McDonald SA, Ehrenkranz RA. Clinical seizures in neonatal hypoxiceischemic encephalopathy have no independentimpact on neurodevelopmental outcome: secondary analyses of date from the neonatal research network hypothermia trial. *J Child Neurol* 2011; 26: 322.
- Knauss TA, Carlson CB. Neonatal paroxysmal monorhythmic alpha activity. *Arch Neurol* 1978; 35: 104-7.

- Kuromori N, Arai H, Ohkubo O, *et al*. A prospective study of epilepsy following neonatal convulsions. *Folia Psychiatr Neurol Jpn* 1976: 379-88.
- Leppert M, Anderson VE, Quattlebaum T, *et al*. Benign familial neonatal convulsions linked to genetic markers on chromosome 20. *Nature* 1989; 337: 647-8.
- Lindsley DB, Schreiner LH, Magoun HW. An electromyographic study of spasticity. *J Neurophysiol* 1949; 12: 197-205.
- Lombroso CT. Seizures in the newborn. In: Vinken PJ, Bruyn GW (eds). *The Epilepsies (Handbook of Clinical Neurology*, vol. 15). Amsterdam: North Holland, 1974, pp. 189-218.
- Lombroso CT. Quantified electrographic scales on 10 pre-term health newborns followed-up to 40-43 weeks of conceptional age by serial polygraphic recordings. *Electroencephalogr Clin Neurophysiol* 1979; 46: 460-74.
- Lombroso CT. Some aspects of EEG polygraphy in newborns at risk from neurological disorders. *Electroencephalogr Clin Neurophysiol* 1982; 36 (suppl): 652-63.
- Lombroso CT. Neonatal seizures: gaps between the laboratory and the clinic. *Epilepsia* 2007; 48 (suppl 2): 83-106.
- Löscher W, Puskarjov M, Kaila K. Cation-chloride cotransporters NKCC1 and KCC2 as potential targets for novel antiepileptic and antiepileptogenic treatments. *Neuropharmacology* 2013; 69: 62-74.
- Lou HC, Friis-Hansen B. Arterial blood pressure elevations during motor activity and epileptic seizures in the newborn. *Acta Pediatr Scand* 1979; 68: 803-6.
- Malone A, Ryan CA, Fitzgerald A, *et al*. Interobserver agreement in neonatal seizure identification. *Epilepsia* 2009; 50: 2097-101.
- Massa T, Niedermeyer E. Convulsive disorders during the first three months of life. *Epilepsia* 1968; 9: 1-9.
- Mastrangelo M, Van Lierde A, Bray M, Pastorino G, Marini A, Mosca F. Epileptic seizures, epilepsy and epileptic syndromes in newborns: a nosological approach to 94 new cases by the 2001 proposed diagnostic scheme for people with epileptic seizures and with epilepsy. *Seizure* 2005; 14: 304-11.
- McInerny TK, Schubert WK. Prognosis of neonatal seizures. *Am J Dis Child* 1969; 117: 261-4.
- Menzies L, Cross JH, Pressler RM. Diagnosis of neonatal seizures: effectiveness of current classification systems. *Epilepsia* 2012; 53 (suppl 5): 66.
- Minkowski A, Sainte-Anne-Dargassies S. [Convulsions in the newborn]. *Évol Psychiatr* (Paris) 1956; 1: 279-89.
- Minkowski A, Ste Anne-Dargassies S, Dreyfus-Brisac C, Samson D. [Convulsive state in the newborn infant]. *Arch Fr Pediatr* 1955; 12: 271-84.
- Mizrahi EM. Neonatal seizures and neonatal epileptic syndromes. *Neurol Clin* 2001; 19: 427-63.
- Mizrahi EM, Clancy RR, Dunn JK, *et al*. Neurologic impairment, developmental delay and post-natal seizures two years after video-EEG documented seizures in near-term and full-term neonates: report of the Clinical Research Centers for Neonatal Seizures. *Epilepsia* 2001; 102: 47.
- Mizrahi EM, Kellaway P. Cerebral concussion in children: assessment of injury by electroencephalography. *Pediatrics* 1984; 73: 419-25.
- Mizrahi EM, Kellaway P. Characterization and classification of neonatal seizures. *Neurology* 1987; 37: 1837-44.
- Mizrahi EM, Kellaway P. *Diagnosis and Management of Neonatal Seizures*. Philadelphia: Lippincott-Raven, 1998.
- Passouant P, Cadilhac J. EEG and clinical study of epilepsy during maturation in man. *Epilepsia* 1962; 3: 14-43.
- Penry JK, Dreifuss FE. A study of automatisms associated with the absence of petit mal. *Epilepsia* 1969; 10: 417-8.

- Penry JK, Porter RJ, Dreifuss RE. Simultaneous recording of absence seizures with video tape and electroencephalography. A study of 374 seizures in 48 patients. *Brain* 1975; 98: 427-40.
- Perlman JM, Volpe JJ. Seizures in the preterm infant: effects on cerebral blood flow velocity, intracranial pressure, and arterial blood pressure. *J Pediatr* 1983; 102: 288-93.
- Pressler RM, Mangum B. Newly emerging therapies for neonatal seizures. *Semin Fetal Neonatal Med* 2013; 18: 216-23.
- Prichard JS. The character and significance of epileptic seizures in infancy. In: Kellaway P, Petersen I (eds). *Neurological and Electroencephalographic Correlative Studies in Infancy*. New York: Grune and Stratton, 1964, pp. 273-86.
- Prior PF, Maynard DE, Sheaff PC, *et al*. Monitoring cerebral function: clinical experience with new device for continuous recording of electrical activity of brain. *Br Med J* 1971; 26: 736-8.
- Quattlebaum TG. Benign familial convulsions in the neonatal period and early infancy. *J Pediatr* 1979; 95: 257-9.
- Proposal for revised clinical and electroencephalographic classification of epileptic seizures. From the Commission on Classification and Terminology of the International League Against Epilepsy. *Epilepsia* 1981; 22: 489-501.
- Rakhade SN, Jensen FE. Epileptogenesis in the immature brain: emerging mechanisms. *Nat Rev Neurol* 2009; 5: 380-91.
- Raol YH, Lapides DA, Keating JG, Brooks-Kayal AR, Cooper EC. A KCNQ channel opener for experimental neonatal seizures and status epilepticus. *Ann Neurol* 2009; 65: 326-36.
- Rennie JM, Chorley G, Boylan GB, Pressler R, Nguyen Y, Hooper R. Non-expert use of the cerebral function monitor for neonatal seizure detection. *Arch Dis Child Fetal Neonatal Ed* 2004; 89: F37-40.
- Ribstein M, Walter M. [Convulsion in the first month of life]. *Rev Neurol* (Paris) 1958; 99: 91-9.
- Ronen GM, Penney S, Andrews W. The epidemiology of clinical neonatal seizures in Newfoundland: a population-based study. *J Pediatr* 1999; 134: 71-5.
- Rose AL, Lombroso CT. A study of clinical, pathological, and electroencephalographic features in 137 full-term babies with a long-term follow-up. *Pediatrics* 1970; 45: 404-25.
- Saint-Anne-Dargassies, Berthault F, Dreyfus-Brisac C, Fischgold H. [Convulsions of the younger nursing infant; electroencephalographic aspects of the problem]. *Presse Med* 1953; 61: 965-6.
- Schulte FJ. Neonatal convulsions and their relation to epilepsy in early childhood. *Dev Med Child Neurol* 1966; 8: 381-92.
- Shah DK, Mackay MT, Lavery S, *et al*. Accuracy of bedside electroencephalographic monitoring in comparison with simultaneous continuous conventional electroencephalography for seizure detection in term infants. *Pediatrics* 2008; 121: 1146-54.
- Shellhaas RA, Soaita AI, Clancy RR. Sensitivity of amplitude-integrated electroencephalography for neonatal seizure detection. *Pediatrics* 2007; 120: 770-7.
- Singh NA, Charlier C, Stauffer D, *et al*. A novel potassium channel gene, KCNQ2, is mutated in an inherited epilepsy of newborns. *Nat Genet* 1998; 18: 25-9.
- Sprague JM, Chambers WW. Control of posture by reticular formation and cerebellum in intact, anesthetized and unanesthetized and in decerebrated cat. *Am J Physiol* 1954; 176: 52-64.
- Tharp BR. Electrophysiological brain maturation in premature infants: An historical perspective. *J Clin Neurophysiol* 1990; 7: 302-14.
- Toet MC, van der Meij W, de Vries LS, Uiterwaal CS, van Huffelen KC. Comparison between simultaneously recorded amplitude integrated electroencephalogram (cerebral function monitor) and standard electroencephalogram in neonates. *Pediatrics* 2002; 109: 772-9.
- Tekgul H, Gauvreau K, Soul J, *et al*. The current etiologic profile and neurodevelopmental outcome of seizures in term newborn infants. *Pediatrics* 2006; 117: 1270-80.
- Volpe JJ. Neonatal seizures. *New Engl J Med* 1973; 289: 413-6.

- Volpe JJ. Neonatal seizures. *Clin Perinatol* 1977; 4: 43-63.
- Volpe JJ. Neonatal seizures: current concepts and revised classification. *Pediatrics* 1989; 84: 422-8.
- Watanabe K. Seizures in the newborn and young infants. *Folia Psychiatr Neurol Jpn* 1981; 35: 275-80.
- Watanabe K, Hara K, Miyazaki S, Hakamada S, Kuroyanagi M. Apneic seizures in the newborn. *Am J Dis Child* 1982; 136: 980-4.
- Watanabe K, Hara K, Miyazaki S, *et al*. Electroclincal studies of seizures in the newborn. *Folia Psychiatr Neurol Jpn* 1977; 31: 381-92.
- Willis J, Gould JB. Periodic alpha seizures with apnea in a newborn. *Dev Med Child Neurol* 1980; 22: 214-22.
- WHO. *Guidelines on Neonatal Seizures*. Geneva: World Health Organization 2011.

EEG monitoring in neonatal seizures: what is done, what could be done?

Sylvie Nguyen The Tich

Child Neurology Unit, Angers University Hospital, France;
LARIS, EA7315, LUNAM University, France

For the brain, birth is a dangerous event. Even after an uneventful pregnancy, full term babies can suffer from brain asphyxia, stroke or meningitis. During the first days or weeks of life other neurological diseases come to light like cerebral malformations, inborn errors of metabolism or early epileptic syndromes (Vasudevan and Levene, 2013).

Seizures are a common final pathway for all these diseases – a non-specific response to any form of injury to the immature brain that has specific physiological properties (Nardou et al., 2013). An understanding of the mechanisms leading to seizures is crucial in order to provide the most accurate treatment and to protect the brain from further insults. In this approach, EEG has a central role in diagnosis, prognosis and treatment.

What is EEG? A brief recall

EEG is an electrical signal recorded by electrodes placed on the scalp. It is a low amplitude signal (from few µV to 1,000 µV) which may be easily overwhelmed by other ambient electrical activity and therefore separating the meaningful signal from noise is a common and difficult part of the EEG analysis. It is even more difficult in the NICU with infants in unstable condition in a hostile electrical environment (André et al., 2010).

The EEG signal originates from the pyramidal cortical cells that are orthogonal to the surface. Neonatal EEG has specific aspects reflecting the cerebral immaturity and part of the electrical signal may come from deeper structures, as the skull is still unfused and the brain still contains much water with a better conductivity than in adults (Nunez and Srinivasan, 2006).

EEG provides information about the basic functioning of the brain (background activity), the presence of non-ictal abnormalities (slow waves, sharp waves, spikes) and the epileptic or non-epileptic nature of the abnormal movements that may have been recorded. The value of EEG for spatial localization is considered low, but this depends on the number of electrodes. The main strength of EEG is its temporal resolution. Metaphorically, it is an open window on the brain with an on-line connection. This implies that the EEG must be carried out at the right time to give the right information. EEG is less useful if performed when events or at risk situations have ended.

The information will vary with the duration of the recording. A very schematic approach could suggest three durations: one minute, one hour and one day.

Within a minute, EEG can immediately reveal a very abnormal background activity, very frequent interictal abnormalities, and whether the child is in status epilepticus or not. Obviously, recording only one minute of EEG would be clinically imprudent but the purpose of this mental exercise is to underline that meaningful information can be obtained on EEG at first glance (Figure 1).

Within an hour, the EEG may confirm that the background activity is normal, and detect non-permanent and infrequent non-ictal features or record frequent seizures.

Within one day, the EEG may detect infrequent seizures and variations of background activity due to modifications of the clinical condition (such as drugs, hypothermia and rewarming, etc.).

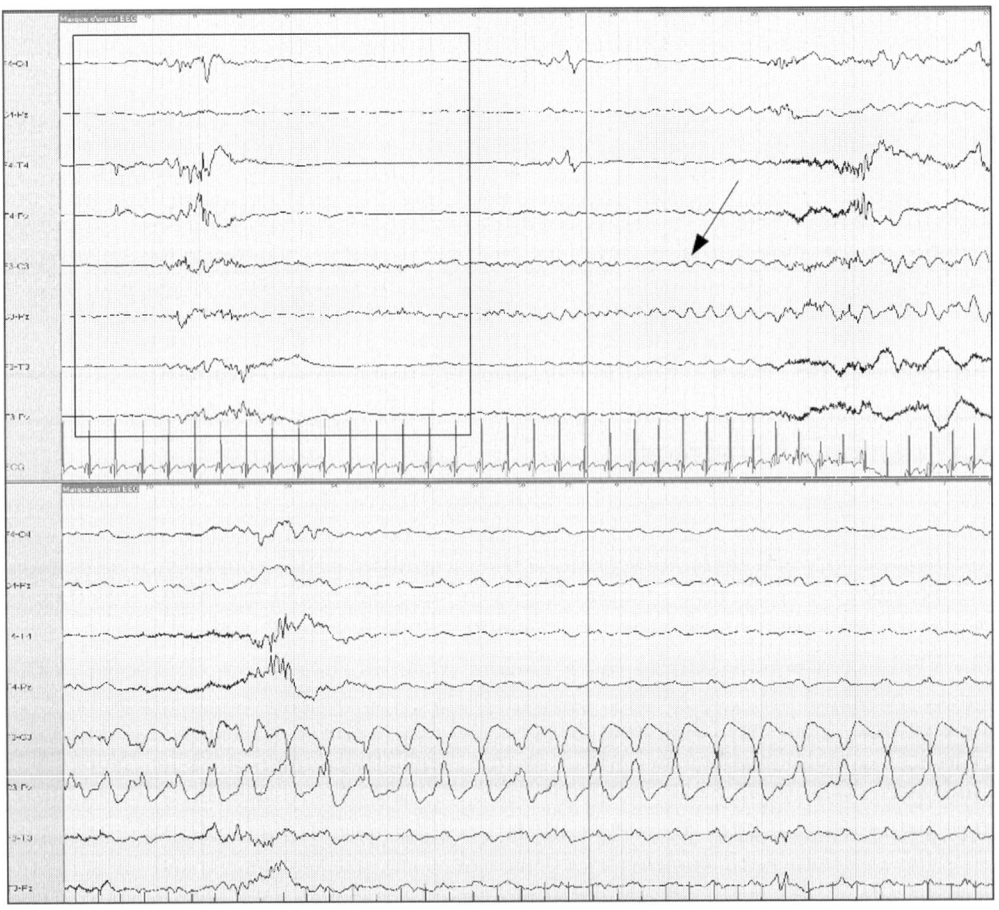

Figure 1. An example of two 20 seconds pages of a clearly abnormal EEG.
Arrow: beginning of a seizure. Frame: discontinuous EEG with abnormal non physiological features.

When a prolonged EEG is required specific methods for displaying the signal are needed to extract the meaningful information from the entire signal. This is the area for signal analysis and digital trend lines. Various mathematical transformations can be applied to the signal. The two mostly used are amplitude EEG (a-EEG) and density spectral array (DSA) (*Figure 2*). The aEEG is based on the amplitude of a filtered signal, and displays the variations of the minimal and maximal values of this signal. The amplitude of this bandwidth and its slow variations reflect the background activity. Rapid variations of the lower margin may indicate a seizure. Neurophysiologists usually prefer DSA because it provides complementary information about the frequency content of the signal (Riviello, 2013).

The precise duration of the monitoring should be individualized based upon the clinical circumstances and a consideration of the purpose of the study. For example, for seizure monitoring after treatment, a 24-hour seizure-free period has been recommended before stopping the EEG (Shellas et al., 2011).

EEG and seizure diagnosis

Diagnosing neonatal seizures based solely upon clinical observations is only as accurate as "flipping a coin" and therefore EEG confirmation is very useful (Malone et al., 2009; Boylan et al., 2013). Without a documented differential diagnosis, some non-epileptic abnormal movements may be inadvertently treated as seizures. On the opposite, non-convulsive seizures may be neglected both before and after drug administration that may ablate only the clinical signs (Murray et al., 2008; McCoy and Hahn, 2013). This phenomenom is known as "electroclinical dissociation" and has been described more frequently in neonates and when the EEG background activity was severely depressed (Pinto and Giliberti, 2001).

An electrographic seizure is defined as "a sudden, abnormal EEG event defined by a repetitive and evolving pattern with a minimum 2μV pp voltage and duration of at least 10 seconds. To be classified as separate seizures, 10 seconds or more must separate two distinct events" (Tsuchida et al., 2013). However, to distinguish seizure from artefacts is not so easy, even with a full montage conventional EEG. For this reason a synchronized video-EEG is recommended (Abend and Wusthoff, 2012; Wusthoff, 2013). It has also become clear from several studies and reports that the diagnosis of seizure should not be based only on digital trend lines and that inspection of raw data is mandatory (Shah DK et al., 2008).

Considering the diagnosis incertitude demonstrated by systematic video-EEG studies, some questions can be raised about the exact frequency of seizures in the NICU and the respective percentages of etiologies reported in studies based only on clinical observation.

EEG and the underlying cause

We widely recognize that a consideration of the causes and the mechanisms of seizures is a critical step in the diagnostic reasoning process but it is often neglected in neonatal seizure management. Two situations can be distinguished. Most commonly, the cause is previously known (birth asphyxia) or evident after routine diagnostic workup (*e.g.* hypoglycemia, hypocalcemia, or meningitis [Cheung et al., 2013]). The relative frequency of the various etiologies varies with the quality of prenatal and obstetrical care (Grünebaum et al., 2013). In this situation the EEG has little impact in the diagnostic decision.

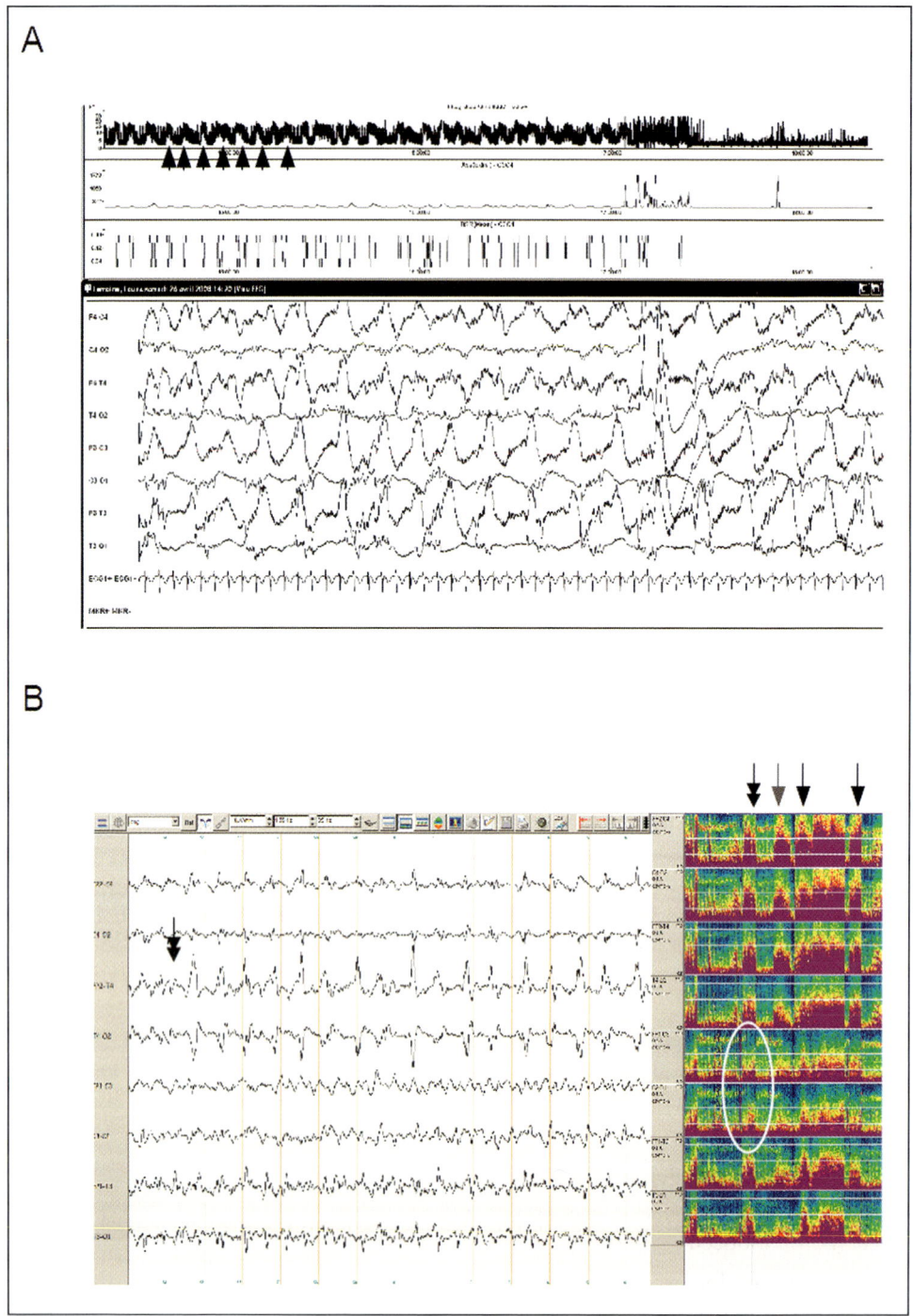

Figure 2. A. aEEG (top) showing repeated seizures (arrow head) with concordance with raw EEG (bottom). **B.** DSA (right) showing repeated focal seizures (arrow), with concordance with the raw EEG (double head arrow). Note that the peak is less pronounced on some derivations (white circle) reflecting the focal character of the seizure.

When these first-line investigations are negative, however, the presence or absence of background abnormalities on EEG will be very helpful in guiding further investigations. A normal background activity in an infant with normal physical examination and clonic seizure evokes benign neonatal seizures, familial or non-familial. A slightly asymmetric background activity with focal sharp waves or spikes and a clonic unilateral seizure is frequent in neonatal stroke and will support the need for a diffusion MRI (Walsh et al., 2011; Selton et al., 2003; Rafay et al., 2009). An abnormal background activity may also confirm HIE when clinical and biological data are insufficiently clear. The so-called "suppression-burst" pattern without birth asphyxia indicates a severe early epileptic syndrome namely early myoclonic epilepsy or Ohtahara syndrome, as well as an inborn error of metabolism.

Early-myoclonic epilepsy and Ohtahara syndrome have been described as two different epileptic syndromes sharing some clinical and electrical characteristics. In Ohtahara syndrome, tonic seizures and early-onset spasms were described as predominant and structural brain abnormalities considered as frequent causes. In early myoclonic epilepsy, the main seizure type is multifocal myoclonias, with less constant suppression-burst pattern and mainly metabolic disturbances. However, recent genetic findings lead to consider those two syndromes as a continuum with clinical forms varying in terms of age onset and/or seizure burden (Ohtahara et al., 2006; Djukic et al., 2006; Beal et al., 2012; Serino et al., 2013; Mastrangelo et al., 2013).

In inborn errors of metabolism, several single cases have been reported with non-specific EEG patterns that could be modified by the treatments used (Agadi et al., 2012; Rossi et al., 2009; Schmitt et al., 2010). Such abnormal patterns should trigger complete genetic and metabolic investigations and systematic treatment by vitamin supplementation (Hallberg et al., 2013).

■ EEG and treatment options

The few antiepileptic drugs available in newborn infants are in reality "anti-seizure" drugs and not "antiepileptic drugs" as they have no effect on aetiology. Most of the seizures in neonates being acute symptomatic, taking care of the underlying condition should be the first-line treatment such as correcting hypoglycaemia or hypocalcemia. In the rare forms of vitamin-dependant epilepsy, supplementation therapy will be the only way to control seizures. In HIE which represents more than half of the etiologies, recent work using video-EEG has shown that seizures were less frequent in a cooled population (Srinivasakumar et al., 2013). Hypothermia should then be considered in the anti-seizure strategy with specific attention on the rewarming period during which rebound of seizures has been observed (Kendall et al., 2012).

On the other hand, if the suspected etiology is an early-onset epileptic syndrome, the objectives of the treatment should not necessarily be a complete control of the seizures. Under certain circumstances a better aim would be to achieve a clinically meaningful reduction of seizure frequency, also avoiding the respiratory and haemodyanmic side effects that could be induced by high doses of anti-seizure drugs.

Whatever the etiology, a rational use of anticonvulsant drugs should be based on seizure burden, monitored by EEG. This is the main interest of digital trendlines, by aEEG or DSA and the scope for automatic detection of seizures. Conventional EEG and aEEG are complementary tools. When signature patterns of the seizures have been identified in cEEG as well as in aEEG or DSA, the trendlines will be more reliable for monitoring.

EEG and prognosis

The term "prognosis" refers to three successive endpoints: the seizures control, the clinical examination and cerebral imaging at discharge, and the long-term development.

Several studies have been conducted to identify predictors for neonatal seizures outcome, among which EEG findings remain a constant along with seizure burden and etiology (Lai et al., 2013; Garfinkkle et al., 2011; Tekgul et al., 2006; Mellits et al., 1982; Khan et al., 2008; Almubarak et al., 2011; Nunes et al., 2005).

To assess the specific role of seizure burden is difficult. Non-convulsive seizures seem to carry a poor prognosis. However, the question to treat or not to treat these subclinical seizures is unresolved and one must balance the potential harmful effects of anticonvulsant drugs on the immature brain with the potential adverse consequences of abnormal sustained electrical activity (McBride et al., 2000; Glass et al., 2011; van des Heide et al., 2012). At a minimum, the first step to resolve this question is to have reliable tools to quantify the number, the duration and the localization of seizure, in other words, a systematic video-EEG monitoring.

The EEG has a specific role in HIE. The need to select infants who will benefit from hypothermia in the first hours of life has significantly changed the practice of EEG in the NICU (Walsh et al., 2011). This first EEG reflects the severity of the insult. A normal background activity in the first hours is reassuring and indicates a good prognosis. Severe background abnormalities at that time may indicate a poor prognosis but have to be confirmed by further recordings. Several classifications of background abnormalities exist with some discrepancies between the criteria and the labels employed. A universal grid for visual analysis is needed. However, severely abnormal EEGs are easily recognized as well as fully normal ones.

The evolution of background activity during the first week will reflect the quality of brain recovery. The persistence of abnormalities after 48 hours of life will confirm a poor prognosis (Murray et al., 2009). Digital analyses are especially useful in this purpose as they may help to quantify the background abnormalities and facilitate long term monitoring.

Hypothermia has to be taken into account when analysing the EEG as it may reduce the amplitude and modify the sleep state cycles (Tsuchida, 2013; Nash et al., 2011). Therefore, beginning the EEG before hypothermia is recommended.

Conclusion

In a landscape dominated by seizures due to HIE, other etiologies and various clinical presentations and evolutions should not be overlooked. EEG plays a major role in this approach and should be the cornerstone of neonatal seizure management.

Despite its reputation of highly skilled technique, EEG is a low-cost and easy to perform investigation when compared to other techniques used in the NICU. The use of digital EEG machines is much simpler than the old paper machines and as a result it is easier to record with modern equipment, although it is still critical to use proper technique for the application of the recording electrodes. The interpretation remains a problem as it requires specific skills and a good knowledge of neonatal pathology including its specific EEG correlates. However, here again, modernization, including digitalized analysis with automated detection along with remote access for analysis has simplified the review process and should facilitate the promotion of this procedure.

In light of clinical situations in which EEG is needed, a rational and pragmatic use would require EEG to be available on a 24/7 basis and for prolonged periods.

In an ideal world, in a neonate with suspected or "expected" seizure, the EEG should be performed as soon as possible by the EEG team or the NICU team with a minimal number of 8 electrodes covering the whole surface of the brain. The electrodes should stay in place for at least 24 hours and be regularly checked. If possible, MRI-compatible electrodes should be used. The first minutes of recording should be rapidly examined, looking for clearly abnormal patterns (flat or very discontinuous tracings, status) that require immediate response. Afterwards, a trend line (aEEG or DSA) could be displayed with a specific teaching for the staff to recognize both the most severe and the fully normal patterns. Any modification of the clinical situation should be noted on the EEG machine by the staff. Reliable detection algorithms should alert the nurses about possible seizures. In case of doubt, a trained neurophysiologist should be contacted to provide an interpretation, on site or by remote access, in emergency and at least once a day. For each 24 hours period, a written report should be produced by a qualified physician.

With around half of the NICU reporting using cEEG or aEEG in international studies (Boylan et al., 2010; Ponnusamy et al., 2010), and more than 80% in France (personal data), this ideal organisation seems reachable shortly but would require a reinforcement in qualified medical and/or nursing staff.

References

- Abend NS, Wusthoff CJ. Neonatal seizures and status epilepticus. *J Clin Neurophysiol* 2012; 29: 441-8.
- Agadi S, Sutton VR, Quach MM, Riviello JJ Jr. The electroencephalogram in neonatal maple syrup urine disease: a case report. *Clin EEG Neurosci* 2012; 43: 64-7.
- Almubarak S, Wong PK. Long-term clinical outcome of neonatal EEG findings. *J Clin Neurophysiol* 2011; 28: 185-9.
- André M, et al. Electroencephalography in premature and full-term infants. Developmental features and glossary. *Neurophysiol Clin* 2010; 40: 59-124.
- Beal JC, Cherian K, Moshe SL. Early-onset epileptic encephalopathies: Ohtahara syndrome and early myoclonic encephalopathy. *Pediatric Neurol* 2012; 47: 317-23.
- Boylan GB, Stevenson NJ, Vanhatalo S. Monitoring neonatal seizures. *Semin Fetal Neonatal Med* 2013; 18: 202-8.
- Boylan G, Burgoyne L, Moore C, O'Flaherty B, Rennie J. An international survey of EEG use in the neonatal intensive care unit. *Acta Paediatr* 2010; 99: 1150-5.
- Djukic A, Fred Lado FA, Shinnar S, Solomon L, Moshé SL. Are early myoclonic encephalopathy (EME) and the Ohtahara syndrome (EIEE) independent of each other? *Epilepsy Res* 2006, 70 (S1): 68-76.
- Garfinkle J, Shevell MI. Prognostic factors and development of a scoring system for outcome of neonatal seizures in term infants. *Eur J Paediatr Neurol* 2011; 15: 222-9.
- Glass HC, Nash KB, Bonifacio SL, et al. Seizures and magnetic resonance imaging-detected brain injury in newborns cooled for hypoxic-ischemic encephalopathy. *J Pediatr* 2011; 159: 731-35.
- Grünebaum A, et al. Apgar score of 0 at 5 minutes and neonatal seizures or serious neurologic dysfunction in relation to birth setting. *Am J Obstet Gynecol* 2013; 209: 323.e1-6.
- Hallberg B, Blennow M. Investigations for neonatal seizures. *Semin Fetal Neonatal Med* 2013; 18: 196-201.

- Kendall GS, Mathieson S, Meek J, Rennie JM. Recooling for rebound seizures after rewarming in neonatal encephalopathy. *Pediatrics* 2012; 130: e451-5.
- Khan RL, Nunes ML, Garcias da Silva LF, da Costa JC. Predictive value of sequential electroencephalogram (EEG) in neonates with seizures and its relation to neurological outcome. *J Child Neurol* 2008; 23: 144-50.
- Khan RL, Nunes ML, Garcias da Silva LF, da Costa JC. Predictive value of sequential electroencephalogram (EEG) in neonates with seizures and its relation to neurological outcome. *J Child Neurol* 2008; 23: 144-50.
- Lai YH, Ho CS, Chiu NC, Tseng CF, Huang YL. Prognostic factors of developmental outcome in neonatal seizures in term infants. *Pediatr Neonatol* 2013; 54: 166-72.
- Malone A, Ryan C, Fitzgerald A, Burgoyne L, Connolly S, Boylan G. Interobserver agreement in neonatal seizure identification. *Epilepsia* 2009; 50: 2097-101.
- Mastrangelo M, Peron A, Spaccini L, *et al*. Neonatal suppression-burst without epileptic seizures: expanding the electroclinical phenotype of STXBP1-related, early-onset encephalopathy. *Epileptic Disord* 2013; 15: 55-61.
- McBride MC, Laroia N, Guillet R. Electrographic seizures in neonates correlate with poor neurodevelopmental outcome. *Neurology* 2000; 55: 506-13.
- Mellits ED, Holden KR, Freeman JM. Neonatal seizures. II. A multivariate analysis of factors associated with outcome. *Pediatrics* 1982; 70: 177-85.
- Murray DM, Boylan GB, Ryan CA, Connolly S. Early EEG findings in hypoxic-ischemic encephalopathy predict outcomes at 2 years. *Pediatrics* 2009; 124: e459-67.
- Murray DM, Boylan GB, Ali I, Ryan CA, Murphy BP, Connolly S. Defining the gap between electrographic seizure burden, clinical expression and staff recognition of neonatal seizures. *Arch Dis Child Fetal Neonatal Ed* 2008; 93: F187-F191.
- Nardou R, Ferrari DC, Ben-Ari Y. Mechanisms and effects of seizures in the immature brain. *Semin Fetal Neonatal Med* 2013; 18: 175-84.
- Nash KB, *et al*. Video-EEG monitoring in newborns with hypoxic-ischemic encephalopathy treated with hypothermia. *Neurology* 2011; 76: 556-62.
- Nunes ML, Giraldes MM, Pinho AP, Costa JC. Prognostic value of non-reactive burst suppression EEG pattern associated to early neonatal seizures. *Arq Neuropsiquiatr* 2005; 63: 14-9.
- Nunez P, Srinivasan R. *Electric Fields of the Brain: The Neurophysics of EEG*, 2nd ed. New York: Oxford University Press, 2006.
- Ohtahara S, Yamatogi Y. Ohtahara syndrome: With special reference to its developmental aspects for differentiating from early myoclonic encephalopathy. *Epilepsy Res* 2006; 70 (S1): 58-67.
- Pinto LC, Giliberti P. Neonatal seizures: background EEG activity and the electroclinical correlation in full-term neonates with hypoxic-ischemic encephalopathy. Analysis by computer-synchronized long-term polygraphic video-EEG monitoring. *Epileptic Disord* 2001; 3: 125-32.
- Ponnusamy V, Nath P, Bissett L, Willis K, Clarke P. Current availability of cerebral function monitoring and hypothermia therapy in UK neonatal units. *Arch Dis Child Fetal Neonatal Ed* 2010; 95: F383-F384.
- Rafay MF, Cortez MA, de Veber GA, *et al*. Predictive value of clinical and EEG features in the diagnosis of stroke and hypoxic ischemic encephalopathy in neonates with seizures. *Stroke* 2009; 40: 2402-7.
- Riviello JJ Jr. Digital trend analysis in the pediatric and neonatal intensive care units. *J Clin Neurophysiol* 2013; 30: 143-55.
- Rossi S, Daniele I, Bastrenta P, Mastrangelo M, Lista G. Early myoclonic encephalopathy and nonketotic hyperglycinemia. *Pediatr Neurol* 2009; 41: 371-4.
- Schmitt B, Baumgartner M, Mills PB, *et al*. Seizures and paroxysmal events: symptoms pointing to the diagnosis of pyridoxine-dependent epilepsy and pyridoxine phosphate oxidase deficiency. *Dev Med Child Neurol* 2010; 52: e133-42.

- Selton D, André M, Hascoët JM. [EEG and ischemic stroke in full-term newborns]. *Neurophysiol Clin* 2003; 33: 120-9.
- Serino D, Specchio N, Pontrelli G, Vigevano F, Fusco L. Video/EEG findings in a KCNQ2 epileptic encephalopathy: a case report and revision of literature data. *Epileptic Disord* 2013; 15: 158-65.
- Shah DK, *et al.* Accuracy of bedside electroencephalographic monitoring in comparison with simultaneous continuous conventional electroencephalography for seizure detection in term infants. *Pediatrics* 2008; 121: 1146-54.
- Shellhaas RA, *et al.* The American Clinical Neurophysiology Society's Guideline on Continuous Electroencephalography Monitoring in Neonates. *J Clin Neurophysiol* 2011; 28: 611-7.
- Srinivasakumar P, Zempel J, Wallendorf M, Lawrence R, Inder T, Mathur A. Therapeutic hypothermia in neonatal hypoxic ischemic encephalopathy: electrographic seizures and magnetic resonance imaging evidence of injury. *J Pediatr* 2013; 163: 465-70.
- Tekgul H, *et al.* The current etiologic profile and neurodevelopmental outcome of seizures in term newborn infants. *Pediatrics* 2006; 117: 1270-80.
- Tsuchida TN, *et al.* American clinical neurophysiology society standardized EEG terminology and categorization for the description of continuous EEG monitoring in neonates: report of the American Clinical Neurophysiology Society critical care monitoring committee. *Clin Neurophysiol* 2013; 30: 161-73.
- Tsuchida TN. EEG background patterns and prognostication of neonatal encephalopathy in the era of hypothermia. *J Clin Neurophysiol* 2013; 30: 122-5.
- van der Heide MJ, Roze E, van der Veere CN, Ter Horst HJ, Brouwer OF, Bos AF. Long-term neurological outcome of term-born children treated with two or more antiepileptic drugs during the neonatal period. *Early Hum Dev* 2012; 88: 33-8.
- Vasudevan C, Levene M. Epidemiology and etiology of neonatal seizures. *Semin Fetal Neonatal Med* 2013; 18: 185-91.
- Walsh BH, Low E, Bogue CO, Murray DM, Boylan GB. Early continuous video electroencephalography in neonatal stroke. *Dev Med Child Neurol* 2011; 53: 89-92.
- Walsh BH, Murray DM, Boylan GB. The use of conventional EEG for the assessment of hypoxic ischaemic encephalopathy in the newborn: a review. *Clin Neurophysiol* 2011; 122: 1284-94.
- Wusthoff CJ. Diagnosing neonatal seizures and status epilepticus. *J Clin Neurophysiol* 2013; 30: 115-21.

Neuro-imaging in neonatal seizures

Lauren C. Weeke, Linda G. van Rooij, Mona C. Toet,
Floris Groenendaal, Linda S. de Vries

Department of Neonatology, Wilhelmina Children's Hospital, UMC Utrecht, Utrecht, The Netherlands

---

Seizures occur more often during the neonatal period than at any other period of life and have a variety of underlying etiologies. The incidence varies between 0.15-3.5 per 1,000 live births, with higher rates in preterm infants and very much depends on the threshold for using continuous aEEG monitoring (Ronen et al., 2007). In previous studies, the mortality has been reported to be as high as 40% but in more recent studies the mortality has come down to 21% (Mastrangelo et al., 2005) and even 7% (Tekgul et al., 2006). However, as opposed to this increase in survival, the prevalence of long-term neurodevelopmental sequelae in survivors has been reported to be about 30% (Bergman et al., 1983). In a more recent study 70 (66%) out of 106 preterm and full-term infants admitted to a neonatal intensive care unit (NICU) had an adverse neurological outcome. Six variables were identified as the most important independent risk factors. Neuro-imaging was one of these six variables, but only cranial ultrasound (cUS) was used (Pisani et al., 2009). Etiologies associated with a poor outcome include cerebral dysgenesis, severe hypoxic-ischemic encephalopathy (HIE), metabolic disorders and infection of the central nervous system. Conversely, infants with focal infarction, transient metabolic disturbances, or idiopathic seizures have been reported to have a favourable outcome.

Most neonatal intensive care units around the world will use cUS as the method of first choice. Computed tomography (CT) is now less commonly used and should only be used in an infant who may acutely need neurosurgical intervention. Magnetic resonance imaging (MRI) is being increasingly used and recognised as the best imaging modality. Looking at the Vermont Oxford neonatal encephalopathy registry 22% of the infants admitted with neonatal encephalopathy still had a CT scan and almost two thirds (65%) had an MRI during the neonatal period (Pfister et al., 2012). In this population, admitted between 2006 and 2010, 65% received anti-epileptic medication during their stay in the NICU. These imaging data are in agreement with data from Tekgul et al. (2006) who studied 89 full-term infants with neonatal seizures. In this study 82% had at least one MRI, whereas 18% only had a CT scan.

Several studies have shown that in the full-term infant, HIE is by far the most common etiology, followed by intracranial haemorrhage and arterial ischemic stroke (*Table I*). These studies were mostly performed before the introduction of therapeutic hypothermia and recent studies have shown that neonatal seizures are less common and better controlled in infants with moderate HIE, treated with hypothermia (Low et al., 2012; Srinivasakumar et al., 2013). Transient metabolic disturbances or inborn errors of metabolism, infection of the central nervous system, cerebral dysgenesis and genetic disorders are less common underlying etiologies for neonatal seizures. Some of these infants may present with encephalopathy and are referred to as "HIE-mimics". Neuro-imaging may help to diagnose an underlying problem, for instance polymicrogyria in Zellweger syndrome, which is important for genetic counselling. In those infants, who die during the neonatal period, and were too unstable to be transported to the MR-unit, a post-mortem MRI should be considered, especially when there is no permission for autopsy. The value of a post-mortem MRI has been shown by several groups (Nicholl et al., 2007; Griffiths et al., 2005). The group of infants with an unknown etiology is becoming smaller as MRI is able to identify lesions, which will not be recognised with cUS or CT, but also because of the advances made in genetics (Weckhuysen et al., 2012 and 2013).

Table I. Etiologic profiles and incidence of neonatal seizures

	Tekgul et al., 2006	Mastrangelo et al., 2005	Yildiz et al., 2012	Ronen et al., 1999	Weeke et al., 2014
HIE	40%	37.1%	28.6%	40%	46%
ICH	17%	4.8%	17%	18%	12.2%
Stroke	18%	11.3%	–	1 case	13.5%
Infection	3% (CNS only)	9.7%	7.2% (+ sepsis)	20% (+ sepsis)	7.6% (+ sepsis)
Cerebral dysgenesis	5%	11.3%	4.5%	10%	2.9%
Metabolic disorders	1%	11.3%	10.7%	19% (including hypoglycaemia)	9% (including hypoglycaemia)
Unknown/ idiopathic	12%	1.6%	8.9%	14%	6.3%

Data on neuro-imaging in newborns presenting with neonatal seizures are scarce and most studies report MRI findings in a specific group of infants, with a diagnosis of either HIE, arterial ischemic stroke or metabolic disorders (Tekgul et al., 2006; Leth et al., 1997). The aim of this review is to discuss the spectrum of neuro-imaging findings in full-term infants with neonatal seizures with different underlying etiologies.

■ Hypoxic-ischemic encephalopathy

Several studies have been reported in the literature about different patterns of injury in relation to HIE. Two main patterns of injury can be recognised. The first one predominantly affects the central grey nuclei (ventrolateral thalami and posterior putamina) and perirolandic cortex bilaterally. Associated involvement of the hippocampus and brain stem is not uncommon. This pattern of injury is most often seen following an acute sentinel event, for instance a ruptured uterus, placental abruption or a prolapsed cord (Miller et al., 2005; Okereafor et al., 2008), and is also referred to as a pattern seen after "acute near total asphyxia". When MRI is performed during the first week, diffusion weighted imaging (DWI) will highlight the abnormalities, which will first become apparent by the end of the first week on conventional imaging (Bednarek et al., 2012).

The second pattern is referred to as the watershed predominant pattern of injury (WS) seen following "prolonged partial asphyxia". The vascular watershed zones (anterior-middle cerebral artery and posterior-middle cerebral artery) are involved, affecting the white matter and in more severely affected infants also the overlying cortex. The lesions can be uni- or bilateral, posterior and/or anterior (Harteman et al., 2013). Although loss of the cortical ribbon and therefore the grey–white matter differentiation can be seen on conventional MRI, DWI highlights the abnormalities and is especially helpful in making an early diagnosis. More widespread punctate lesions in the white matter (PWML) have also been reported within the HIE population. Li et al. (2009) found these PWML in 23% of their infants with neonatal encephalopathy and pointed out that infants with this type of injury had a significantly lower gestational age at birth with a milder degree of encephalopathy and fewer clinical seizures relative to other newborns in their cohort, who were diagnosed to have the two more common patterns of injury. This pattern of brain injury is also seen in newborn infants with congenital heart defects (Li et al., 2009; Galli et al., 2004).

Perinatal arterial ischemic stroke

Neonatal seizures and especially hemiconvulsions often suggest the diagnosis of perinatal arterial ischemic stroke (PAIS). Compared to those who develop seizures due to HIE, seizures related to PAIS tend to develop significantly later and are more often focal (Rafay et al., 2009). It is important to use at least a 2-channel aEEG recording in infants presenting with hemiconvulsions (van Rooij et al., 2010). cUS will be able to recognise the larger middle cerebral artery infarcts and lenticulostriate infarcts which are well within the field of view, but in general it will take 24-72 hours before the increase in echogenicity becomes apparent (Ecury-Goosens et al., 2013). cUS may not be able to recognise cortical infarcts or infarcts in the territory of the posterior cerebral artery, unless the posterior fontanelle is used as an acoustic window (Cowan et al., 2005; van der Aa et al., 2013). MRI and especially diffusion weighted imaging (DWI) enables detection of PAIS within hours after the onset and allows prediction of development of subsequent unilateral spastic cerebral palsy, by assessing involvement of the corticospinal tracts (de Vries et al., 2005 and Kirton et al., 2007).

Cerebrosinovenous thrombosis

Cerebrosinovenous thrombosis (CSVT) may also present with neonatal seizures. The presence of an intraventricular haemorrhage associated with a unilateral thalamic haemorrhage suggests the presence of a CSVT (Wu et al., 2003). Doppler ultrasound may help to diagnose occlusion of the superior sagittal sinus but is less reliable for other sinuses, and an MRI and magnetic resonance venography (MRV) are often required to confirm CSVT. Making the correct diagnosis is important, as anticoagulant therapy is increasingly being used (Moharir et al., 2010). The presence of a neonatal thalamic haemorrhage is strongly associated with later development of electrical status epilepticus in slow wave sleep (Kersbergen et al., 2013).

Intracranial haemorrhage

An intracranial haemorrhage (ICH) in the full-term infant is not as common as in the preterm infant, but does occur (Bruno et al., 2013). Blood in the *posterior fossa* is common, which can be a chance finding (Whitby et al., 2004) and does not often lead to neonatal seizures. An *intraventricular haemorrhage* can be associated with CSVT, but can also occur without a good explanation. Neonatal seizures in a full-term with an IVH may be difficult to control (Toet et al., 2005). A parenchymal haemorrhage can also be diagnosed in the absence of a complicated delivery. A frontal lobe haemorrhage is most common and in the presence of a midline shift neurosurgical intervention may be considered (Brouwer et al., 2010). An infant with a temporal lobe haemorrhage often presents with apneic episodes, which prove to be of epileptic origin, when continuous aEEG monitoring is used (Hoogstrate et al., 2009). Epileptic apneic episodes are thought to originate from the limbic system (Watanabe et al., 1982).

Central nervous system infection

Any infection of the central nervous system (CNS) can present with seizures. Both bacterial and viral CNS infections can occur in the neonatal period, but severe CNS infections are not so common. Early gram negative bacterial infection as well as late onset group B streptococcus infection may be associated with severe brain injury (de Vries et al., 2006). The neuro-imaging pattern may be very characteristic, for instance in *Bacillus cereus* septicaemia, where the white matter may show cystic evolution within hours after the onset of the infection (Lequin et al., 2005). In infants with an *Escherichia coli* infection, hydrocephalus may only become apparent weeks after the acute illness, and isolated dilatation of the fourth ventricle is often an associated finding.

A wide spectrum of viral infections can present with neonatal seizures. Some infants present with a fever and/or a rash and the PCR in the cerebrospinal fluid (CSF) will confirm the diagnosis of an enterovirus or parechovirus encephalitis (Verboon et al., 2006 and 2008). Changes on DWI may be extensive, but the outcome may be better than expected on the basis of these findings in the majority of infants (van Zwol et al., 2009). Herpes simplex virus encephalitis is rare. Severe lesions in the temporal lobes, but also elsewhere in the neonatal brain, are best seen with MRI, and once again more clearly and earlier with DWI (Vossough et al., 2008).

Other infections, for instance *Toxoplasmosis gondii*, can also present with neonatal seizures, in the presence of hydrocephalus and extensive white matter injury.

Inborn errors of metabolism

Inborn errors of metabolism can be difficult to diagnose, and recognition of characteristic neuro-imaging features is very helpful in the diagnostic process. It is beyond the scope of this review to describe all potential metabolic disorders, which may present with neonatal seizures. A useful review was published by Prasad and Hoffmann (2010). A specific imaging pattern can suggest the diagnosis in some disorders and the additional use of ^{1}H-magnetic resonance spectroscopy (^{1}H-MRS) may also aid in making the diagnosis (Leijser et al., 2007).

Newborn infants with nonketotic hyperglycinaemia (NKH) often present with neonatal seizures and/or hiccups which may have been felt by the mother in-utero. The aEEG typically shows a burst suppression pattern without a history of HIE. The diagnosis may already be suspected using cUS, as the corpus callosum is often dysplastic, associated with a so-called bull-horn shape of the ventricles. MRI will be able to confirm this, but DWI will also show restricted diffusion of the posterior limb of the internal capsule and of the dorsal aspect of midbrain and pons due to vacuolating myelinopathy (Kanekar et al., 2013). Using ^{1}H-MRS, the high glycine peak will also suggest NKH.

Newborn infants with *molybdenum cofactor deficiency* or sulphite oxidase deficiency are often considered to have HIE, but the history is often atypical in which case these metabolic disorders should be considered. Typically, the onset of seizures is rather earlier than would be expected from HIE, the seizures are very difficult to control and the background activity tends to deteriorate over time (Sie et al., 2010). An MRI during the first week will show extensive DWI abnormalities preceding extensive cystic evolution which can be seen when the MRI is performed again several weeks later (Stence et al., 2013).

Those with *peroxisomal biogenesis disorders* do not invariably present with neonatal seizures. cUS will recognise ventricular dilation, germinolytic cysts, lenticulostriate vasculopathy. As the fontanelle is large in newborn infants with Zellweger syndrome, polymicrogyria may be recognised with cUS and confirmed with MRI. In addition, MRI will show signal intensity changes in the white matter and delayed myelination of the posterior limb of the internal capsule (PLIC). Using ^{1}H-MRS with a short TE, a reduced N-Acetyl Aspartate peak at 2 parts per million (ppm), a lactate peak at 1.33 ppm and an abnormal peak at 0.9 ppm can be seen, the latter being due to the resonances of the methyl residues of mobile lipids (Groenendaal et al., 2001).

Hypoglycaemia can be considered as a transient metabolic disturbance and newborn infants may present with seizures due to severe hypoglycaemia, usually with a value below 1 mmol/L. cUS tends to miss the abnormalities which are typically located in the occipital white matter, unless the posterior fontanelle is also used. MRI is a better technique to identify the lesions, which are often not restricted to the occipital regions (Burns et al., 2008) (*Table II*).

Table II. Neuro-imaging findings in metabolic disorders

Transient metabolic disorders	Neuro-imaging findings
Hypoglycaemia	Predominant occipital abnormalities
Hyperbilirubinemia (kernicterus)	Increased signal intensity in the globus pallidus on T2 weighted sequence
Inborn errors of metabolism	
Pyridoxine deficiency	Abnormalities of the white matter and corpus callosum; haemorrhage in the white matter.
Biotinidase deficiency	DWI abnormalities of the PLIC, corpus callosum, corona radiata (vacuolating myelinopathy)
Glutaric aciduria type 1	Widened anterior temporal, Sylvian and frontal CSF spaces an T2 hyperintensity of the pallidus
Nonketotic hyperglycinaemia	Dysplastic corpus callosum, DWI abnormalities and lack of myelination of the PLIC (vacuolating myelinopathy)
Molybdenum cofactor deficiency/ sulphite oxidase deficiency	Extensive DWI changes of white matter with cystic evolution
Zellweger syndrome	Germinolytic cysts, lenticulostriate vasculopathy, polymicrogyria; ^{1}H-MRS: abnormal mobile lipid peak at 0.9 ppm

Cerebral dysgenesis/Genetic disorders

Infants with migrational disorders can present with neonatal seizures, but this is rather uncommon and most of the infants will develop seizures later during the first year. In most of these infants, there are associated findings, leading to a diagnosis for instance migrational disorders may be encountered in children with a metabolic disorder (polymicrogyria in Zellweger syndrome) or congenital cytomegalovirus infection. There is a considerable overlap here with genetic disorders and this overlap is increasing with advances in genetics (Yang et al., 2013). Neurocutaneous syndromes (linear naevus syndrome, incontinentia pigmenti, tuberous sclerosis) may also present with neonatal seizures (Merks et al., 2003; Hennel et al., 2003; Isaacs 2009; Wortmann et al., 2008).

Refractory neonatal seizures can increasingly be explained by an underlying genetic problem. Weckhuysen et al. (2012, 2013) recently showed mutations in KCNQ2, which encode the voltage-gated potassium channels Kv7.2 previously associated with benign familial neonatal seizures, in children with unexplained neonatal or early-infantile seizures and associated psychomotor retardation. Early MRI showed characteristic hyperintensities in the basal ganglia and thalamus that later resolved in a subgroup of their patients.

Early infantile epileptic encephalopathy (EIEE, Ohtahara syndrome) is a diagnosis made when intractable seizures are seen in the neonatal period. Many infants with Ohtahara syndrome have an associated underlying cerebral malformation, EIEE has been associated with several gene mutations, including Aristaless-related homeobox (ARX), cyclin-dependent kinase-like 5 (CDKL5), and syntaxin-binding protein 1 (STXBP1). No specific neuroimaging findings have been reported in these children (Pavone et al., 2012).

Aicardi-Goutières syndrome is a genetically determined early-onset encephalopathy with a variable phenotype, including neurological manifestations such as dystonia, spasticity, epileptic seizures, progressive microcephaly, severe developmental delay and calcification within. Aicardi-Goutières syndrome is a genetically heterogeneous disorder with five disease-associated genes (AGS1-5) accounting for 83% of cases that fulfil the clinical diagnostic criteria. In a recent study, 25% percent of the infants were reported to have seizure onset within the first month after birth. cUS will detect calcification better than MRI, but MRI will show delayed myelination, grey and white matter atrophy, ventricular enlargement and cystic degeneration over time, often quite marked in the temporal lobes and the periventricular white matter (Ramantani et al., 2013).

■ Unknown

Although not so common anymore, every now and then neonatal seizures may occur without an explanation on either neuro-imaging or extensive genetic and metabolic investigations. More and more infants can however subsequently be diagnosed at a later stage. Sometimes a second MRI, using higher resolution and thinner slices can detect an area of cortical dysplasia (Wang et al., 2013). In others a new mutation may be identified (Mastrangelo and Leuzzi, 2012).

■ Conclusion

Neuro-imaging is very helpful to identify the underlying etiology of neonatal seizures in full-term infants. cUS should be used in the acute phase and will show severe and centrally located lesions as well as calcification, which will not be recognised with MRI. More detailed information will subsequently be obtained with MRI, provided that thin (2 mm) slices will be made, and sequences suitable for imaging neonates are used. MRI will then be superior in diagnosing migrational disorders and lesions in the posterior fossa. When

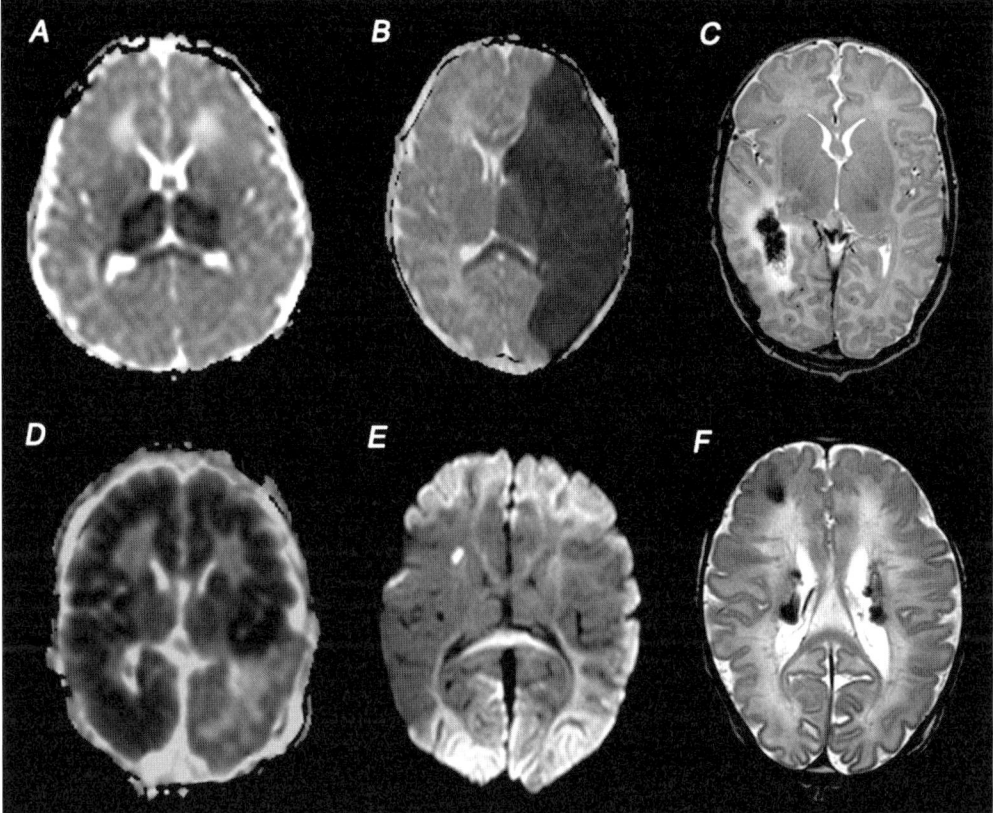

Figure 1. Examples of axial MR images (Apparent Diffusion Coefficient (ADC) map, A, B, D; T2 weightes sequence, C, F; DWI, E) performed during the first week after birth in infants presenting with neonatal seizures (A-E). A. Hypoxic-ischemic injury to the thalami, optic radiation and splenium of the corpus callosum; B. PAIS of the main branch of the left middle cerebral artery; C. Haemorrhage in the right temporal lobe; D. extensive areas of restricted diffusion throughout the white matter with sparing of the left parieto-occipital lobe in molybdenum cofactor deficiency; E. Extensive restricted diffusion of the cortex and subcortical white matter in group B streptococcus encephalitis, also note small infarct in right caudate nucleus; F. Antenatal diagnosis of tuberous sclerosis (cardiac rhabdomyoma), periventricular subependymal nodules and right sided subcortical tuber.

MRS is added to the imaging protocol, metabolic disorders may be suspected prior to full results from metabolic investigations being available. Information on the type and severity of brain lesions may help to give a more accurate prognosis, and in some families, will aid with genetic counselling.

References

- Bednarek N, Mathur A, Inder T, Wilkinson J, Neil J, Shimony J. Impact of therapeutic hypothermia on MRI diffusion changes in neonatal encephalopathy. *Neurology* 2012 1; 78(18): 1420-7.
- Bergman I, Painter M, Hirsch R, Crumrine P, David R. Outcome in neonates with convulsions treated in an intensive care unit. *Ann Neurol* 1983; 14: 642-7.

- Brouwer AJ, Groenendaal F, Koopman C, Nievelstein RJ, Han SK, de Vries LS. Intracranial hemorrhage in full-term newborns: a hospital-based cohort study. *Neuroradiology* 2010; 52(6): 567-76.
- Bruno CJ, Beslow LA, Witmer CM, Vossough A, Jordan LC, Zelonis S, et al. Haemorrhagic stroke in term and late preterm neonates. *ADC-FNN*. Epub 2013.
- Burns CM, Rutherford MA, Boardman JP, Cowan FM. Patterns of cerebral injury and neurodevelopmental outcomes after symptomatic neonatal hypoglycemia. *Pediatrics* 2008; 122(1): 65-74.
- Cowan F, Mercuri E, Groenendaal F, Bassi L, Ricci D, Rutherford M, et al. Does cranial ultrasound imaging identify arterial cerebral infarction in term neonates? *Arch Dis Child Fetal Neonatal Ed.* 2005; 90(3): F252-6.
- de Vries LS, Van der Grond J, Van Haastert IC, Groenendaal F. Prediction of outcome in new-born infants with arterial ischaemic stroke using diffusion-weighted magnetic resonance imaging. *Neuropediatrics* 2005; 36(1): 12-20.
- de Vries LS, Verboon-Maciolek MA, Cowan FM, Groenendaal F. The role of cranial ultrasound and magnetic resonance imaging in the diagnosis of infections of the central nervous system. *Early Hum Dev* 2006; 82(12): 819-25.
- Ecury-Goossen GM, Raets MM, Lequin M, Feijen-Roon M, Govaert P, Dudink J. Risk factors, clinical presentation, and neuroimaging findings of neonatal perforator stroke. *Stroke* 2013; 44(8): 2115-20.
- Galli KK, Zimmerman RA, Jarvik GP, Wernovsky G, Kuypers MK, Clancy RR, et al. Periventricular leukomalacia is common after neonatal cardiac surgery. *J Thorac Cardiovasc Surg* 2004; 127: 692-704.
- Griffiths PD, Paley MN, Whitby EH. Post-mortem MRI as an adjunct to fetal or neonatal autopsy. *Lancet* 2005; 365(9466): 1271-3.
- Groenendaal F, Bianchi MC, Battini R, Tosetti M, Boldrini A, de Vries LS, et al. Proton magnetic resonance spectroscopy (1H-MRS) of the cerebrum in two young infants with Zellweger syndrome. *Neuropediatrics* 2001; 32(1): 23-7.
- Harteman JC, Groenendaal F, Toet MC, Benders MJ, Van Haastert IC, Nievelstein RA, et al. Diffusion-weighted imaging changes in cerebral watershed distribution following neonatal encephalopathy are not invariably associated with an adverse outcome. *Dev Med Child Neurol* 2013; 55(7): 642-53.
- Harting I, Neumaier-Probst E, Seitz A, Maier EM, Assmann B, Baric I, et al. Dynamic changes of striatal and extrastriatal abnormalities in glutaric aciduria type I. *Brain* 2009; 132(Pt 7): 1764-82.
- Hennel SJ, Ekert PG, Volpe JJ, Inder TE. Insights into the pathogenesis of cerebral lesions in incontinentia pigmenti. *Pediatr Neurol* 2003; 29(2): 148-50.
- Hoogstraate SR, Lequin MH, Huysman MA, Ahmed S, Govaert PP. Apnoea in relation to neonatal temporal lobe haemorrhage. *Eur J Paediatr Neurol* 2009; 13(4): 356-61.
- Isaacs H. Perinatal (fetal and neonatal) tuberous sclerosis: a review. *Am J Perinatol* 2009; 26(10): 755-60.
- Kanekar S, Byler D. Characteristic MRI findings in neonatal nonketotic hyperglycinemia due to sequence changes in GLDC gene encoding the enzyme glycine decarboxylase. *Metab Brain Dis* 2013; 28(4): 717-20.
- Kersbergen KJ, de Vries LS, Leijten FS, Braun KP, Nievelstein RA, Groenendaal F, et al. Neonatal thalamic hemorrhage is strongly associated with electrical status epilepticus in slow wave sleep. *Epilepsia* 2013; 54(4): 733-40.
- Kirton A, Shroff M, Visvanathan T, deVeber G. Quantified corticospinal tract diffusion restriction predicts neonatal stroke outcome. *Stroke* 2007; 38(3): 974-80.

- Leijser L, de Vries LS, Rutherford MA, Manzur AY, Groenendaal F, de Koning TJ, et al. Cranial Ultrasound in Metabolic Disorders Presenting in the Neonatal Period: Characteristic Features and Comparison with MR Imaging. *AJNR Am J Neuroradiol* 2007; 28: 1223-31.
- Leth H, Toft PB, Herning M, Peitersen B, Lou HC. Neonatal seizures associated with cerebral lesions shown by magnetic resonance imaging. *Arch Dis Child Fetal Neonatal Ed.* 1997; 77: F105-F10.
- Lequin MH, Vermeulen JR, van Elburg RM, Barkhof F, Kornelisse RF, Swarte R, et al. Bacillus cereus meningoencephalitis in preterm infants: neuroimaging characteristics. *AJNR Am J Neuroradiol* 2005; 26(8): 2137-43.
- Li AM, Chau V, Poskitt KJ, Sargent MA, Lupton BA, Hill A, et al. White matter injury in term newborns with neonatal encephalopathy. *Pediatr Re* 2009; 65(1): 85-9.
- Low E, Boylan GB, Mathieson SR, Murray DM, Korotchikova I, Stevenson NJ, et al. Cooling and seizure burden in term neonates: an observational study. *Arch Dis Child Fetal Neonatal Ed.* 2012; 97(4): F267-72.
- Mastrangelo M, Van Lierde A, Bray M, Pastorino G, Marini A, Mosca F. Epileptic seizures, epilepsy and epileptic syndromes in newborns: a nosological approach to 94 new cases by the 2001 proposed diagnostic scheme for people with epileptic seizures and with epilepsy. *Seizure* 2005; 14(5): 304-11.
- Mastrangelo M, Leuzzi V. Genes of early-onset epileptic encephalopathies: from genotype to phenotype. *Pediatr Neurol* 2012; 46(1): 24-31.
- Merks JH, de Vries LS, Zhou XP, Nikkels P, Barth PG, Eng C, et al. PTEN hamartoma tumour syndrome: variability of an entity. *J Med Genet* 2003; 40(10): e111.
- Miller SP, Ramaswamy V, Michelson D, Barkovich AJ, Holshouser B, Wycliffe N, et al. Patterns of brain injury in term neonatal encephalopathy. *J Pediatr* 2005; 146(4): 453-60.
- Moharir MD, Shroff M, Stephens D, Pontigon AM, Chan A, MacGregor D, et al. Anticoagulants in pediatric cerebral sinovenous thrombosis: a safety and outcome study. *Ann Neurol* 2010; 67(5): 590-9.
- Nicholl RM, Balasubramaniam VP, Urquhart DS, Sellathurai N, Rutherford MA. Postmortem brain MRI with selective tissue biopsy as an adjunct to autopsy following neonatal encephalopathy. *Eur J Paediatr Neurol* 2007; 11(3): 167-74.
- Okereafor A, Allsop J, Counsell SJ, Fitzpatrick J, Azzopardi D, Rutherford MA, et al. Patterns of brain injury in neonates exposed to perinatal sentinel events. *Pediatrics* 2008; 121: 906-14.
- Pavone P, Spalice A, Polizzi A, Parisi P, Ruggieri M. Ohtahara syndrome with emphasis on recent genetic discovery. *Brain Dev* 2012; 34(6): 459-68.
- Pfister RH, Bingham P, Edwards EM, Horbar JD, Kenny MJ, Inder T, et al. The Vermont oxford neonatal encephalopathy registry: rationale, methods, and initial results. *BMC Ped* 2012; 22; 12: 84.
- Pisani F, Sisti L, Seri S. A scoring system for early prognostic assessment after neonatal seizures. *Pediatrics* 2009; 124(4): e580-7.
- Prasad AN, Hoffmann GF. Early onset epilepsy and inherited metabolic disorders: diagnosis and management. *Can J Neurol Sci* 2010; 37(3): 350-8.
- Rafay MF, Cortez MA, de Veber GA, Tan-Dy C, Al-Futaisi A, Yoon W, et al. Predictive value of clinical and EEG features in the diagnosis of stroke and hypoxic ischemic encephalopathy in neonates with seizures. *Stroke* 2009; 40(7): 2402-7.
- Ramantani G, Maillard LG, Bas T, Husain RA, Niggemann P, Kohlhase J, et al. Epilepsy in Aicardi-Goutières syndrome. *Eur J Paediatr Neurol* 2013 Sep 4. [Epub ahead of print].
- Ronen GM, Buckley D, Penney S, Streiner DL. Long-term prognosis in children with neonatal seizures: a population-based study. *Neurology* 2007 6; 69(19): 1816-22.

- Sie SD, de Jonge RC, Blom HJ, Mulder MF, Reiss J, Vermeulen RJ, et al. Chronological changes of the amplitude-integrated EEG in a neonate with molybdenum cofactor deficiency. *J Inherit Metab Dis* 2010; 33 (suppl 3): 401-7.
- Soares-Fernandes JP, Magalhães Z, Rocha JF, Barkovich AJ. Brain diffusion-weighted and diffusion tensor imaging findings in an infant with biotinidase deficiency. *Am J Neuroradiol* 2009; 30(9): E128.
- Srinivasakumar P, Zempel J, Wallendorf M, Lawrence R, Inder T, Mathur A. Therapeutic hypothermia in neonatal hypoxic ischemic encephalopathy: electrographic seizures and magnetic resonance imaging evidence of injury. *J Pediatr* 2013; 163(2): 465-70.
- Stence NV, Coughlin CR 2nd, Fenton LZ, Thomas JA. Distinctive pattern of restricted diffusion in a neonate with molybdenum cofactor deficiency. *Pediatr Radiol* 2013; 43(7): 882-5.
- Tekgul H, Gauvreau K, Soul J, Murphy L, Robertson R, Stewart J, et al. The Current Etiologic Profile and Neurodevelopmental Outcome of Seizures in Term Newborn Infants. *Pediatrics* 2006; 117(4): 1270-80.
- Toet MC, Groenendaal F, Osredkar D, van Huffelen AC, de Vries LS. Postneonatal epilepsy following amplitude-integrated EEG-detected neonatal seizures. *Pediatr Neurol* 2005; 32(4): 241-7.
- van der Aa NE, Dudink J, Benders MJ, Govaert P, van Straaten HL, Porro GL, et al. Neonatal posterior cerebral artery stroke: clinical presentation, MRI findings, and outcome. *Dev Med Child Neurol* 2013; 55(3): 283-90.
- van Rooij LG, de Vries LS, van Huffelen AC, Toet MC. Additional value of two-channel amplitude integrated EEG recording in full-term infants with unilateral brain injury. *Arch Dis Child Fetal Neonatal Ed* 2010; 95(3): F160-8.
- van Zwol AL, Lequin M, Aarts-Tesselaar C, van der Eijk AA, Driessen GA, de Hoog M, et al. Fatal neonatal parechovirus encephalitis. *BMJ Case Rep* 2009; doi: 10.1136/bcr.05.2009.1883.
- Verboon-Maciolek MA, Groenendaal F, Cowan F, Govaert P, van Loon AM, de Vries LS. White matter damage in neonatal enterovirus meningoencephalitis. *Neurology* 2006; 66(8): 1267-9.
- Verboon-Maciolek MA, Groenendaal F, Hahn CD, Hellmann J, van Loon AM, Boivin G, et al. Human parechovirus causes encephalitis with white matter injury in neonates. *Ann Neurol* 2008; 64(3): 266-73.
- Vossough A, Zimmerman RA, Bilaniuk LT, Schwartz EM. Imaging findings of neonatal herpes simplex virus type 2 encephalitis. *Neuroradiology* 2008; 50(4): 355-66.
- Watanabe K, Hara K, Miyazaki S, Hakamada S, Kuroyanagi M. Apneic seizures in the newborn. *Am J Dis Child* 1982; 136: 980-4.
- Wang DD, Deans AE, Barkovich AJ, Tihan T, Barbaro NM, Garcia PA, et al. Transmantle sign in focal cortical dysplasia: a unique radiological entity with excellent prognosis for seizure control. *J Neurosurg* 2013; 118(2): 337-44.
- Weckhuysen S, Mandelstam S, Suls A, Audenaert D, Deconinck T, Claes LR, et al. KCNQ2 Encephalopathy: Emerging Phenotype of a Neonatal Epileptic Encephalopathy. *Ann Neurol* 2012; 71(1): 15-25.
- Weckhuysen S, Ivanovic V, Hendrickx R, Van Coster R, Hjalgrim H, Møller RS, et al. On behalf of the KCNQ2 Study Group. Extending the KCNQ2 encephalopathy spectrum: Clinical and neuroimaging findings in 17 patients. *Neurology* 2013; 81(19): 1697-703.
- Weeke LC, Groenendaal F, Toet MC, Benders MJ, Nievelstein RA, van Rooij LG, et al. The aetiology of neonatal seizures and the diagnostic contribution of neonatal cerebral magnetic resonance imaging. *Dev Med Child Neurol* 2014; doi: 10.1111/dmcn.12629.
- Whitby EH, Griffiths PD, Rutter S, Smith MF, Sprigg A, Ohadike P, et al. Frequency and natural history of subdural haemorrhages in babies and relation to obstetric factors. *Lancet* 2004; 363(9412): 846-51.

- Wortmann SB, Reimer A, Creemers JW, Mullaart RA. Prenatal diagnosis of cerebral lesions in Tuberous sclerosis complex (TSC). Case report and review of the literature. *Eur J Paediatr Neurol* 2008; 12(2): 123-6.
- Wu YW, Hamrick SE, Miller SP, Haward MF, Lai MC, Callen PW, et al. Intraventricular hemorrhage in term neonates caused by sinovenous thrombosis. *Ann Neurol* 2003; 54(1): 123-6.
- Yang Y, Muzny DM, Reid JG, Bainbridge MN, Willis A, Ward PA, et al. Clinical Whole-Exome Sequencing for the Diagnosis of Mendelian Disorders. *N Engl J Med* 2013; 369: 1502-11; doi: 10.1056/NEJMoa1306555.
- Yildiz EP, Tatli B, Ekici B, Eraslan E, Aydinli N, Caliskan M, et al. Evaluation of etiologic and prognostic factors in neonatal convulsions. *Pediatr Neurol* 2012; 47(3): 186-92; doi: 10.1016/j.pediatrneurol.2012.05.015.

Clinical and electrographical neonatal seizures: to treat or not to treat

Lena Hellström-Westas

Department of Women's and Children's Health, Uppsala University and University Hospital, Uppsala, Sweden

The question whether clinical and electrographical neonatal seizures should be treated or not is complicated and cannot be answered with a straight yes or no. For a long time, general recommendations for newborn infants with clinical seizures have been that they should receive antiepileptic treatment. Whether also electrographic seizures without clinical manifestations, *i.e.* subclinical seizures, should be treated with antiepileptic medications has been a matter of debate for more than two decades. A major contributing factor for these discussions is that the overall scientific evidence for the management of neonatal seizures is not very strong.

Around 1-3 per 1,000 newborn infants are affected by neonatal seizures. A majority of these seizures appear during the first three days of life, commonly after a previous insult affecting cerebral blood flow, oxygenation, and/or metabolism (Ronen *et al.*, 1989). Neonatal seizures due to epileptic syndromes, malformations or hereditary diseases are less common. Neonatal seizures are consequently associated with acute brain injury, increased mortality and risk for epilepsy and neurocognitive handicaps in survivors.

Previously, neonatal seizures were mainly diagnosed when clinical seizures were observed. However, it has been known for almost three decades that many clinically recognized seizures in newborns do not have electrographic correlates (Mizrahi and Kellaway, 1987). Furthermore, several studies have demonstrated that a majority of neonatal seizures are entirely subclinical, *i.e.* electrographic without obvious clinical symptoms.

Clinical manifestations of neonatal seizures were previously classified according to Volpe as *clonic*, *tonic*, *myoclonic*, and *subtle* according to the dominating symptoms, and this classification is still very much used in neonatal departments (Volpe, 1989). The seizures could further be described as *focal*, *multifocal* or *generalized*. However, *subclinical* seizures were not included in this classification. The revised report of the International League Against Epilepsy (ILAE) defines an epileptic seizure as "a transient occurrence of signs and/or symptoms due to abnormal excessive or synchronous neuronal activity in the brain" (Berg *et al.*, 2009). The latest revision also included some changes of the previous classification from 1981, including the notion that neonatal seizures should no longer be regarded as a separate entity, furthermore that seizures in neonates should be classified within the same scheme as other seizures as: *generalized seizures* (including tonic-clonic, absence, myoclonic, clonic, tonic, atonic), *focal seizures* and *unknown* (epileptic spasms) (Berg et al., 2009). However, since a majority of neonatal seizures are subclinical, these seizures do not fit very well in this classification.

Clinical seizures

Clinical recognition of abnormal movements and behaviours is the dominating mode of diagnosing seizures in newborn infants. However, studies using video-EEG have shown that a majority of clinically suspected seizures do not have corresponding electrographic seizure activity (Mizrahi and Kellaway, 1987; Murray et al., 2009). Still, abnormal clinical behaviours suggestive of being seizures, although no EEG was recorded to verify the epileptic nature, were also shown to be independently associated with adverse neurodevelopmental outcome in both term asphyxiated infants and in preterm infants (Glass et al., 2009; Davis et al., 2010). Some of these clinical seizures probably represent electroclinical seizures, while others are symptoms of neurological compromise. Increased severity of clinically recognized seizures has also been associated with more severe morphologic brain injury and signs of metabolic derangement, as demonstrated by MRI and MR spectroscopy (Millet et al., 2002). Little is known about the semiology of neonatal seizures, although it is well known that the duration and clinical symptoms may be grossly affected by administration of antiepileptic medications. Infants with subtle and generalized tonic seizures, or two or more clinical seizure-types, seem to have a higher risk for adverse outcome such as epilepsy, mental retardation and cerebral palsy (Brunquell et al., 2002). Nagarajan and coworkers showed that many infants exhibit multiple (average 2.7) clinical features during a seizure, and suggested a semiologic classification based on the initial feature (Nagarajan et al., 2012).

Traditionally, antiepileptic medications to newborn infants has been administered according to the presence or absence of clinical seizures, and the response of the medication on the clinical seizures was also a major determinant for assessing efficacy in many earlier studies.

Phenobarbital is the preferred first drug of choice by many clinicians, and several pharmacokinetic and dosing studies have been performed. According to the Cochrane review on antiepileptic treatment in newborns, published in 2004, only two randomized studies have evaluated antiepileptic medications in newborns in relation to EEG response (Booth and Evans, 2004). One of these studies included a follow up to one-year while the other study assessed effect of the treatment on EEG. Consequently, there is almost no information available on possible long-term benefits, or adverse effects, of antiepileptic treatment related to neonatal effects.

Phenobarbital was given to infants in a few randomized trials with the main goal to improve long-term outcomes after perinatal asphyxia (Hall et al., 1998; Evans et al., 2007). The primary goal of these studies was consequently not to control seizures, although some studies did show a reduction of clinical seizures. Two studies (one published as an abstract) also included long-term follow up, but according to a Cochrane review published in 2007, there was no reduction in mortality or severe neurodevelopmental disability in term asphyxiated infants receiving phenobarbital as compared to controls (Evans et al., 2007).

What happens if an infant with recurrent clinical seizures does not receive antiepileptic treatment? There is a high risk for hypoxia, hypoventilation, nutritional problems, hypoglycemia, and with intense and prolonged seizures an increased risk for cardiovascular collapse and death. There is also a high risk that repeated hypoxia and muscle activity from the clinical seizures may cause the infant distress and pain. Cerebral high-energy phosphate balance was assessed by ^{31}P- MR spectroscopy in eight infants with EEG verified seizures. Seizures occurred during the examination in four infants and were associated with a 50% decrease in the phosphocreatine to inorganic phosphate (PCr/Pi) ratio, with focal seizures causing lateralized decreases in the PCr/Pi ratio. One infant with seizures received phenobarbital i.v. (10 mg/kg), resulting in an immediate increase in the PCR/Pi ratio from 0.7 to 1.2 (Younkin et al., 1986). Several studies have also demonstrated relatively large changes in cerebral blood flow and arterial blood pressure during both subtle clinical and subclinical seizures (see below). Induced bicuculline status epilepticus for 30 minutes in anesthetized, neonatal monkeys with stable blood pressure, plasma glucose and oxygenation, was associated with high energy phosphate and glucose depletion and elevated lactate in cortex and thalamus (Fujikawa et al., 1988). Neonatal rats seem to be relatively resistant to the acute effects of induced seizures, although they may experience alteration of synaptic plasticitiy and later suboptimal cognitive performance (Isaeva et al., 2013).

Electrographic seizures

Neonatal electrographic seizure activity is often defined as: "sudden repetitive, evolving and stereotyped ictal pattern with a clear beginning, middle and ending and a minimum duration of (5-) 10 sec"; the duration of the ictal discharge may range from 10 seconds to several minutes (Boylan et al., 2002; André et al., 2010). More recently, the American Clinical Neurophysiology Society defined an electrographic seizure as "a sudden, abnormal EEG event defined by a repetitive and evolving pattern with a minimum 2 mV pp voltage and duration of at least 10 seconds" (Tsuchida et al., 2013). A majority of investigators require that a seizure has a duration of at least 10 seconds, although there are studies showing that also brief rhythmic discharges (BRD or BIRD, brief ictal/interictal discharges) are associated with hypoxic-ischemic brain injury and white matter injury (Oliveira et al., 2000). The evolving pattern is one of the characteristics of neonatal seizures, but is usually not evident in periodic lateralized epileptic discharges (PLED) (Scher and Beggarly, 1989). Neonatal status epilepticus is usually defined as seizure duration of more than 30 minutes, or more than 50% of the duration of an EEG recording.

Electrographic seizures may be "electroclinical", i.e. the seizures have simultaneous clinical manifestations, or they may be "subclinical", i.e. the seizures have no obvious concomitant clinical signs. In practice, the delineation between electroclinical and electrographic (subclinical) seizures is not entirely sharp since it is likely that subtle clinical symptoms may be present in some seizures considered to be electrographic only, and an infant may have a combination of clinical, electroclinical and electrographic (subclinical) seizures.

Electrographic seizures have been increasingly recognized with the introduction and increasing use of various methods for continuous EEG monitoring. It was consequently shown with amplitude-integrated EEG already in the mid 1980s that subclinical seizures are common in NICU-treated infants and may persist for many hours (Hellström-Westas et al., 1985). It was also shown by Clancy and co-workers that a majority (80%) of seizures in EEG recordings were "occult", i.e. without clinical manifestations (Clancy et al., 1988). With the increasing use of EEG-monitoring also the phenomena called "uncoupling" has become ingcreasingly recognized, i.e. that administration of antiepileptic treatment is associated with abolished clinical seizures but that epileptic activity continues as subclinical seizures (Connell et al., 1989; Boylan et al., 2002).

Effects of seizures

Neonatal seizures are associated with increased arterial blood pressure even if the clinical seizure manifestations are subtle (Lou and Friis-Hansen, 1979; Perlman and Volpe, 1983). The study by Lou and Friis-Hansen included nine infants who were either term-asphyxiated infants or preterm infants with respiratory distress. Clinical seizures were associated with 50-100% increase in mean arterial blood pressure. In the study by Perlman and Volpe, 12 preterm infants had subtle or generalized tonic seizures. In some, but not in all infants, seizures were confirmed by EEG while in others a positive clinical response to antiepileptic treatment counted as an indicator of seizures. In spite of the relatively subtle seizure symptoms, mean arterial blood pressure rose with an average of 13.8 mm Hg during seizures; also cerebral blood flow velocity and intracranial pressure increased during seizures (Perlman and Volpe, 1983).

In a cohort of extremely preterm infants, who had continuous two-channel aEEG/EEG monitoring, 11 infants had seizures that were verified by the two-channel EEG. Seizures were accompanied by a brief increase in heart rate and decrease in respiratory rate. A majority of the infants had subclinical seizures and two had clinical seizures (Shah et al., 2010).

Also using continuous EEG, Boylan and coworkers demonstrated a mean increase of 15.6% in cerebral blood flow velocity, as measured by Doppler, in 11 term born infants with both electroclinical and subclinical seizures (Boylan et al., 1999). With positron emission tomography (PET, focal increases in cerebral blood flow were associated with clinical and subclinical seizures in 12 newborn infants (Börch et al., 1998).

To treat or not to treat

There is a long-standing clinical tradition that newborn infants with both clinical and electrographical seizures should receive antiepileptic treatment but the scientific evidence for this recommendation is not very strong. Only a few studies have investigated the effects of antiepileptic medications in a randomized way, and evaluated these effects on electrographic seizures and outcome. Phenobarbital and phenytoin were compared in a randomized study with a cross-over design, and were found to be equally effective with around 45% of term born infants responding to a single loading dose of either drug, and around 60% responding when both drugs were combined (Painter et al., 1999). No long-term follow up was performed in this study. A smaller study compared lignocaine and benzodiazepines as second line drugs (after phenobarbitone) in a randomized way. Only a few infants required second-line medications, which was associated with a high risk for adverse neurodevelopment at one year. Three out of five infants responded to lignocaine while none of six infants receiving benzodiazepines responded (Boylan et al., 2004).

Two randomized studies compared efficacy of seizure treatment in encephalopathic infants with continuous aEEG/EEG in whom the monitor screen was either blank or visible, i.e. in one group electrographical seizures were treated and in the other group only clinical seizures were treated but the EEG was recorded for later analysis (Lawrence et al., 2009; van Rooij et al., 2010). In both studies, the overall seizure burden and the proportion of subclinical seizures was high. One study included 40 infants, 20 with visible screen and 20 with blinded screen. There were non-significant trends that the seizure burden (p = 0.114) and global MRI injury score (p = 0.11) were reduced in the group with visible screen (Lawrence et al., 2009). The other study included 33 infants, and also in this study there was a non-significant trend that infants with visible screen had lower duration of seizures (van Rooij et al., 2010). In this study the duration of the seizure pattern correlated with the severity of brain injury on MRI, and this association was significant in the group with blinded screen but not in the group with visible screen and seizures.

Outcome in infants with neonatal seizures

Many studies have shown associations between neonatal seizures, high mortality and increased risks for neurodevelopmental impairments and epilepsy in survivors. Miller and collaborators performed MRIs in term infants with HI, 33/90 infants developed seizures. Severity of seizures correlated independently with signs of metabolic injury (MRS) on cerebral MRIs, performed at a median age of 6 days, indicating that seizures per se may have adverse effects (Miller et al., 2002).

The effects of seizures on outcome in very preterm infants seem to differ somewhat as compared to term infants. In a large (n = 6,499) epidemiological study of extremely low birthweight infants (401-1,000 grams), 414 infants had clinical seizures which were associated with higher mortality and neurodevelopmental impairment (Davis et al., 2010). However, in two clinical studies evaluating electrographic seizures the association with adverse long-term outcome was not so clear. In a cohort of 49 very preterm infants (gestational age < 32 weeks) with a majority being extremely preterm (GA < 28 w) electrographic seizures were detected by aEEG/EEG monitoring during the first three days of life in 43%. The median seizure burden during the first 72 hours in infants affected by seizures was 4 min and 14 sec. Seizures were associated with presence of intraventricular hemorrhages but not with long-term outcome at 2 years (Wikström et al., 2012). None of these infants received antiepileptic treatment. In a study of 95 very preterm infants with GA 24-30 weeks, electrographic seizures were identified in 48% of the infants. Seizures were subclinical in all but 3 of the 46 infants affected by seizures. The median seizure burden during the first 72 hours was 104 seconds. Seizures were associated with IVH and mortality, and in a subgroup also with poorer language performance at 2 years (Vesoulis et al., 2014).

There is little animal data that includes models comparable to the clinical situation, including electroclinical and electrographical seizures. Wirrell et al. demonstrated increased brain injury in 10-day old rats subjected to a combination of hypoxia-ischemia and induced seizures with kainic acid, as compared to rats who also underwent hypoxia-ischemia but who did not receive kainic acid (Wirrell et al., 2001). These findings indicate that the added seizures contributed to increase the injury. More recently, a similar animal model was presented using the Rice-Vannucci method with unilateral carotid ligation followed by hypoxia in 12-day old rats. The EEG was recorded in these rats and demonstrated clinical as well as subclinical seizures (Cuaycong et al., 2011).

Conclusion

Currently, neonatal seizures are treated, or not treated, according to therapeutic traditions and individual opinions but without strong scientific support for the management. There are no indications that electroclinical seizures and electrographic seizures differ in physiological characteristics or effects, and seizure-expression may also vary from time to time in the same infant. The rationales for administering antiepileptic treatment are several: seizures look unpleasant and may be experienced as distressing and painful for the affected infant; seizures are associated with cerebral hemodynamic and metabolic effects even when infants have subclinical or subtle clinical seizures; animal data indicate that neonatal epileptic seizures also in well oxygenated animals are associated with adverse cerebral metabolic effects. Neonatal seizures are often markers of perinatal brain injury and there is a risk that untreated neonatal seizures may increase preexisting brain injury due to, for instance, metabolic demands that are exceeded or excitotoxic injury. Several studies demonstrate that the seizure burden is associated with the severity of brain injury. Data from one small randomized study indicates that treatment of subclinical seizures may interrupt this association, and this finding therefore supports the view that acute antiepileptic treatment is beneficial (van Rooij et al., 2010). Although no results from controlled studies are available, data from two studies using aEEG/EEG monitoring with the aim to also abolish subclinical seizures showed that these populations seemed to have a lower risk for postnatal epilepsy (8-9%) compared to other studies (Pisani et al., 2012), even when few infants received prophylactic treatment (Hellström-Westas et al., 1995; Toet et al., 2007; Pisani et al., 2012).

New data indicate that brief subclinical seizures are prevalent in very preterm infants and may affect almost half of these infants (Wikström et al., 2012; Vesoulis et al., 2014). A majority of the very preterm infants having seizure did not receive antiepileptic treatment, and although the presence of seizures was associated with intraventricular haemorrhages and short term outcome, seizures did not seem to exert major effects on long-term outcomes in survivors. Consequently, the optimal antiepileptic treatment management may differ according to the aetiology of the seizures, and also to the gestational age of the infant not least due to the maturation of neurotransmitters that occurs during the third trimester (Herlenius and Lagercrantz, 2001). Furthermore, several studies have demonstrated that some of the commonly used antiepileptic drugs may exert adverse effects on the immature brain including increased apoptosis (Bittigau et al., 2002). Long-term prophylactic antiepileptic medication, usually with phenobarbital, is frequently administered in newborn infants who developed seizures. The necessity of this strategy has been questioned (Guillet and Kwon, 2008). Unfortunately, one of the few controlled studies to investigate this in a prospective randomized fashion, and with long-term follow up, was terminated because of inadequate rate of enrollment (NCT01089504) which also reflects the difficulties encountered when performing this kind of clinical studies in neonates.

Both electroclinical and electrographic seizures in newborn seem to result in measurable physiological effects, although very little is known about the effects on the brain. The clinical expressions of neonatal seizures vary but there seems to be no fundamental difference between electroclinical and subclinical seizures. There is evidence from both human and animal data that neonatal seizures affect cerebral blood flow and metabolism, which indicates that they should be treated. Furthermore, prolonged and untreated seizures are associated with brain injury. The risk for postnatal epilepsy may be reduced if also subclinical seizures are treated, as indicated from a few observational studies, but this should be assessed in controlled studies. The vulnerability of newborn brains to seizures differs from that of older individuals. Consequently, it is necessary to continue to develop adequate experimental models for neonatal seizures. Only a few studies have investigated the efficacy of antiepileptic medications on electrographic seizures, and only a few studies on antiepileptic treatment have assessed long-term effects on neurodevelopment. More research on neonatal seizures, including both clinical studies and animal models is urgently needed!

References

- André M, Lamblin MD, d'Allest AM, et al. Electroencephalography in premature and full-term infants. Developmental features and glossary. *Neurophysiol Clin* 2010; 40: 59-124.
- Berg AT, Berkovic SF, Brodie MJ, et al. Revised terminology and concepts for organization of seizures and epilepsies: report of the ILAE Commission on Classification and Terminology, 2005-2009. *Epilepsia* 2010; 51: 676-85.
- Bittigau P, Sifringer M, Genz K, et al. Antiepileptic drugs and apoptotic neurodegeneration in the developing brain. *Proc Natl Acad Sci USA* 2002; 99: 15089-94.
- Booth D, Evans DJ. Anticonvulsants for neonates with seizures. *Cochrane Database Syst Rev* 2004: CD004218.
- Børch K, Pryds O, Holm S, Lou H, Greisen G. Regional cerebral blood flow during seizures in neonates. *J Pediatr* 1998; 132: 431-5.
- Boylan GB, Panerai RB, Rennie JM, Evans DH, Rabe-Hesketh S, Binnie CD. Cerebral blood flow velocity during neonatal seizures. *Arch Dis Child Fetal Neonatal* 1999; 80: F105-10.
- Boylan GB, Rennie JM, Pressler RM, Wilson G, Morton M, Binnie CD. Phenobarbitone, neonatal seizures, and video-EEG. *Arch Dis Child Fetal Neonatal* 2002; 86: F165-70.
- Boylan GB, Rennie JM, Chorley G, et al. Second-line anticonvulsant treatment of neonatal seizures: a video-EEG monitoring study. *Neurology* 2004; 62: 486-8.
- Brunquell PJ, Glennon CM, DiMario FJ Jr, Lerer T, Eisenfeld L. Prediction of outcome based on clinical seizure type in newborn infants. *J Pediatr* 2002; 140: 707-12. Erratum in: *J Pediatr* 2002; 141: 452.
- Clancy RR, Legido A, Lewis D. Occult neonatal seizures. *Epilepsia* 1988; 29: 256-61.
- Connell J, Oozeer R, de Vries L, Dubowitz LM, Dubowitz V. Clinical and EEG response to anticonvulsants in neonatal seizures. *Arch Dis Child* 1989; 64 (4 Spec No): 459-64.
- Cuaycong M, Engel M, Weinstein SL, et al. A novel approach to the study of hypoxia-ischemia-induced clinical and subclinical seizures in the neonatal rat. *Dev Neurosci* 2011; 33: 241-50.
- Davis AS, Hintz SR, Van Meurs KP, et al. Seizures in extremely low birth weight infants are associated with adverse outcome. *J Pediatr* 2010; 157: 720-5.e1-2.
- Evans DJ, Levene MI, Tsakmakis M. Anticonvulsants for preventing mortality and morbidity in full term newborns with perinatal asphyxia. *Cochrane Database Syst Rev* 2007; 18: CD001240.
- Fujikawa DG, Vannucci RC, Dwyer BE, Wasterlain CG. Generalized seizures deplete brain energy reserves in normoxemic newborn monkeys. *Brain Res* 1988; 454: 51-9.
- Glass HC, Glidden D, Jeremy RJ, Barkovich AJ, Ferriero DM, Miller SP. Clinical neonatal seizures are independently associated with outcome in infants at risk for hypoxic-ischemic brain injury. *J Pediatr* 2009; 155: 318-23.
- Guillet R, Kwon JM. Prophylactic phenobarbital administration after resolution of neonatal seizures: survey of current practice. *Pediatrics* 2008; 122: 731-5.
- Hall RT, Hall FK, Daily DK. High-dose phenobarbital therapy in term newborn infants with severe perinatal asphyxia: a randomized, prospective study with three-year follow-up. *J Pediatr* 1998; 132: 345-8.
- Hellström-Westas L, Rosén I, Swenningsen NW. Silent seizures in sick infants in early life. Diagnosis by continuous cerebral function monitoring. *Acta Paediatr Scand* 1985; 74: 741-8.
- Hellström-Westas L, Blennow G, Lindroth M, Rosén I, Svenningsen NW. Low risk of seizure recurrence after early withdrawal of antiepileptic treatment in the neonatal period. *Arch Dis Child Fetal Neonatal Ed* 1995; 72: F97-101.
- Herlenius E, Lagercrantz H. Neurotransmitters and neuromodulators during early human development. *Early Hum Dev* 2001; 65: 21-37.

- Isaeva E, Isaev D, Holmes GL. Alteration of synaptic plasticity by neonatal seizures in rat somatosensory cortex. *Epilepsy Res* 2013; 106: 280-3.
- Lawrence R, Mathur A, Nguyen The Tich S, Zempel J, Inder T. A pilot study of continuous limited-channel aEEG in term infants with encephalopathy. *J Pediatr* 2009; 154: 835-41.
- Lou HC, Friis-Hansen B. Arterial blood pressure elevations during motor activity and epileptic seizures in the newborn. *Acta Paediatr Scand* 1979; 68: 803-6.
- McCutchen CB, Coen R, Iragui VJ. Periodic lateralized epileptiform discharges in asphyxiated neonates. *Electroencephalogr Clin Neurophysiol* 1985; 61: 210-7.
- Miller SP, Weiss J, Barnwell A, et al. Seizure-associated brain injury in term newborns with perinatal asphyxia. *Neurology* 2002; 58: 542-8.
- Mizrahi EM, Kellaway P. Characterization and classification of neonatal seizures. *Neurology* 1987; 37: 1837-44.
- Murray DM, Boylan GB, Ali I, Ryan CA, Murphy BP, Connolly S. Defining the gap between electrographic seizure burden, clinical expression and staff recognition of neonatal seizures. *Arch Dis Child Fetal Neonatal Ed* 2008; 93: F187-91.
- Nagarajan L, Palumbo L, Ghosh S. Classification of clinical semiology in epileptic seizures in neonates. *Eur J Paediatr Neurol* 2012; 16: 118-25.
- Oliveira AJ, Nunes ML, Haertel LM, Reis FM, da Costa JC. Duration of rhythmic EEG patterns in neonates: new evidence for clinical and prognostic significance of brief rhythmic discharges. *Clin Neurophysiol* 2000; 111: 1646-53.
- Painter MJ, Scher MS, Stein AD, et al. Phenobarbital compared with phenytoin for the treatment of neonatal seizures. *N Engl J Med* 1999; 341: 485-9.
- Perlman JM, Volpe JJ. Seizures in the preterm infant: effects on cerebral blood flow velocity, intracranial pressure, and arterial blood pressure. *J Pediatr* 1983; 102: 288-93.
- Pisani F, Piccolo B, Cantalupo G, et al. Neonatal seizures and postneonatal epilepsy: a 7-y follow-up study. *Pediatr Res* 2012; 72: 186-93.
- Ronen GM, Penney S, Andrews W. The epidemiology of clinical neonatal seizures in Newfoundland: a population-based study. *J Pediatr* 1999; 134: 71-5.
- Scher MS, Beggarly M. Clinical significance of focal periodic discharges in neonates. *J Child Neurol* 1989; 4: 175-85.
- Shah DK, Zempel J, Barton T, Lukas K, Inder TE. Electrographic seizures in preterm infants during the first week of life are associated with cerebral injury. *Pediatr Res* 2010; 67: 102-6.
- Stafstrom CE, Chronopoulos A, Thurber S, Thompson JL, Holmes GL. Age-dependent cognitive and behavioral deficits after kainic acid seizures. *Epilepsia* 1993; 34: 420-32.
- Toet MC, Groenendaal F, Osredkar D, van Huffelen AC, de Vries LS. Postneonatal epilepsy following amplitude-integrated EEG-detected neonatal seizures. *Pediatr Neurol* 2005; 32: 241-7.
- Tsuchida TN, Wusthoff CJ, Shellhaas RA, et al. American Clinical Neurophysiology Society Standardized EEG Terminology and Categorization for the Description of Continuous EEG Monitoring in Neonates: Report of the American Clinical Neurophysiology Society Critical Care Monitoring Committee. *J Clin Neurophysiol* 2013; 30: 161-73.
- van Rooij LG, Toet MC, van Huffelen AC, et al. Effect of treatment of subclinical neonatal seizures detected with aEEG: randomized, controlled trial. *Pediatrics* 2010; 125: e358-66.
- Vesoulis ZA, Inder TE, Woodward LJ, Buse B, Vavasseur C, Mathur AM. Early electrographic seizures, brain injury, and neurodevelopmental risk in the very preterm infant. *Pediatr Res* 2014; 75: 564-9.
- Volpe JJ. Neonatal seizures: current concepts and revised classification. *Pediatrics* 1989; 84: 422-8.
- Wikström S, Pupp IH, Rosén I, et al. Early single-channel aEEG/EEG predicts outcome in very preterm infants. *Acta Paediatr* 2012; 101: 719-26.

- Wirrell EC, Armstrong EA, Osman LD, Yager JY. Prolonged seizures exacerbate perinatal hypoxic-ischemic brain damage. *Pediatr Res* 2001; 50: 445-54.
- Younkin DP, Delivoria-Papadopoulos M, Maris J, Donlon E, Clancy R, Chance B. Cerebral metabolic effects of neonatal seizures measured with *in vivo* 31P NMR spectroscopy. *Ann Neurol* 1986; 20: 513-9.

Genetics of neonatal epilepsies and the forgotten epilepsy phenotypes

Maria Roberta Cilio, Michael S. Oldham

*Department of Neurology, Pediatric Epilepsy Center,
University of California, San Francisco, San Francisco, USA*

Epileptic seizures have their highest incidence in the neonatal period. When considering seizures in the neonates, one of the first issues of importance is recognizing that not all seizures have the same etiology. Early distinction and differentiation of acute seizures *versus* neonatal-onset epilepsies have significant therapeutic and prognostic implications. Acute seizures are often the only sign in the neonate of an infection, hypoxic-ischemic brain injury, hemorrhage of the central nervous system, or transient metabolic disturbance, and may require no pharmacologic intervention, or only a very short course of treatment. Furthermore, searching for the cause of seizures may be limited to basic serum labs, a lumbar puncture, and/or head imaging (head ultrasound or MRI).

On the other hand, neonatal-onset epilepsies are rare, although often overlooked because their phenotype may be difficult to characterize. This is, in part, due to the fact that pediatricians or neonatologists frequently manage seizures in neonates without access to specialists with detailed knowledge of seizure semiology, epilepsy syndromes, and specific etiologies in this age group. Recognition is paramount, though, because these epilepsies may require targeted diagnostic evaluations, and prolonged treatment with anti-epileptic drugs. Furthermore, appropriate characterization of the epilepsy may lead to more rapid and focused diagnosis, and consideration of specific pharmacologic therapy.

There are certain questions to answer when faced with a neonate having seizures. The neurological exam (*i.e.*, normal *versus* abnormal between seizures) and the actual age of onset of seizures (*i.e.*, first day *versus* first week *versus* within the first month of life) can help provide clues to the diagnosis. The specific semiology of the seizures and the ictal and interictal EEG are also vital pieces of information. However, given the high incidence of acute seizures in the neonate, and often the lack of an accurate family history at the time of the evaluation in the neonatal intensive care unit, the diagnosis of neonatal-onset epilepsy remains, in most cases, a diagnosis of exclusion and many of these babies will have other basic diagnostic studies already completed that will help guide the thought-process.

Neonatal-onset epilepsies unrelated to prenatal, perinatal or postnatal lesions present a major diagnostic and therapeutic challenge. However, genetic etiologies are being discovered for a growing proportion of these disorders, helping elucidate their molecular mechanisms (Nabbout and Dulac, 2012). Neonatal-onset epilepsies have a broad spectrum phenotype: from relatively benign to much more severe. The development of the brain is an extremely complex process, which depends on genetically determined factors and on the electrical activity of the brain. Electrical activity emerges during the third trimester of pregnancy and plays an important role in the construction of the cortical maps. Many studies have shown that fundamental changes in patterns of brain activity could have deleterious consequences. The association of epilepsy with the deterioration of cognitive functions forms a group of diseases known as "epileptic encephalopathies", entities for which the EEG epileptiform abnormalities themselves are considered to have a major impact on brain development (Engel, 2001; Berg et al., 2010).

This chapter will focus on three specific genetically determined neonatal-onset epilepsies: benign familial neonatal seizures (BFNS), *KCNQ2* encephalopathy, and the epileptic encephalopathy associated with *CDKL5* mutation. These particular epilepsies are chosen because they exquisitely illustrate (1) the role of accurate phenotyping and seizure characterization at onset in achieving an early diagnosis and (2) the possibility of targeted treatment in order to change the outcome, not only regarding seizures but also neurologic development.

■ Benign familial neonatal seizures

BFNS is an autosomal-dominant epilepsy syndrome of the newborn which has a favorable prognosis with respect to seizures and psychomotor development. Rett and Teubel (1964) first described a boy with a strong positive family history of seizures in the neonatal period, with 7 cases over 3 generations. The seizures in the proband were characterized by an initial tonic phase accompanied by cyanosis, followed by bilateral clonic movements of the limbs, face and eyes. Normal interictal EEGs were reported for the patient and his affected brother, as well as for other affected individuals in the family. In addition, they all had good outcome of seizure control and normal psychomotor development.

Numerous other families have been reported since the initial case series, being defined by a favorable outcome, specifically normal psychomotor development and the absence of subsequent epilepsy in most patients.

Typically, the seizures start on day of life 2 or 3, with the majority in the first week of life. The seizures are typically brief (1-2 minutes in duration), but can occur up to 30 times per day, sometimes evolving into status epilepticus. There are often reports from the child's parents (or more often grandmother) about other family members with similar seizures. These newborns can continue to have seizures for several weeks before spontaneous remission, although seizures usually respond well to antiepileptic drugs. There are a few reports of seizures lasting more than several months (Bjerre and Corelius, 1968; Soldovieri et al., 2014).

Seizures are usually brief and the semiology is most often of a mixed type, with a typical sequence being onset of asymmetric tonic posturing, often accompanied by autonomic features (apnea or tachypnea), then a progression to focal clonic jerks. Myoclonic seizures and epileptic spasms have not been reported in this type of epilepsy. The ictal EEG is consistent with the clinical semiology, characterized by an electrodecremental pattern, superimposed muscle artifact during the tonic phase, and then rhythmic focal spike and wave discharges during the clonic phase (*Figure 1*).

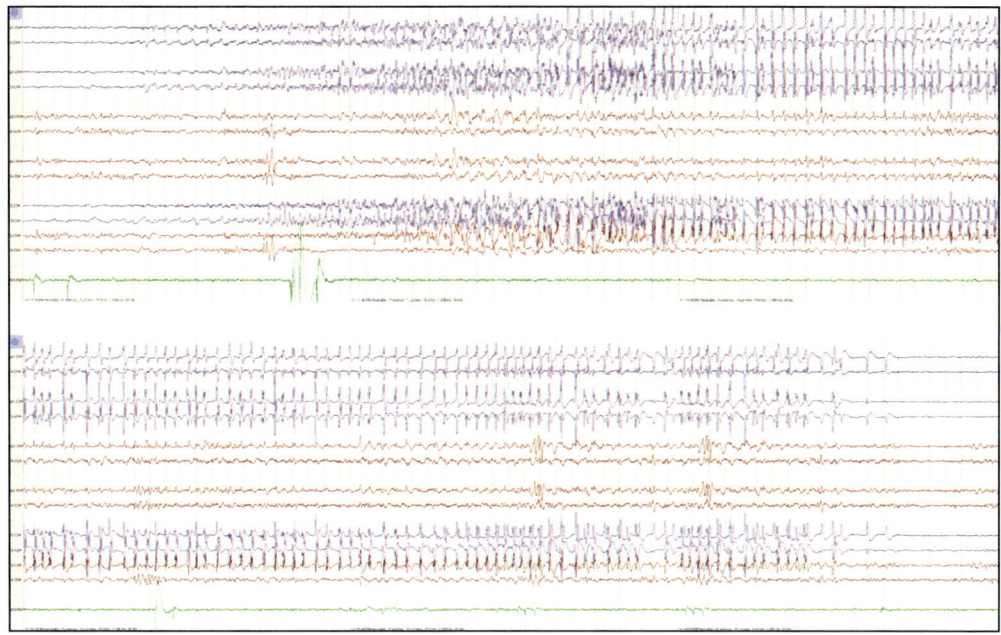

Figure 1. EEG in a 4-day old neonate showing left focal seizure, which starts with a tonic phase of low-amplitude fast activity, followed by rhythmic, high-amplitude spikes over the left hemisphere, after which there is a period of complete attenuation over the left hemisphere.

The interictal EEG in babies with BFNS is either normal or shows some bilateral independent epileptiform abnormalities mainly over the central regions (personal observation). The previously reported pattern of "theta pointu alternant" (De Weerd et al., 1999) – dominant theta activity, intermixed with sharp waves – although present in almost 60% of cases, is actually non-specific. Poor prognostic patterns, such as burst-suppression, have never been reported in patients with BFNS. Clinically, the patients have a normal neurologic examination between seizures, and are able to be breast- or bottle-feed without difficulty. All metabolic, infectious, hematologic studies, as well as brain imaging, are normal. The natural course of the seizures is self-limited, as seizures stop spontaneously within a few days or weeks. However, about 10 to 15% of patients have febrile or afebrile seizures later in life (Ronen et al., 1993) while showing a normal psychomotor development.

The genes associated with BFNS are *KCNQ2* on chromosome 20q13.3 and *KCNQ3* on chromosome 8q24, and encode the voltage-gated potassium channel subunits KV 7.2 (Q2) and KV 7.3 (Q3), respectively (Singh et al., 1998; Biervert et al., 1998; Charlier et al., 1998). There are over 80 different mutations reported on *KCNQ2* and 6 mutations on *KCNQ3*. The Q2 and Q3 subunits of the potassium channel help mediate the M-current and play a key role in repolarizing action potentials by allowing flow of potassium out of the cell. This process leads to hyperpolarization and decreased excitability. Reduction of the activity of these channels will cause increased neuronal excitability and the increased risk of seizures. Between 60-80% of families with BFNS will have a mutation or a deletion in either of these genes, the vast majority in *KCNQ2*. The majority of mutations are substitutions, insertions or deletions; however, a few missense mutations have recently been identified (Soldovieri et al., 2014). In addition, the mutations are largely located in the long C-terminus region of Q2.

In the acute setting of the seizures, there is significant variability in medication usage – phenobarbital, valproate, phenytoin, levetiracetam, or combinations of these medications have all been reported (Soldovieri et al., 2014). The duration of therapy after cessation of seizures, and how prolonged pharmacologic therapy may impact the risk of seizure recurrence and epilepsy, is also unclear.

KCNQ2 encephalopathy

More recently, the genetic screening for *KCNQ2/KCNQ3* mutations of patients with unexplained neonatal-onset epileptic encephalopathy led to the recognition of *de novo* *KCNQ2* mutations in patients with severe neonatal epileptic encephalopathy. This new entity has been named "*KCNQ2* encephalopathy," and is characterized by intractable seizures of neonatal onset and severe psychomotor impairment. Within the last two years, multiple papers with several dozen patients have been reported, but many of these patients were diagnosed well after the neonatal period and their electroclinical phenotype was not clearly differentiated from early myoclonic encephalopathy (EME) or Ohtahara syndrome (Weckhuysen et al., 2012; Kato et al., 2013; Milh et al., 2013; Weckhuysen et al., 2013).

Several common features are seen in patients with *KCNQ2* encephalopathy when compared with BFNS. The onset of seizures is almost always in the first week of life. The seizure semiology also is very similar to BFNS – a prominent tonic component with or without associated clonic jerking of the face or limbs, and often associated with autonomic features such as apnea and desaturation (Serino et al., 2013). However, the burden of seizure frequency in *KCNQ2* encephalopathy is quite high, with 10 or more seizures per day or even per hour, which tend to be therapy-resistant for weeks to months. In many cases, a tendency to resolve after the first year or two of life has been observed. All babies will have a severely abnormal interictal EEG pattern, either of burst suppression or multifocal epileptiform activity.

A recent report on three new cases of *KCNQ2* encephalopathy, diagnosed in the neonatal period and studied with continuous video-EEG recording, describes a distinct electroclinical phenotype with a dramatic response to oral carbamazepine in terms of seizures, but still severe neurological impairment on follow-up (Numis et al., 2014). In a typical seizure, the ictal EEG shows the onset of low voltage fast activity over a single hemisphere followed by focal spike and wave complexes. While the seizures are quite short in duration, the post ictal phase is characterized by marked and prolonged diffuse voltage attenuation (*Figure 2*).

The interictal EEG of the same patient as above clearly lacks physiological patterns and is characterized by multifocal epileptiform abnormalities, intermixed with random, asynchronous attenuations (*Figure 3*).

While the age of onset, seizure semiology and ictal pattern are similar to BFNS, the interictal EEG and clinical exam in babies with *KCNQ2* encephalopathy is extremely different. These babies have a severely abnormal neurologic exam already in the neonatal period, usually with lack of visual fixation or following, decreased spontaneous movements, and axial hypotonia with poor head control. However, given the very frequent seizures and the resistance to antiepileptic drugs, these patients are almost invariably treated with high doses of medications, including phenobarbital and benzodiazepines very early after onset, which could, at least in part, contribute to the initial clinical neurological findings.

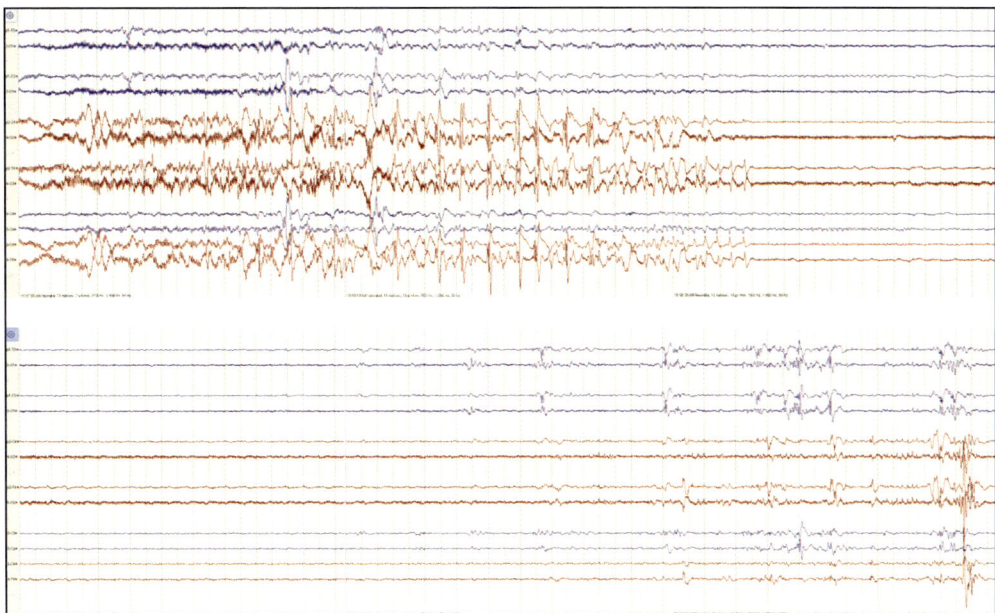

Figure 2. EEG in a 6-week old infant (ex-preterm born at 34 weeks, 40 weeks corrected age at the time of this recording) with KCNQ2-encephalopathy and seizures onset showing a typical seizure – short focal seizure over the right hemisphere, followed by severe, prolonged voltage attenuation.

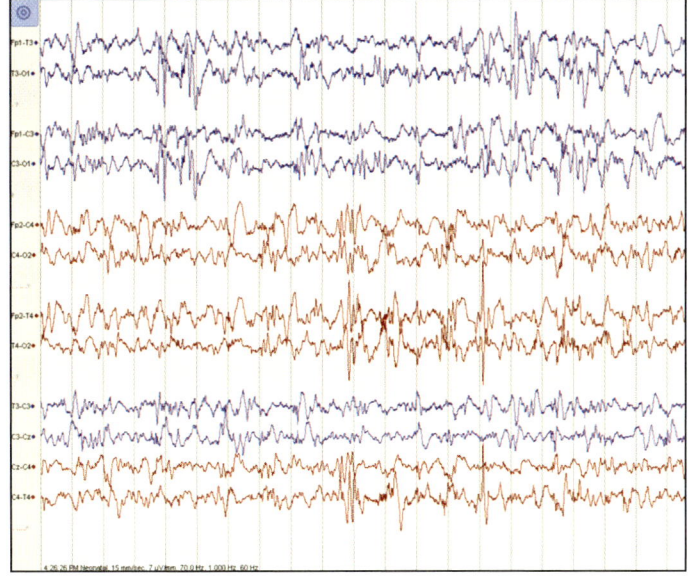

Figure 3. Interictal EEG in the same patient as *Figure 2*, characterized by multifocal epileptiform abnormalities and periods of asynchronous random attenuation.

Many children with *KCNQ2* encephalopathy are able to achieve seizure freedom; however, psychomotor development, for the most part, remains profoundly impaired. At follow-up, almost all have moderate to severe mental retardation, accompanied by abnormal tone and a lack of any appreciable gross or fine motor skills. As a result of a relatively large cohort of children with *KCNQ2* encephalopathy, one research group was able to characterize 3 different phenotypes: (1) frequent, therapy-resistant seizures initially, but a high rate of seizure-freedom, with severe to profound intellectual disability and axial hypotonia, along with fronto-temporal atrophy and/or white matter loss on brain MRI; (2) relatively well-controlled seizures and only mild to moderate intellectual disability at follow-up; (3) a lower seizure frequency at onset, but the ultimate development of moderate to severe intellectual disability (Weckhuysen et al., 2013).

The fact that mutations in the same gene can give rise either to benign or severe epilepsies accompanied by neurological impairment demonstrates the importance of *KCNQ2* in brain development and suggests that the resulting potassium current may be differently affected in the two diseases. For any voltage-gated channel, it is thought that heterozygous mutations disrupting electromechanical coupling are more deleterious than a gene deletion because the mutated subunit(s) can have an adverse effect on the normal subunits from the wild-type gene. Explaining the mechanisms by which a mutation in the same gene can lead to both benign and severe epilepsies has been challenging. One study (Miceli et al., 2013) compared the impact of two mutations at the same position in *KCNQ2* found in children with BFNS (R213W mutation) and in children with neonatal epileptic encephalopathy (R213Q mutation), and showed that the R213Q caused a more pronounced functional defect, possibly reflected in the more severe phenotype. More recent data by Orhan and colleagues (2014) supported and extended this finding. In order for the *KCNQ* channel to properly allow ion flow, all four gates of the tetramer must work in tandem. If one of the subunits has a mutation leading to electromechanical uncoupling or pore-blocking, the tetramer becomes non-conducting, despite 3 normal wild-type subunits. This phenomenon, called a dominant-negative effect, is exhibited by many of the mutations leading to *KCNQ2* encephalopathy (Orhan et al., 2014).

Peters et al. (2005) showed in a mouse model that structural disorganization in the brain, increased neuronal excitability, and abnormal behavior can be avoided by restricting function of the mutant *KCNQ2* subunit in early development, even if only for a short period of time. Retigabine is a medication that binds to a hydrophobic pocket near the gate of the potassium channel, stabilizing and maintaining the open form of the channels. Thus, in the setting of depolarization or increased neuronal excitability, the cell is more ready to respond, and the ability to inhibit burst firing is augmented. With over 100 published studies in the preclinical setting, retigabine was shown to be effective in multiple clinical phase trials as well (Barrese et al., 2010). Unfortunately, the medication has been marred by the after-market appearance of potentially permanent changes to the retina, vision loss and blue skin discoloration. This led, in the spring of 2013, the European Medicines Agency (EMA) to recommend restricting use to last-line therapy, and to a black box warning by the US Food and Drug Administration (FDA) in late 2013.

The severe phenotype seen in *KCNQ2* encephalopathy may be further explained by the separation of the mutated potassium channels from their usual axonal partner, the voltage-gated sodium channels. In a typical cell, ankyrin-G is a submembranous framework that binds potassium and sodium channels together in the axon initial segment (AIS). The failure of appropriate clustering of channels in the membrane can lead to abnormal excitability (Yue et al., 2006; Soldovieri et al., 2007; Shah et al., 2008). This theory provides further grounds for the development of pharmacologic interventions that could reconnect or bind the channels and prevent the excessive or sustained firing of action potentials seen with seizures.

While *KCNQ2* encephalopathy results in a refractory seizure disorder, carbamazepine and oxcarbazepine have been shown to be effective, resulting in a dramatic reduction in seizure frequency and ultimately to seizure freedom (Numis et al., 2014). This is unlikely attributable to evolution of the syndrome alone, as just one of eight infants with *KCNQ2* encephalopathy in a prior series had seizure freedom by three months of age (Weckhuysen et al., 2012). Interestingly, two of three children in the Weckhuysen cohort (2012) had a response to carbamazepine or oxcarbazepine when trialed at various ages.

Low-dose carbamazepine has been found to be dramatically effective in benign infantile seizures (Matsufuji et al., 2005). Carbamazepine and its derivatives stabilize the inactive state of voltage-gated sodium channels, while *KCNQ2* mutations decrease the inhibitory potassium current on membranes. Seemingly disparate, voltage-gated sodium channels and *KCNQ* potassium channels typically co-localize; modulation of one channel may significantly impact the function of the channel-complex. Accordingly, phenytoin (an inhibitor of the voltage-gated sodium channel) may also be of benefit in *KCNQ2* encephalopathy. However, if the channels are abnormally clustered, as discussed above, it is not clear if sodium channel blockers would work in all patients.

Epileptic encephalopathy associated with *CDKL5* mutations

Seen most frequently in females, with a 12:1 female to male ratio, the epileptic encephalopathy associated with *CDKL5* mutations can arise in the neonatal period, with the majority of patients having onset of seizures within the first 3 months of life. This form of epilepsy was first identified in two females with severe intellectual disability and early-onset seizures in 2003 (Kalscheuer et al., 2003), then in four additional females diagnosed with Rett syndrome in 2004 (Weaving et al., 2004).

Patients have severe psychomotor impairment, specifically hypotonia, poor visual fixation, and lack of development of language or fine motor skills already evident at onset, but there is no developmental regression as seen with Rett syndrome. Much like girls with typical Rett syndrome, a significant proportion of children with epileptic encephalopathy associated with a *CDKL5* mutation will have deceleration of head growth and hand stereotypies of some form. However, an excellent review by Fehr et al. (2013) with a large cohort (over 80 children – 77 females and 9 males), advocates for the *CDKL5* disorder to be a separate clinical entity, rather than a "Rett variant". They found a subtle facial, limb, and hand phenotype (prominent forehead, deep-set eyes, tapered fingers) amongst those with *CDKL5* mutations, and the high incidence of early-onset, treatment-resistant seizures and lack of developmental regression as compared to children with a *MECP2* mutation was very strongly significant.

Seizures in those with the epileptic encephalopathy associated with *CDKL5* mutations can occur in the first few weeks of life, and almost always in the first 3 months. Often at the onset of epilepsy, the interictal EEG can be normal. A three-stage electroclinical course was described in 2008 by Bahi-Buisson and colleagues. Initially, the effected individual will have frequent, albeit brief, seizures. Some of these children will have success with seizure control after several weeks to months, with some even achieving a "honeymoon period" of seizure freedom. Regardless of ultimate epilepsy course, all patients at this stage already exhibit hypotonia and poor eye contact. The second stage is characterized by a failure of developmental progression, and the appearance of epileptic spasms with or without hypsarrhythmia on EEG. Finally, in the third stage, children suffer from severe refractory epilepsy with multiple seizure types, including tonic, myoclonic, and spasms, occurring frequently and multiple times per day. By this point, the interictal EEG also remains abnormal, with high-amplitude slow waves and bursts of spikes and polyspikes (*Figure 4*).

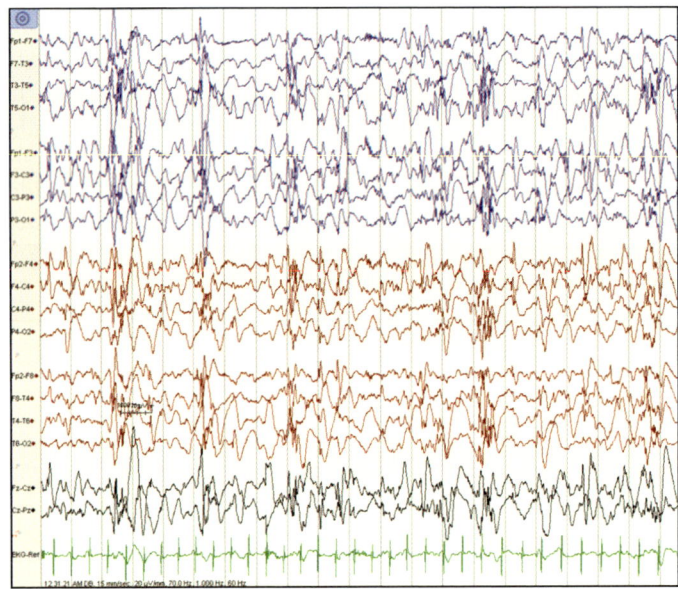

Figure 4. EEG in a 2-year old girl with epileptic encephalopathy associated with CDKL5 mutation showing diffuse slowing with poor organization, high-amplitude slow waves, and frequent bursts of generalized spikes and polyspikes.

A distinctive seizure type seen during the course of this epileptic encephalopathy is the hypermotor-tonic-spasms sequence (Klein *et al.*, 2011), and the recognition of this quite specific sequence may lead the clinician to consider the diagnosis of a *CDKL5* encephalopathy. However, the hypermotor-tonic-spasms sequence may appear later in the course, during the second stage of *CDKL5* encephalopathy (Klein *et al.*, 2011). Identifying this disorder at presentation in the very first weeks of life can be challenging and most patients are still diagnosed only later in life. Nevertheless, the onset of brief tonic-spasms seizures in a girl with no interictal EEG abnormalities (*Figure 5*) should suggest a *CDKL5* mutation.

The *CDKL5* gene (cyclin-dependent kinase-like 5), also known as serine/threonine kinase 9 (STK9), is found at position 22 on the short arm of the X chromosome (Xp22). Many mutations have been found in the *CDKL5* gene, and as the clinical entity is more greatly recognized, some variability in phenotype does exist. In Bahi-Buisson's cohort (2008), there was trend toward clinical severity (earlier onset of epilepsy, intractable spasms, and worse psychomotor impairment) and mutations that impaired the catalytic domain, as opposed to truncating mutations that were downstream from the catalytic domain. Further research continues on pathogenicity and phenotypic variability as greater numbers of mutations are being found.

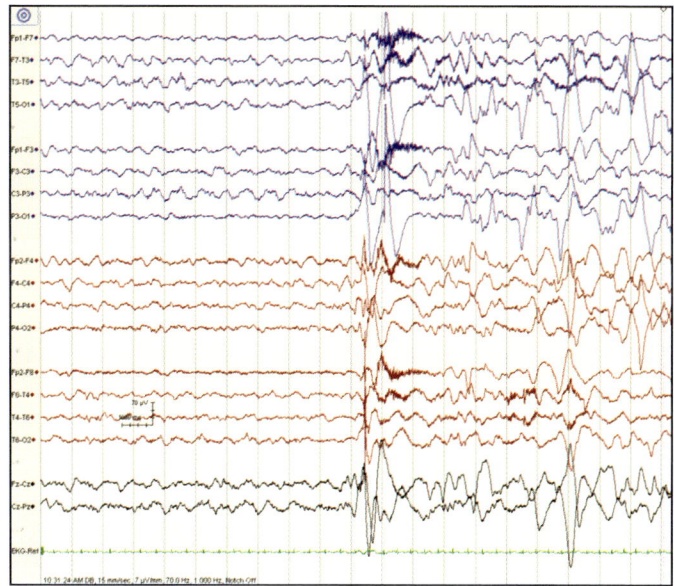

Figure 5. EEG recorded at 3 weeks of age in the same patient as *Figure 4* showing a brief tonic seizure, preceded by a normal background.

It is also unclear exactly how or why a mutation in the *CDKL5* gene leads to the severe phenotype of early onset epileptic encephalopathy. A function of the CDKL5 protein is to add a phosphate group to specific positions on other proteins, a major target being MeCP2 which is known to be involved in neuronal function and synaptic maintenance. The association of these proteins and how it may play a role in epilepsy has not yet been fully defined. Another link stems from the finding that a specific mutation in the green algae *Chlamydomonas* leads to a protein similar to the human CDKL kinase protein (Tam et al., 2013). This protein is involved in appropriate flagellar length in the algae species, interesting due to the fact that a greater number of human diseases are being attributed to abnormal cilia (Badano et al., 2006). Research continues to explore these relationships and how they may result in an epileptic encephalopathy.

To date, no specific antiepileptic drugs have been shown to have greater efficacy for seizure control in this particular epileptic encephalopathy. In addition, the medications chosen during the clinical course which includes infantile spasms are no different than other idiopathic or cryptogenic spasms, with most clinicians using ACTH or another steroid derivative, and vigabatrin. Carbamazepine, valproate, and clobazam, have also been trialed in order to control the tonic seizures with different results. At present, there are no specific treatments for children with *CDKL5* epileptic encephalopathy.

■ Potential for targeted therapies

The gene discovery efforts of the past decade for severe epilepsies, particularly early onset epileptic encephalopathies, have shown that genetic mutations play a major role, and, although monogenic epileptic channelopathies are rare, they must be considered in the differential diagnosis of seizures in newborns and infants. However, many unresolved questions remain. The electroclinical presentation in the neonatal period of neonatal-onset epilepsies is not yet well defined since many patients are diagnosed later in life, and clinical and EEG findings related to the neonatal period may be scarce. Additionally, mutations in the same gene can be linked to both severe and benign neonatal epilepsies within a given family (Borgatti et al., 2004). In conclusion, even in the midst of an exciting period of genetic discoveries, the electroclinical phenotype remains an important piece of information for a correct diagnosis, management, and prognosis. In the context of early diagnosis and targeted treatment, an accurate characterization of the neonatal phenotype is key to determine the best strategy to manage and treat neonatal-onset epilepsies, especially if the goal is not only seizures control but also a normal developmental outcome. The past twenty years have seen the development of prolonged video-EEG monitoring as a method for characterizing seizures in infants and children, providing the basis for a precise diagnosis of epilepsy type and syndrome and targeted therapy. We believe that similar care should be applied in neonates with seizures, considering that a number of them may benefit from an epileptological approach.

References

- Badano JL, Mitsuma N, Beales PL, Katsanis N. The ciliopathies: an emerging class of human genetic disorders. *Annu Rev Genomics Hum Genet* 2006; 7: 125-48.
- Bahi-Buisson N, Kaminska A, Boddaert N, et al. The three stages of epilepsy in patients with *CDKL5* mutations. *Epilepsia* 2008; 49: 1027-37.
- Barrese V, Miceli F, Soldovieri MV, et al. Neuronal potassium channel openers in the management of epilepsy: role and potential of retigabine. *Clin Pharmacol* 2010; 2: 225-36.
- Berg AT, Berkovic SF, Brodies MJ, et al. Revised terminology and concepts for organization of seizure and epilepsies: report of the ILAE Commission on Classification and Terminology, 2005-2009. *Epilepsia* 2010; 51: 676-85.
- Biervert C, Schroeder BC, Kubisch C, et al. A potassium channel mutation in neonatal human epilepsy. *Science* 1998; 279: 403-04.
- Bjerre I, Corelius E. Benign neonatal familial convulsions. *Acta Paediat Scand* 1968; 57: 557-61.
- Charlier C, Singh, NA, Ryan SG, Lewis TB, Reus BE, Leach RJ, Leppert M. A pore mutation in a novel KQT-like potassium channel gene in an idiopathic epilepsy family. *Nat Genet* 1998; 18: 53-55.
- De Weerd AW, Despland PA, Plouin P. Neonatal EEG. The International Federation of Clinical Neurophysiology. *Electroencephalogr Clinical Neurophysiol* 1999; 52 (suppl); 149-57.
- Engel J Jr. ILAE Commission Report. A Proposed Diagnostic Scheme for People with Epileptic Seizures and with Epilepsy: Report of the ILAE Task Force on Classification and Terminology. *Epilepsia* 2001; 42: 796-803.
- Fehr S, Wilson M, Downs J, et al. The *CDKL5* disorder is an independent clinical entity associated with early-onset encephalopathy. *Eur J Hum Genet* 2013; 21: 266-73.
- Kalscheuer VM, Tao J, Donnelly A, Hollway G, Schwinger E, Kubart S, et al. Disruption of the serine/threonine kinase 9 gene causes severe X-linked infantile spasms and mental retardation. *Am J Hum Genet* 2003; 72: 1401-11.
- Klein KM, Yendle SC, Harvey AS, et al. A distinctive seizure type in patients with *CDKL5* mutations: hypermotor-tonic-spasms sequence. *Neurology* 2011; 76: 1436-38.
- Matsufuji H, Ichiyama T, Isumi H, Furukawa S. Low-dose carbamazepine therapy for benign infantile convulsions. *Brain Dev* 2005; 27: 554-57.
- Miceli F, Soldovieri MV, Ambrosino P, et al. Genotype-phenotype correlations in neonatal epilepsies caused by mutations in the voltage sensor of Kv7.2 potassium channel subunits. *Proc Natl Acad Sci USA* 2013; 110: 4386-91.

- Milh M, Boutry-Kryza N, Sutera-Sardo J, et al. Similar early characteristics but variable neurological outcomes of patients with a de novo mutation of KCNQ2. *Orphanet J Rare Dis* 2013; 8: 80.
- Nabbout R, Dulac O. Genetics of early-onset epilepsy with encephalopathy. *Nat Rev Neurol* 2012; 8: 129-30.
- Orhan G, Bock M, Schepers D, et al. Dominant-negative effects of KCNQ2 mutations are associated with epileptic encephalopathy. *Ann Neurol* 2014; 75: 382084.
- Peters HC, Hu H, Pongs O, Storm JF, Isbrandt D. Conditional transgenic suppression of M channels in mouse brain reveals functions in neuronal excitability, resonance and behavior. *Nat Neurosci* 2005; 8: 51-60.
- Rett A, Teubel R. Neugeborenkrampfe in Rahmen einer epileptisch belasteten familie. *Wien Klin Worschr* 1964; 76: 609-13.
- Ronen GM, Rosales TO, Connolly M, Anderson VE, Leppert M. Seizure characteristics in chromosome 20 benign familial neonatal convulsions. *Neurology* 1993; 43: 1355-60.
- Serino D, Specchio N, Pontrelli G, Vigevano F, Fusco L. Video/EEG findings in a KCNQ2 epileptic encephalopathy: a case report and revision of literature data. *Epileptic Disord* 2013; 15(2): 158-65.
- Shah MM, Migliore M, Valencia I, Cooper EC, Brown DA. Functional significance of axonal Kv7 channels in hippocampal pyramidal neurons. *Proc Natl Acad Sci USA* 2008; 105: 7869-74.
- Singh NA, Charlier C, Stauffer D, et al. A novel potassium channel gene, KCNQ2, is mutated in an inherited epilepsy of newborns. *Nat Genet* 1998; 18: 23-9.
- Soldovieri MV, Cilio MR, Miceli F, et al. Atypical gating of M-type potassium channels conferred by mutations in uncharged residues in the S4 region of KCNQ2 causing benign familial neonatal convulsions. *J Neurosci* 2007; 27: 4919-28.
- Soldovieri MV, Boutry-Kryza N, Milh M, et al. Novel KCNQ2 and KCNQ3 Mutations in a large cohort of families with benign neonatal epilepsy: first evidence for an altered channel regulation by syntaxin-1A. *Hum Mutat* 2014; 35: 356-67.
- Tam LW, Ranum PT, Lefebvre PA. CDKL5 regulates flagellar length and localizes to the base of the flagella in Chlamydomonas. *Mol Biol Cell* 2013; 24: 588-600.
- Yue C, Yaari Y. Axo-somatic and apical dendritic Kv7/M channels differentially regulate the intrinsic excitability of adult rat CA1 pyramidal cells. *J Neurophysiol* 2006; 95: 3480-95.
- Weaving LS, Christodolou J, Williamson SL, et al. Mutations of CDKL5 cause a severe neurodevelopmental disorder with infantile spasms and mental retardation. *Am J Hum Genet* 2004; 75: 1079-93.
- Weckhuysen S, Mandelstam S, Suls A, et al. KCNQ2 encephalopathy: emerging phenotype of a neonatal epileptic encephalopathy. *Ann Neurol* 2012; 71: 15-25.
- Weckhuysen S, Ivanovic V, Hendrickx R, et al. Extending the KCNQ2 encephalopathy spectrum: Clinical and neuroimaging findings in 17 patients. *Neurology* 2013; 81: 1697-1703.

Genetic basis of epileptic encephalopathy

Lucia Fusco[1], Domenico Serino[1], Giulia Barcia[2], Rima Nabbout[2]

[1] Neurology Division, Ospedale Pediatrico Bambino Gesù, Rome, Italy
[2] Reference Centre for Rare Epilepsies, Department of Pediatric Neurology, Necker Enfants Malades Hospital, Paris, France

An epileptic encephalopathy (EE) is an electroclinical syndrome associated with a high probability of encephalopathic features that present or worsen after the onset of epilepsy. The term "epileptic encephalopathy" embodies the notion that "[...] the epileptic activity itself may contribute to severe cognitive and behavioral impairments, above and beyond what might be expected from the underlying pathology alone, and that these can worsen over time" (Berg *et al.*, 2010). The severity of such impairment is variable and not syndrome specific: even though certain syndromes are often referred to as epileptic encephalopathies, the encephalopathic effects of seizures and epilepsy may potentially occur in association with any form of epilepsy (Berg *et al.*, 2010). Also, while the concept of EE implies the presence of psychomotor impairment which is potentially reversible once seizures are controlled, an obvious relationship between seizures and cognitive impairment is not always clear cut. This is especially true in relation to genetic etiologies, where a "cause-effect" relationship is often overshadowed by the presence of a common denominator affecting both seizure onset and cognitive decline. In these cases we come across the subtle difference between *epileptic* encephalopathies and epilepsy *with* encephalopathy. The scope of this work is to hopefully clarify the approach towards EE by outlining genetic abnormalities which are known to be associated with classical EE phenotypes but also by outlining different phenotypes which are variably associated with single gene mutations.

▪ Ohtahara syndrome

Also known as early infantile encephalopathic epilepsy (EIEE) or early onset encephalopathic epilepsy (EOEE), Ohtahara syndrome (OS) is a disorder characterized by onset in infancy, tonic spasms and a suppression-burst pattern on the electroencephalogram (EEG) (Mizrahi and Milh, 2012). Onset is within the first 3 months of life. Infants show reduced responsiveness, hypo- or hypertonia and sometimes focal neurological features. Seizures are predominantly characterized by tonic spasms, isolated or in clusters, during both wake and sleep. Partial seizures with variable focality or hemiconvulsive seizures may also be present but are less frequent, while myoclonic seizures are rare. The typical suppression-burst EEG pattern is characterized by bursts of high voltage slow waves lasting from 2 to 6 seconds mixed with multifocal and generalized spike discharges, and inter-burst intervals lasting between 5 and 10 seconds (Ohtahara et al., 1992) (*Figure 1*). There is typically no significant pattern change between wakefulness and sleep until the evolution towards hypsarhythmia.

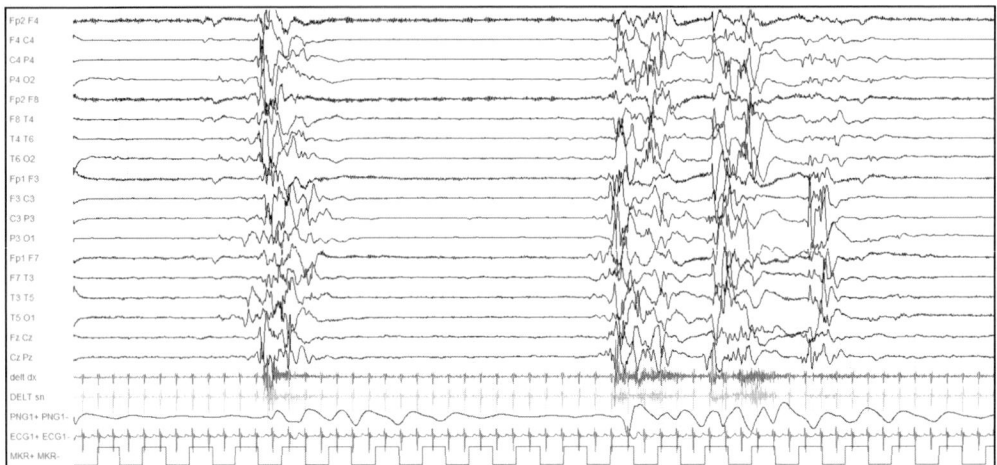

Figure 1. EEG of a patient with Ohtahara syndrome, showing a typical suppression-burst pattern.

Structural brain abnormalities represent the most frequent etiological factors related to OS, while metabolic disorders have been reported to occur in only a few cases. The first report of a genetic mutation associated with OS involved the *ARX* gene (Aristaless-related Homeobox Gene) (Kato et al., 2007). This gene is located in the human chromosome Xp22 region and is a transcription factor involved in the development of cerebral interneurons. Mutations of the *ARX* gene had been already described in relation to a wide variety of phenotypes, ranging from lissencephaly to non-syndromic mental retardation; however, this was the first report in which such a mutation was found in relation to epilepsy.

Several other mutations of the *ARX* gene have been later reported in association with OS (Fullston et al., 2010; Ekşioğlu et al., 2011). In 2008 Saitsu and coworkers, found a *de novo* micro-deletion at 9q22.2-q34.11 in a girl with OS. The deleted region included more than 40 genes, among which was also *STXBP1*, better known as *MUNC18-1*, which encodes for syntaxin binding protein 1, essential for synaptic vescicle release. The authors screened the *STXPB1* gene in 13 unrelated patients with OS and found that four out of 13 carried a missense mutation (Saitsu et al., 2008). In 2010 the same authors screened 29 patients with OS and 54 with West syndrome and found seven patients with an *STXPB1* mutation among the first group (Saitsu et al., 2010). The use of whole exome sequencing and copy number variant analysis allowed the possibility of extending the search for candidate genes. Two years later the same research group identified a new mutation in 2 boys with OS and cerebellar hypoplasia, which involved the *CASK* gene (Saitsu et al., 2012). Meanwhile, mutations of two genes previously associated with other epileptic phenotypes were found in patients with OS. In 2013 Nakamura and coworkers screened 328 patients with EOEE, including 67 patients with OS and 150 with West syndrome, for *SCN2A* mutations. Fourteen novel *SCN2A* missense mutations were found among nine OS patients, one patient with West syndrome and five patients with unclassified EOEEs (Nakamura et al., 2013a). Differentiation in phenotype-genotype correlation among patients with benign and malign mutations of the *SCN2A* gene was explained by differences in mutation sites which give way to abnormalities in different domains of the encoded protein. The same situation applies to mutations of the *KCNQ2* gene, previously thought to be associated only with benign familial infantile spasms but now also reported in association with OS (Kato *et al.*, 2013; Weckhuysen *et al.*, 2013) (*Table I*).

Table I. Genetic mutations in Ohtahara syndrome phenotype

ARX
STXBP1
CASK (associated with cerebellar hypoplasia)
SCN2A
KCNQ2

■ West syndrome

WS is an age-dependent epileptic syndrome characterized by epileptic spasms and chaotic EEG abnormalities, frequently associated with modification of behavior or cognitive decline (Fusco *et al.*, 2012). Epileptic spasms consist in sudden and brief contractions of axial and proximal limb muscles. The associated ictal EEG is characterized by usually diffuse high amplitude slow waves (Fusco and Vigevano, 1993). The typical interictal EEG of WS is represented by hypsarrhythmia: a chaotic cerebral activity characterized by asynchronous, arrhythmic, high-voltage slow-waves variably intermingled with multifocal spikes (Fusco *et al.*, 2012) (*Figure 2*).

Etiology of WS is variable. Structural etiologies are a major cause, including both malformations and acquired lesions, while a cryptogenic etiology may be found in about 20% of patients. Metabolic causes may also be present but are less frequent. Genetic etiology represents about 13% of prenatal etiologies of WS (Auvin *et al.*, 2009). While WS has been reported as associated with several chromosomal abnormalities (Osborne *et al.*, 2010),

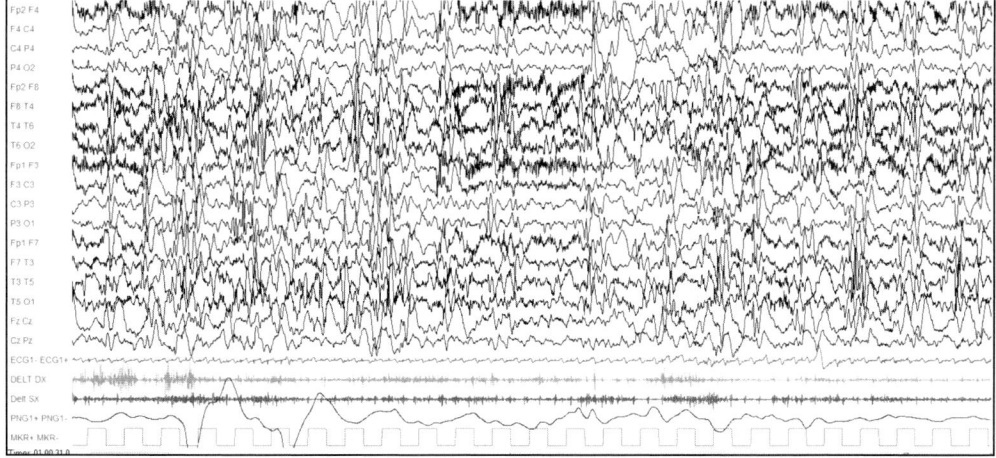

Figure 2. Typical hypsarrhythmic EEG pattern in a patient with West Syndrome.

in the early stages of genetic analysis the clinicians' attention was mainly focused on mutations in X-linked genes, specifically ARX in boys and CDKL5 in girls (Mei et al., 2010; Shoubridge et al., 2010).

In the past the role of single gene mutations in WS was considered to be limited and the diagnostic approach was more protocol based than clinically based. In this light, in 2010 a US consensus report was published, proposing a three-step diagnostic algorithm for WS (Pellock et al., 2010). The authors affirmed that 70% of cases of WS could be diagnosed based on the analysis of clinical context, semeiology of spasms, EEG features, and MRI findings, while among the remaining 30%, half were referable to a rare metabolic disorder. Only in the remaining 15% another etiology should have been suspected. For these patients, the authors suggested an undifferentiated work-up consisting of further metabolic screenings and, on a genetic level, screening limited to ARX (in males) and CDKL5 (in females) mutations, CGH-array and karyotyping. By 2010 however, the technological leap in genetic testing prompted several new studies which brought to light a number of new genes associated with WS.

A Japanese cohort study by Otsuka and colleagues (Otsuka et al., 2010) was the first report showing that mutations in the STXBP1 gene may cause epilepsy that features WS as its onset. Among the 43 screened patients with WS, none had mutations of the ARX and CDKL5 genes. These new advances in genetic analysis, among other things, prompted a more selective, cost-effective and time-effective diagnostic approach, taking advantage of a more precise etiology-phenotype correlation. Such an approach, proposed by Dulac and colleagues (Dulac et al., 2010), is based on the concept that in WS, specific etiologies result in specific clinical, neurophysiologic, and imaging pictures, with different outcome. Different etiologies may be suspected since the very beginning of symptoms, thus narrowing the field of investigations (Table II).

Following this publication, several more gene mutations characterized by specific phenotypes were found to be associated with WS, underscoring even more the importance of a selective diagnostic approach. In a published series of 38 patients diagnosed with cryptogenic WS, CGH-array screening found a mutation of the FOXG1 in 2 (Striano et al., 2011). It was later confirmed that duplications of FOXG1 in 14q12 are associated with developmental epilepsy, mental retardation and severe speech impairment (Brunetti-Pierri

Table II. Etiology based approach in WS (Dulac et al., 2010)

Phenotype	Etiology
Motor and cognitive delay preexisting the onset of spasms, with or without dysmorphisms.	Genetic disorder (trisomy, 1p36 deletion, etc.)
Association of spasms and movement disorder in a male.	ARX mutations
Early onset of tonic seizures in a girl with no interictal EEG abnormality, followed by spasms and hypsarrhythmia.	CDKL5 mutation
Focal interictal slow waves	Focal brain lesion
Asymmetric spasms or focal seizures preceding or combined with the spasms	Focal or multifocal malformations, including Aicardi syndrome, hemimegalencephaly, tuberous sclerosis complex, or cortical dysplasia

et al., 2011; Bertossi et al., 2013). Writzl and colleagues (2012) reported a mutation of the *SPTAN1* gene in a girl with WS, severe hypomielination and coloboma-like optic disks. The association was later confirmed by another publication (Nonoda et al., 2013).

A recently published work reported the results of exome sequencing in four infants, three offspring of consanguineous parents and their second degree cousin, with a clinical phenotype characterized by onset of infantile spasms with hypsarhythmia at 3-7 months of age, revealing mutations of the *ST3Gal-III* gene (Edvardson et al., 2013).

Some of the new genetic mutations found in association with WS might also shed some light on the pathogenetic mechanisms underlying infantile spasms. A recently published brief report showed an association between a 17q21.31 microdeletion and WS (Wray, 2013). This region includes the corticotropin release hormone receptor 1 gene (*CRHR1*), which encodes for the receptor for the corticotropin release hormone (CRH), a hypothalamic hormone that mediates stress-induced endocrine, behavioral, autonomic and immune responses. CRH seems particularly important in the pathogenesis of infantile spasms and the association between the reported genetic mutation and WS might support the existence of this key role.

Another important chapter in the genetic etiology of WS is represented by the study of copy number variants (CNV), which may also contribute in clarifying the pathogenesis of WS. In 2011 Paciorkowski and coworkers reported on chromosomal abnormalities detected by CNV analysis (personal cases and review of literature data) and on the analysis of the gene content in patients with WS (Paciorkowski et al., 2011). Using bioinformatics tools, the authors analyzed the gene content of these CNVs for enrichment in pathways of pathogenesis. Through this method they were able to determine that the gene content was enriched for the gene regulatory network involved in ventral forebrain development, underscoring the role played by the ventral forebrain in the pathogenesis of epileptic spasms. Also, they found that genes in pathways of synaptic function were overrepresented, significantly those involved in synaptic vesicle transport.

Table III. Genes associated with West syndrome at onset

ARX
CDKL5
STXBP1
FOXG1 (14q12 duplication)
SCN2A
KCNQ2
ST3Gal-III
SPTAN1 (with hypomyelinization)
CNV

Dravet syndrome

Dravet syndrome (DS), also known as severe myoclonic epilepsy in infancy (SMEI), is an epileptic encephalopathy with onset in the first year of life, in previously healthy children, and characterized by febrile and afebrile, generalized seizures, focal seizures, or both. Family history of epilepsy and/or febrile seizures is frequent. The course is characterized by recurrent polymorphic seizures (myoclonic, focal, atypical absences, and generalized and unilateral clonic and tonic-clonic seizures) slowing of psychomotor development, and appearance of neurologic signs (Dravet, 1978; Arzimanoglou, 2009). Around 80% of all DS cases are caused by mutation in the *SCN1A* gene with 95% of these occurring *de novo*, most often on the paternal allele. Approximately half of the mutations are missense and most of the remainders are point mutations predicting truncation of the protein, with a minority being deletions of one or more exons or mutations affecting the promoter region (Marini *et al.*, 2011). There seems to be no difference with regard to the presence and type of mutations in relation to the neurological (Brunklaus *et al.*, 2012) and neuropsychological (Ragona *et al.*, 2011) phenotype.

Other genetic mutations associated with epileptic encephalopathies

The advent of exome sequencing has uncovered a number of previously unknown genetic mutations associated with peculiar types of epileptic encephalopathy with their own characteristic phenotype. Of note are a reported pathogenic mutation of the SCN8A channel, which is responsible for a form of infantile epileptic encephalopathy associated with SUDEP (Veeramah *et al.*, 2012) and a biallelic SZT2 mutation, associated with infantile epileptic encephalopathy and dysmoprhic corpus callosum (Basel-Vanagaite *et al.*, 2013). Among the growing list of genes associated with infantile encephalopathy, CHD2, SYN-GAP1 (Carvill *et al.*, 2013) and GNAO1 (Nakamura *et al.*, 2013b) have also been added; however, these are only a few of a number which is sure to significantly increase in the coming years.

Table IV. Genetic heterogeneity of epileptic encephalopathies

Gene	Epileptic encephalopathy
ARX	Ohtahara syndrome, West syndrome
STXBP1	Ohtahara syndrome, West syndrome Focal epilepsies
CDKL5	West syndrome, Ohtahara syndrome
KCNQ2	BNFS, Ohtahara syndrome
FOXG1	West syndrome

Malignant migrating partial seizures of infancy

Migrating malignant partial seizures in infancy (MMPSI) is a rare and severe epileptic syndrome first reported in 1995 by Coppola and colleagues (Coppola *et al.*, 1995) and included among the childhood epilepsy syndromes in the proposal of the revision of the International League against Epilepsy (ILAE) (Engel, 2006).

MMPSI is characterized by: i) seizures onset during the first 6 months of life, ii) focal seizures arising and randomly migrating from one cortical region to another (*Figure 3*), iii) marked pharmacoresistance, and iv) severe cognitive long-term outcome (Coppola *et al.*, 1995). MMPSI prognosis is poor, with a third of patients dying before the end of the second year of age, mainly due to the prolonged status epilepticus and/or respiratory

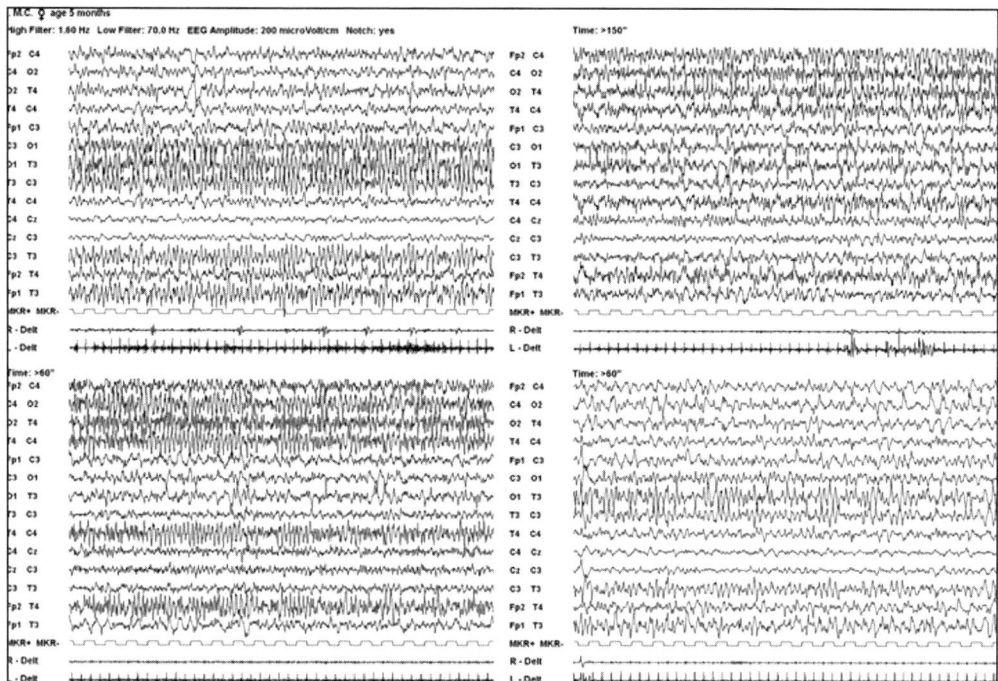

Figure 3. Ictal pattern of a patient with MMPSI, characterized by high-voltage polyspike activity migrating from the left central and temporal regions (upper left corner) to the controlateral counterparts (upper right and bottom left corners) and then back again to the left hemisphere (bottom right corner).

insufficiency. The genetic basis of MMPSI is heterogeneous with one major gene, *KCNT1* encoding a K+ channel depending by the intracellular concentration in Na+, with *de novo* mutations identified by exome sequencing in 50% of sporadic patients with MMPSI (Barcia *et al.*, 2012; McTague *et al.*, 2013; Ishii *et al.*, 2013). The first report by Barcia *et al.* was based on three trios study by exome sequencing technique and *KCNT1* variants were identified in 2 patients (Barcia *et al.*, 2012). The functional studies of these mutations showed an increased K current with a constitutive activation of mutated channels compared to wild type (Barcia *et al.*, 2012). A few other genes are reported in isolated cases. Two reports identified 2 missense mutations and one deletion of the sodium channel gene *SCN1A* (Freilich *et al.*, 2011; Carranza Rojo *et al.*, 2011). Poduri *et al.* (2012) described a homozygous deletion in *PLCB1* (phospholipase C, beta 1) in a child with MMPSI and Milh *et al.* (2013) reported compound heterozygous mutations in the gene encoding the TBC1 domain protein *TBC1D24*, in 2 affected siblings. Poduri *et al.* (2013) also reported a mutation in the *SLC25A22* channel in 2 sibs and Damhija *et al.* (2013) a *de novo* mutation in *SCN2A* in one patient with MMPSI (*Table V*). In sporadic patients with MMPSI, *KCNT1* should be analyzed first. *PLCB1*, *TBC1D24* and *SLC25A22* screening should be appropriated in familial cases or if an autosomal recessive inheritance is suspected. *SCN1A* and *SCN2A* should be screened in sporadic patients with a negative *KCNT1* study (Striano *et al.*, 2013).

Table V. Genes associated with Migrating Malignant Partial Seizures of Infancy

Gene/locus	Authors	Inheritance	Number of patients with MMPSI	Other associated phenotypes	Authors
KCNT1	Barcia, 2012 McTague, 2013 Ishii, 2013	Autosomal dominant	16	ADNFLE EOEE Infantile spasms	Heron, 2012 Dahmijia, 2013 Carvill, 2013
SCN2A	Dahmijia, 2013	Autosomal dominant	1	Dravet syndrome GEFS+ Infantile spasms	Shi, 2009 Carvill, 2013
SCN1A	Freilich, 2011 Carranza-Rojo, 2011	Autosomal dominant	2	Dravet syndrome GEFS+ Infantile spasms	Depienne, 2009 Carvill, 2013
PLCB1	Poduri, 2012	Autosomal recessive	2	–	–
TBC1D24	Milh, 2012	Autosomal recessive	1	Idiopathic myoclonic epilepsy	Falace, 2010
SLC25A22	Poduri, 2013	Autosomal recessive	2	EIEE	Molinari, 2005

References

- Arzimanoglou A. Dravet syndrome: from electroclinical characteristics to molecular biology. *Epilepsia* 2009; 50 (suppl 8): 3-9.
- Auvin S, Holder-Espinasse M, Lamblin MD, Andrieux J. Array-CGH detection of a *de novo* 0.7-Mb deletion in 19p13.13 including *CACNA1A* associated with mental retardation and epilepsy with infantile spasms. *Epilepsia* 2009; 50: 2501-3.
- Barcia G, Fleming MR, Deligniere A, *et al*. De novo gain-of-function KCNT1 channel mutations cause malignant migrating partial seizures of infancy. *Nat Genet* 2012; 44: 1255-9.
- Basel-Vanagaite L, Hershkovitz T, Heyman E, *et al*. Biallelic *SZT2* mutations cause infantile encephalopathy with epilepsy and dysmorphic corpus callosum. *AmJ Hum Genet* 2013; 93: 524-9.
- Berg AT, Berkovic SF, Brodie MJ, *et al*. Revised terminology and concepts for organization of seizures and epilepsies: report of the ILAE Commission on Classification and Terminology, 2005-2009. *Epilepsia* 2010; 51: 676-85.
- Bertossi C, Cassina M, De Palma L, *et al*. 14q12 duplication including FOXG1: Is there a common age-dependent epileptic phenotype? *Brain Dev* 2014; 36: 402-7.
- Brunetti-Pierri N, Paciorkowski AR, Ciccone R, *et al*. Duplications of *FOXG1* in 14q12 are associated with developmental epilepsy, mental retardation, and severe speech impairment. *Eur J Hum Genet* 2011; 19: 102-7.
- Brunklaus A, Ellis R, Reavey E, Forbes GH, Zuberi SM. Prognostic, clinical and demographic features in SCN1A mutation-positive Dravet syndrome. *Brain* 2012; 135: 2329-36.
- Carranza Rojo D, Hamiwka L, McMahon JM, *et al*. De novo *SCN1A* mutations in migrating partial seizures of infancy. *Neurology* 2011; 77: 380-3.

- Carvill GL, Heavin SB, Yendle SC, et al. Targeted resequencing in epileptic encephalopathies identifies de novo mutations in CHD2 and SYNGAP1. *Nature Genet* 2013; 45: 825-30.
- Coppola G, Plouin P, Chiron C, Robain O, Dulac O. Migrating partial seizures in infancy: a malignant disorder with developmental arrest. *Epilepsia* 1995; 36: 1017-24.
- Depienne C, Trouillard O, Saint-Martin C, et al. Spectrum of SCN1A gene mutations associated with Dravet syndrome: analysis of 333 patients. *J Med Genet* 2009; 46: 183-91.
- Dhamija R, Wirrell E, Falcao G, Kirmani S, Wong-Kisiel LC. Novel de novo SCN2A mutation in a child with migrating focal seizures of infancy. *Pediatr Neurol* 2013; 49: 486-8.
- Dravet C. Les épilepsies graves de l'enfant. *Vie Med* 1978; 8: 543-8.
- Dulac O, Bast T, Dalla Bernardina B, Gaily E, Neville B. Infantile spasms: toward a selective diagnostic and therapeutic approach. *Epilepsia* 2010; 51: 2218-9; author reply 2221.
- Edvardson S, Baumann AM, Mühlenhoff M, et al. West syndrome caused by ST3Gal-III deficiency. *Epilepsia* 2013; 54: e24-7.
- Engel J Jr. Report of the ILAE classification core group. *Epilepsia* 2006; 47: 1558-68.
- Ekşioğlu YZ, Pong AW, Takeoka M. A novel mutation in the aristaless domain of the ARX gene leads to Ohtahara syndrome, global developmental delay, and ambiguous genitalia in males and neuropsychiatric disorders in females. *Epilepsia* 2011; 52: 984-92.
- Falace A, Filipello F, La Padula V, et al. TBC1D24, an ARF6-interacting protein, is mutated in familial infantile myoclonic epilepsy. *Am J Hum Genet* 2010; 87: 365-70.
- Freilich ER, Jones JM, Gaillard WD, et al. Novel SCN1A mutation in a proband with malignant migrating partial seizures of infancy. *Arch Neurol* 2011; 68: 665-71.
- Fullston T, Brueton L, Willis T, et al. Ohtahara syndrome in a family with an ARX protein truncation mutation (c.81C>G/p.Y27X). *Eur J Hum Genet* 2010; 18: 157-62.
- Fusco L, Vigevano F. Ictal clinical electroencephalographic findings of spasms in West syndrome. *Epilepsia* 1993; 34: 671-8.
- Fusco L, Chiron C, Trivisano M, Vigevano F. Infantile spasms. In: Bureau M, Genton P, Dravet C, Delgado-Escueta AV, Tassinari CA, Thomas P, Wolf P (eds). *Epileptic Syndromes in Infancy, Childhood and Adolescence*, 5th ed. Paris: John Libbey Eurotext, 2012, pp. 99-113.
- Heron SE, Smith KR, Bahlo M, et al. Missense mutations in the sodium-gated potassium channel gene KCNT1 cause severe autosomal dominant nocturnal frontal lobe epilepsy. *Nat Genet* 2012; 44: 1188-90.
- Ishii A, Shioda M, Okumura A, et al. A recurrent KCNT1 mutation in two sporadic cases with malignant migrating partial seizures in infancy. *Gene* 2013; 531: 467-71.
- Kato M, Saitoh S, Kamei A, et al. A longer polyalanine expansion mutation in the ARX gene causes early infantile epileptic encephalopathy with suppression-burst pattern (Ohtahara syndrome). *Am J Hum Genet* 2007; 81: 361-6.
- Kato M, Yamagata T, Kubota M, et al. Clinical spectrum of early onset epileptic encephalopathies caused by KCNQ2 mutation. *Epilepsia*. 2013; 54: 1282-7.
- Marini C, Scheffer IE, Nabbout R, Suls A, De Jonghe P, Zara F, et al. The genetics of Dravet syndrome. *Epilepsia* 2011; 52 (suppl 2): 24-9.
- McTague A, Appleton R, Avula S, et al. Migrating partial seizures of infancy: expansion of the electroclinical, radiological and pathological disease spectrum. *Brain* 2013; 136: 1578-91.
- Mei D, Marini C, Novara F, et al. Xp22.3 genomic deletions involving the CDKL5 gene in girls with early onset epileptic encephalopathy. *Epilepsia* 2010; 51: 647-54.
- Milh M, Falace A, Villeneuve N, et al. Novel compound heterozygous mutations in TBC1D24 cause familial malignant migrating partial seizures of infancy. *Hum Mutat* 2013; 34: 869-72.
- Mizrahi EM, Milh M. Early severe neonatal and infantile epilepsies. In: Bureau M, Genton P, Dravet C, Delgado-Escueta AV, Tassinari CA, Thomas P, Wolf P (eds). *Epileptic Syndromes in Infancy, Childhood and Adolescence*, 5th ed. Paris: John Libbey Eurotext, 2012, pp. 89-98.

- Molinari F, Raas-Rothschild A, Rio M, et al. Impaired mitochondrial glutamate transport in autosomal recessive neonatal myoclonic epilepsy. *Am J Hum Genet* 2005; 76: 334-9.
- Nakamura K, Kato M, Osaka H, et al. Clinical spectrum of SCN2A mutations expanding to Ohtahara syndrome. *Neurology* 2013a; 81: 992-8.
- Nakamura K, Kodera H, Akita T, et al. De novo mutations in GNAO1, encoding a Gαo subunit of heterotrimeric G proteins, cause epileptic encephalopathy. *Am J Hum Genet* 2013b; 93: 496-505.
- Nonoda Y, Saito Y, Nagai S, et al. Progressive diffuse brain atrophy in West syndrome with marked hypomyelination due to SPTAN1 gene mutation. *Brain Dev* 2013; 35: 280-3.
- Osborne JP, Lux AL, Edwards SW, et al. The underlying etiology of infantile spasms (West syndrome): information from the United Kingdom Infantile Spasms Study (UKISS) on contemporary causes and their classification. *Epilepsia* 2010; 51: 2168-74.
- Otahara S, Ohtsuka Y, Yamatogi Y, et al. Early epileptic encephalopathy with suppression-bursts. In: Roger J, Bureau M, Dravet C, Dreifuss FE, Perret A, Wolf P (eds). *Epileptic Syndromes in Infancy, Childhood and Adolescence*, 2nd ed. London: John Libbey Eurotext, 1992, pp. 25-34.
- Otsuka M, Oguni H, Liang JS, et al. STXBP1 mutations cause not only Ohtahara syndrome but also West syndrome–result of Japanese cohort study. *Epilepsia* 2010; 51: 2449-52.
- Paciorkowski AR, Thio LL, Rosenfeld JA, et al. Copy number variants and infantile spasms: evidence for abnormalities in ventral forebrain development and pathways of synaptic function. *Eur J Hum Genet* 2011; 19: 1238-45.
- Pellock JM, Hrachovy R, Shinnar S, et al. Infantile spasms: a US consensus report. *Epilepsia* 2010; 51: 2175-89.
- Poduri A, Chopra SS, Neilan EG, et al. Homozygous PLCB1 deletion associated with malignant migrating partial seizures in infancy. *Epilepsia* 2012; 53: e146-50.
- Ragona F, Granata T, Dalla Bernardina B, et al. Cognitive development in Dravet syndrome: a retrospective, multicenter study of 26 patients. *Epilepsia* 2011; 52: 386-92.
- Saitsu H, Kato M, Mizuguchi T, et al. De novo mutations in the gene encoding STXBP1 (MUNC18-1) cause early infantile epileptic encephalopathy. *Nature Genet* 2008; 40: 782-8.
- Saitsu H, Kato M, Okada I, et al. STXBP1 mutations in early infantile epileptic encephalopathy with suppression-burst pattern. *Epilepsia* 2010; 51: 2397-405.
- Saitsu H, Kato M, Osaka H, et al. CASK aberrations in male patients with Ohtahara syndrome and cerebellar hypoplasia. *Epilepsia* 2012; 53: 1441-9.
- Shi X, Yasumoto S, Nakagawa E, Fukasawa T, Uchiya S, Hirose S. Missensemutation of the sodium channel gene SCN2A causes Dravet syndrome. *Brain Dev* 2009; 31: 758-62.
- Shoubridge C, Fullston T, Gécz J. ARX spectrum disorders: making inroads into the molecular pathology. *Human Mut* 2010; 31: 889-900.
- Striano P, Coppola G, Zara F, Nabbout R. Genetic heterogeneity in malignant migrating partial seizures of infancy. *Ann Neurol* 2014; 75: 324-6.
- Striano P, Paravidino R, Sicca F, et al. West syndrome associated with 14q12 duplications harboring FOXG1. *Neurology* 2011; 76: 1600-2.
- Veeramah KR, O'Brien JE, Meisler MH, et al. De novo pathogenic SCN8A mutation identified by whole-genome sequencing of a family quartet affected by infantile epileptic encephalopathy and SUDEP. *Am J Hum Genet* 2012; 90: 502-10.
- Weckhuysen S, Ivanovic V, Hendrickx R, et al. Extending the KCNQ2 encephalopathy spectrum: Clinical and neuroimaging findings in 17 patients. *Neurology* 2013; 81: 1697-703.
- Wray CD. 17q21.31 microdeletion associated with infantile spasms. *Eur J Med Genet* 2013; 56: 59-61.
- Writzl K, Primec ZR, Straiar BG, et al. Early onset West syndrome with severe hypomyelination and coloboma-like optic discs in a girl with SPTAN1 mutation. *Epilepsia* 2012; 53: e106–10.

Treatment of neonatal seizures with antiepileptic drugs

Chrysanthy Ikonomidou

Department of Neurology, University of Wisconsin-Madison, Wisconsin, USA

Neonatal seizures have an incidence of 3.5/1,000 in infants of all birth weights and gestational ages. Of the term infants who experience neonatal seizures between 20-30% die, 30% develop epilepsy and up to 40% develop cerebral palsy. Seizures are thought to be harmful. In fact, a positive correlation between the amount of electrographic seizure activity and subsequent morbidity and mortality has been reported (Painter at al., 2012; Uria-Avellanal *et al.*, 2013). Thus, infants with recurrent seizures or status epilepticus are treated aggressively with anti-epileptic drugs (AEDs) at doses sufficient to induce deep sedation in order to arrest seizures.

Pharmacological treatment of neonatal seizures: current standards and challenges

Despite the introduction of several new antiepileptic drugs over the past two decades, the medications routinely used for neonatal seizure management are limited and treatment protocols vary. Phenobarbital and phenytoin/fosphenytoin are the first line drugs but only demonstrate approximately 50% efficacy (Booth and Evans, 2004; Pressler and Mangum, 2013). Levetiracetam and topiramate are increasingly being used (Silverstein and Ferriero 2008) but clinical data on efficacy and safety of these compounds in neonates are limited. Levetiracetam and topiramate are thought to have fewer side effects and are easy to use as they do not require frequent blood draws and level monitoring (for review see Slaughter *et al.*, 2013).

Slaughter *et al.* (2013) systematically reviewed the published literature to determine which medication(s) are most effective for treating neonatal seizures, by retrieving trials and observational investigations *via* PubMed that focused on pharmacological seizure treatment of neonates and utilized continuous or amplitude-integrated EEG to confirm seizure diagnosis and cessation. They identified 557 initial articles and 14 additional studies after reference reviews, with 16 meeting inclusion criteria. Of these, only two were randomized trials while three additional investigations included comparison groups. Of those only one was large enough to enable statistical analysis (Painter *et al.*, 1999). Only three other studies, including a prospective nonrandomized experimental study (Hellstroem-Westas et al., 1988) and two retrospective cohort investigations (Castro-Conde et al., 2005; Shany et al., 2007) allowed comparison of between-group treatment effects. The authors were able to devise a treatment algorithm from available data. They recommended phenobarbital as first-line treatment given its inclusion in the only randomized controlled trial of first line treatment of neonatal seizures (Painter et al., 1999), the fact that it is the most studied antiepileptic medication in animals, and its historical use as the first-line antiepileptic drug for neonates (Clancy, 2006). They cautioned that there is extremely limited evidence on the effect of phenobarbital on long-term neonatal neurodevelopment. Until today, no neonatal antiepileptic has been shown superior to phenobarbital in a well-designed investigation (Slaughter et al., 2013).

Levetiracetam, phenytoin/fosphenytoin, and lidocaine all appear potentially effective as second-line treatments for neonatal seizures that are unresponsive to phenobarbital. Based on their systematic review findings alone, Slaughter et al. (2013) concluded that there is not strong evidence to recommend the use of any one of the medications over the others for second-line seizure control. Phenytoin/fosphenytoin was shown to only provide about a 10% to 15% increase in seizure control. Lidocaine is effective but has a narrow therapeutic window. Levetiracetam reportedly reduced seizure burden, but there were no within-study comparison groups (Abend et al., 2011; Khan et al., 2011). The authors caution that its efficacy and safety profile has not been adequately studied in term or preterm neonates.

Thus, there is limited evidence regarding the best pharmacologic treatment for neonatal seizures. The challenges of efficacy and safety of emerging treatments remain and need to be systematically addressed in carefully designed prospective randomized trials.

Emerging therapies for neonatal seizures

Bumetanide

Bumetanide is a diuretic which inhibits the chloride co-transporter and consequently reduces intracellular chloride and reverses the depolarizing action of GABA, resulting in reduced neuronal firing (Dzhala et al., 2005). When given under hypothermic conditions, bumetanide augments phenobarbital bioactivity in neonatal rodents (Liu et al., 2012; Cleary et al., 2013). Thus, the combination of phenobarbital and bumetanide may provide a more effective therapy for neonatal seizures than phenobarbital alone.

Currently two clinical studies are ongoing:

- Pilot Study of Bumetanide for Newborn Seizures, Massachusetts, USA (http://www.clinicaltrials.gov/ct2/show/NCT00830531). This is a randomized, double-blind, controlled, dose escalation study of bumetanide as add-on therapy to treat refractory seizures caused by HIE, focal or multi-focal stroke, or intracranial hemorrhage not controlled by an initial loading dose of phenobarbital.
  The primary outcome is determination of the pharmacokinetics and safety of bumetanide in newborn babies with refractory seizures. Secondary outcome is to determine the feasibility of a novel study design to test AEDs to treat neonatal seizures.

- NEMO1: An open label exploratory dose finding and pharmacokinetic clinical trial of bumetanide for the treatment of NEonatal Seizure using Medication Off-patent, EU (http://www.clinicaltrials.gov/ct2/show/NCT01434225). This is a two-stage trial with the following primary outcomes: stage I is to estimate the optimal dose of bumetanide for the treatment of neonatal seizures not responding to an initial loading dose of phenobarbital; stage II is to determine the pharmacokinetics at an optimal dose level.

Levetiracetam

Levetiracetam interacts with the synaptic vesicle protein 2A, which is implicated in the control of synaptic vesicle fusion, exocytosis, and neurotransmitter release (Lynch et al., 2004). Levetiracetam alters epileptiform burst firing but not normal neuronal excitability (Margineanou and Klitgaard, 2000). Levetiracetam does no cause neuronal apoptosis in the immature brain (Manthey et al., 2005) or disrupt synaptic development (Forcelli et al., 2012).

Currently two clinical trials with levetiracetam in neonatal seizures are ongoing:

- Efficacy of Intravenous Levetiracetam in Neonatal Seizures: A Phase 2 Randomized Blinded Controlled Study of the Efficacy of Intravenous Levetiracetam as First Line Treatment for Neonatal Seizures, San Diego, USA (http://www.clinicaltrials.gov/ct2/show/NCT01720667). The goal is to determine the efficacy of intravenous levetiracetam in terminating neonatal seizures when given as first-line therapy compared with phenobarbital. Primary outcome is efficacy.

- Efficacy of Levetiracetam for Neonatal Seizures, Cincinnati, USA (http://www.clinicaltrials.gov/ct2/show/record/NCT01475656). This is an observational study comparing levetiracetam and phenobarbital as a first-line AED. The primary outcome is the proportion of neonates who achieve electrographic seizure freedom as measured by continuous EEG monitoring for 24 h after intravenous levetiracetam administration. Secondary outcomes are safety, tolerability and pharmacokinetics.

Topiramate

Topiramate has good efficacy and safety profiles in children and adults (Connock et al., 2006; Glier et al., 2004). It has received FDA approval in adults and children with partial-onset seizures, primary generalized tonic clonic seizures and for seizures associated with Lennox Gastaut syndrome (Guerrini and Parmeggiani, 2006).

Currently, two trials are evaluating neuroprotective properties of topiramate in hypoxic ischemic encephalopathy (HIE), one of which has seizures as an outcome measure.

- Topiramate as an Adjuvant to Therapeutic Hypothermia for Infants with Hypoxic Ischemic Encephalopathy, California, USA (http://www.clinicaltrials.gov/ct2/show/NCT01765218). This is a randomized placebo-controlled trial to evaluate the neuroprotective properties of oral topiramate at a dose of 5 mg/kg/day. The primary outcomes are clinical or electrical seizures occurring before hospital discharge or before 4 weeks postnatal age (whichever is earlier) compared between the topiramate and control groups. Secondary outcome is HIE scores at birth and 4 weeks as well as normalisation of amplitude integrated EEG, serum and urine S100beta levels (a marker of neuronal injury), neonatal magnetic resonance imaging scores and developmental outcome at 9, 18 and 27 months of age.

- Safety and Efficacy of Oral Topiramate in Neonates with Hypoxic Ischemic Encephalopathy Treated with Hypothermia: a Pilot Study of the Neonatal Neuroprotection of Asphyxiated Tuscan Infants (NeoNATI) Network, Italy (http://www.clinicaltrials.gov/

ct2/show/NCT01241019). This is a randomized, single-blind trial to evaluate whether topiramate enhances the neuroprotective properties of hypothermia for the treatment of neonatal HIE (Filippi et al., 2012). The primary outcome is the neurological outcome at 6, 12, 18 months of life in the treatment group compared with the control group. The secondary outcome measures are neuroradiological outcomes at 3 and 12 months of life.

Xenon

Xenon, a monoatomic gas with very high tissue solubility, is a non-competitive inhibitor of the N-methyl-D-aspartate (NMDA) glutamate receptor (Franks et al., 1998). It is an anesthetic with a minimum alveolar concentration of approximately 60% in humans and lower concentrations of xenon are neuroprotective following hypoxic ischemic injury (Faulkner et al., 2011). Anticonvulsant effect of xenon in infants suffering perinatal asphyxial encephalopathy has recently been reported (Azzopardi et al., 2013).

Azzopardi and colleagues examined seizure activity on the real time and amplitude integrated EEG records of 14 full-term infants with perinatal HIE treated within 12 h of birth with 30% inhaled xenon for 24 h combined with 72 h of moderate systemic hypothermia. Seizures were identified on 5 of 14 infants. Seizures stopped during xenon therapy but recurred within a few minutes of withdrawing xenon and stopped again after xenon was restarted. These data show that subanesthetic levels of xenon may have an anticonvulsant effect.

■ Hypothermia for treatment of neonatal seizures

Low et al. (2012) conducted a study to investigate any possible effect of cooling on seizure burden. In a retrospective observational study, they quantified the recorded electrographic seizure burden based on multichannel video-EEG recordings in term neonates (> 37 weeks gestation) with hypoxic ischemic encephalopathy (HIE) who received cooling and in those who did not. Off-line analysis of prolonged continuous multichannel video-EEG recordings was performed independently by two experienced encephalographers. Comparison between the recorded electrographic seizure burden in non-cooled and cooled neonates was assessed (see also next chapter in this volume, by Boylan and Low).

Of 107 neonates with HIE who underwent prolonged continuous multichannel EEG monitoring 37 neonates had electrographic seizures, of whom 31 had EEG recordings that were suitable for the analysis (16 non-cooled and 15 cooled). The recorded electrographic seizure burden in the cooled group was significantly lower than in the non-cooled group (60 [39-224] vs 203 [141-406] min). Further exploratory analysis showed that the recorded electrographic seizure burden was only significantly reduced in cooled neonates with moderate HIE (49 [26-89] vs 162 [97-262] min). In conclusion, a decreased seizure burden was seen in neonates with moderate HIE who received cooling.

In a separate study, Mathur and colleagues (Srinivasakumar et al., 2013) evaluated the electrographic seizure burden in neonates with HIE treated with or without therapeutic hypothermia and stratified results by severity of HIE and severity of injury as assessed by magnetic resonance imaging (MRI). Sixty-nine neonates with moderate or severe HIE were prospectively enrolled, including 51 who received therapeutic hypothermia and 18 who did not. The therapeutic hypothermia group had a lower electrographic seizure burden (log units) after controlling for injury, as assessed by MRI. A reduction in seizure burden was seen in neonates with moderate HIE, but not in those with severe HIE. Among neonates with injury assessed by MRI, seizure burden was lower in those with mild and moderate injury, but not in those with severe injury.

Safety concerns: Antiepileptic drugs may injure the developing brain

Physiological cell death, a phenomenon by which unsuccessful neurons are deleted by apoptosis (cell suicide) from the central nervous system occurs in the developing brain.

It has been shown that compounds which are used as sedatives, anesthetics or anticonvulsants in medicine, trigger widespread apoptotic neurodegeneration throughout the developing brain when administered to immature rodents (Bittigau et al., 2002; Ikonomidou et al., 1999; 2000). Such compounds include antagonists of N-methyl-D-aspartate (NMDA) receptors (ketamine, nitrous oxide), agonists of γ-amino-butyric acid subtype A (GABA$_A$) receptors (barbiturates, benzodiazepines, propofol) and/or sodium channel blockers (phenytoin, valproate).

Rodents are vulnerable to this phenomenon during the first two postnatal weeks of life, a period which coincides with the brain growth spurt, described by Dobbing and Sands (1979). The comparable period in humans extends from the sixth month of pregnancy to several years after birth.

Neurotoxic effects of antiepileptic drugs (AEDs) have been systematically studied in infant rodents (Bittigau et al., 2002). These studies revealed that the majority of AEDs may cause apoptotic neurodegeneration in the developing rat brain at doses and plasma concentrations relevant for anticonvulsant treatment. The threshold dose for triggering an apoptotic response was 20 mg/kg for phenytoin, which resulted in phenytoin plasma concentrations ranging between 10-15 µg/ml over 4 h. Phenobarbital, diazepam, clonazepam, valproate and vigabatrin elicited similar neurotoxic effects in a dose-dependent manner.

Neurotoxicity of common AEDs was assessed in relationship to their effective anticonvulsant dose-range in rodents. For barbiturates, benzodiazepines, phenytoin, valproate, vigabatrin or sulthiame neurotoxicity was present within their reported anticonvulsant dose ranges in rodent seizure models. Interestingly, topiramate elicited a neurotoxic effect in infant rat brain beginning at a dose of 50 mg/kg which is higher than the reported effective anticonvulsant doses in infant rodent seizure models (Glier et al., 2004), suggesting a rather beneficial profile. Levetiracetam showed no neurotoxicity in the infant rat brain at all doses tested (Manthey et al., 2005).

Morphological changes in the brains of subjects exposed *in utero* to AEDs were analyzed. For this purpose, a group of healthy young adults with prenatal exposure to AEDs (PAE) and a group of age-matched unexposed healthy controls were subjected to magnetic resonance imaging (MRI) of the brain and structural differences between the two groups were studied by means of voxel based morphometry (Ikonomidou et al., 2007). Regional decreases of grey matter volumes were found in PAE subjects in the area of the lentiform nucleus, including both pallidum and putamen bilaterally, and the hypothalamus. The conclusion was drawn that prenatal exposure to AEDs causes subtle morphological changes in grey matter of the human brain consisting of lower grey matter volumes in the basal ganglia and the hypothalamus. It is possible that AED-induced neurodegeneration within the basal ganglia may partly account for the lower grey matter volumes measured in this area.

In addition to their proapoptotic effects in the developing brain, sedatives and AEDs may also impair cell proliferation and differentiation, neurogenesis, synaptogenesis, synaptic plasticity, cell migration and axonal arborization. A disruption of these developmental processes may potentially account for neurological deficits seen in humans exposed to AEDs pre- or postnatally (Stefovska et al., 2008; Ikonomidou and Turski, 2010).

■ Neuroprotective strategies in the horizon

Lithium

Lithium has long been used as a first-line maintenance therapy for bipolar and other psychiatric disorders. There is evidence from *in vitro* and *in vivo* animal studies suggesting that it may have neuroprotective properties in adult neurological disorders such as Alzheimer's disease and stroke (Bian et al., 2007; Chuang and Priller, 2006).

Zhong et al., 2006 and Olney and colleagues reported that lithium protects the infant mouse brain against neurodegeneration induced by ethanol. Similar neuroprotective effects of lithium were documented against anesthesia-induced neuroapoptosis (Straiko et al., 2009; Creeley and Olney, 2010). Olney and colleagues found that subanesthetic doses of ketamine and propofol do cause neurodegeneration, and lithium prevents this action and completely eliminates the neuroapoptosis reaction induced by these anesthetic drugs (Creeley and Olney, 2010).

Lithium's toxicity potential for immature humans has been studied primarily in the context of lithium being administered chronically to pregnant women who have bipolar disorder. It has weak teratogenic properties in that exposure during the first trimester may be associated with an increase in cardiac anomalies. Chronic exposure during later stages of pregnancy is considered safe (Gilles and Bannigan, 2006; Yacobi and Ornoy, 2008). No studies have addressed neuroprotective effects of lithium against apoptosis induced by antiepileptic drugs and clearly, before lithium could be recommended as a protective therapy, it would have to be evaluated much more thoroughly for both efficacy and safety. Studies in nonhuman primates are necessary to evaluate lithium's potential as an adjunctive neuroprotectant in the treatment of seizures in the neonatal period. There is realistic hope that a pharmacological means for controlling this neurotoxic process can be developed. It is also realistic to believe that further research aimed at understanding the intracellular mechanisms underlying lithium's protective action will lead to the development of other drugs that might be superior to lithium for this therapeutic purpose.

Hypothermia

In addition to its antiepileptic potential, there is recent evidence to suggest that hypothermia can prevent neuronal degeneration induced in the developing brain by anesthetic drugs.

So far only pilot experiments have been conducted but the results are very encouraging. Creeley and Olney (2010) conducted experiments to determine how changes in ambient temperature (AT) influence brain temperature (BT) in 4-day-old (P4) infant mice. To test the influence of BT on the neuroapoptogenic action of anesthetic drugs, they compared two temperature extremes, the 34.7° C condition (normothermia) *versus* the 29.7° C condition (hypothermia). They exposed some groups of P4 mice (n = 8 per group) to isoflurane, ketamine, or no anesthesia at normothermia (34.7° C) and other groups to the same treatment conditions at hypothermia (29.7° C). All pups were killed 5 h after initiation of treatment for histological evaluation of their brains for mapping and quantifying neurons undergoing apoptosis. Pups treated with either isoflurane or ketamine under the normothermic condition had a significantly increased neuroapoptosis response compared with the normothermic controls. The density of apoptotic profiles after treatment with these drugs under the hypothermic condition was very significantly reduced, signifying that under the hypothermic condition, isoflurane and ketamine did not induce a neuroapoptosis response. These results clearly support the conclusion that brain cooling to only a moderate degree markedly suppressed the neuroapoptosis response to either isoflurane or ketamine in the infant mouse brain. Thus, hypothermia warrants further investigation as a potentially safe and effective means for preventing antiepileptic and anesthetic drugs from injuring the developing brain.

Melatonin

Melatonin is a sleep-promoting agent and antioxidant known to inhibit apoptotic-type neuronal damage by improving mitochondrial homeostasis and stabilizing the inner mitochondrial membrane. Yon *et al.* reported that melatonin protects the developing rat brain from anesthesia induced neuroapoptosis (Yon *et al.*, 2006). Forcelli and colleagues described in a more recent paper that melatonin prevented the phenobarbital-induced disruption of synaptic maturation in the striatum (Forcelli *et al.*, 2012) and potentiated the anticonvulsant effect of phenobarbital in infant rats (Forcelli *et al.*, 2013). These findings are encouraging in that melatonin could be a useful adjunctive medication which might prevent adverse effects of AED on the neonatal brain.

Conclusion

Current treatments of neonatal seizures continue to be unsatisfactory despite the introduction of multiple new AEDs in the past two decades. Developing approaches with higher efficacy and safety for neonates remains a major challenge. There are encouraging developments, both in terms of the use of newer antiepileptic drugs and hypothermia to improve antiepileptic efficacy as well as novel measures to prevent AED neurotoxicity. Lithium and melatonin are promising agents that may help prevent adverse effects of AEDs and improve neurodevelopmental outcomes. Hypothermia is a potentially unique approach which may help increase both efficacy and safety of AED therapy and ought to be investigated with high priority in that respect.

References

- Abend NS, Gutierrez-Colina AM, Monk HM, Dlugos DJ, Clancy RR. Levetiracetam for treatment of neonatal seizures. *J Child Neurol* 2011; 26: 465-70.
- Azzopardi D, Robertson NJ, Kapetanakis A, Griffiths J, Rennie JM, Mathieson SR, Edwards AD. Anticonvulsant effect of xenon on neonatal asphyxial seizures. *Arch Dis Child Fetal Neonatal Ed* 2013; 98: F437-9.
- Bian Q, Shi T, Chuang DM, Qian Y. Lithium reduces ischemia-induced hippocampal CA1 damage and behavioral deficits in gerbils. *Brain Res* 2007; 1184: 270-6.

- Bittigau P, Sifringer M, Genz K, Reith E, Pospischil D, Govindarajalu S, *et al.* Antiepileptic drugs and apoptotic neurodegeneration in the developing brain. *Proc Natl Acad Sci USA* 2002; 99: 15089-94.
- Booth D, Evans DJ. Anticonvulsants for neonates with seizures. *Cochrane Database Syst Rev* 2004 Oct 18; (4): CD004218.
- Castro-Conde JR, Borges AAH, Martinez ED, González Campo C, Perera Soler R. Midazolam in neonatal seizures with no response to phenobarbital. *Neurol* 2005; 64: 876-9.
- Chuang DM, Priller J. Potential use of lithium in neurodegenerative disorders. In: Bauer M, Grof P, Müller-Oerlingausen B, eds. *Lithium in neuropsychiatry: the comprehensive guide*. London: Taylor & Francis Books Ltd, 2006, pp. 381-97.
- Clancy RR. Summary proceedings from the neurology group on neonatal seizures. *Pediatrics* 2006; 117: S23-7.
- Cleary RT, Sun H, Huynh T, Manning SM, Li Y, Rotenberg A, Talos DM, *et al.* Bumetanide enhances phenobarbital efficacy in a rat model of hypoxic neonatal seizures. *PLoS One* 2013; 8: 57148.
- Connock M, Frew ME, Evans B-W, Bryan S, Cummins C, Fry-Smith A, *et al.* The clinical effectiveness and cost-effectiveness of newer drugs for children with epilepsy. A systematic review. *Health Technol Assess* 2006; 10: iii, ix-118.
- Creeley CE, Olney JW. The young: neuroapoptosis induced by anesthetics and what to do about it. *Anesth Analg* 2010; 110: 442-8.
- Dobbing J, Sands J. The brain growth spurt in various mammalian species. *Early Hum Dev* 1979; 3: 79-84.
- Dzhala VI, Talos DM, Sdrulla DA, Brumback AC, Mathews GC, Benke TA, *et al.* NKCC1 transporter facilitates seizures in the developing brain. *Nat Med* 2005; 11: 1205-13.
- Faulkner S, Bainbridge A, Kato T, Chandrasekaran M, Kapetanakis AB, Hristova M, *et al.* Xenon augmented hypothermia reduces early lactate/N-acetylaspartate and cell death in perinatal asphyxia. *Ann Neurol* 2011; 70: 133-50.
- Forcelli PA, Janssen MJ, Vicini S, Gale K. Neonatal exposure to antiepileptic drugs disrupts striatal synaptic development. *Ann Neurol* 2012 Sep; 72: 363-72.
- Forcelli PA, Soper C, Duckles A, Gale K, Kondratyev A. Melatonin potentiates the anticonvulsant action of phenobarbital in neonatal rats. *Epilepsy Res* 2013; 107: 217-23.
- Franks NP, Dickinson R, de Sousa SL, Hall AC, Lieb WR. How does xenon produce anaesthesia? *Nature* 1998; 396: 324.
- Glier C, Dzietko M, Bittigau P, Jarosz B, Korobowicz E, Ikonomidou C. Therapeutic doses of topiramate are not toxic to the developing brain. *Exp Neurol* 2004; 185: 403-9.
- Guerrini R, Parmeggiani L. Topiramate and its clinical applications in epilepsy. *Expert Opin Pharmacother* 2006; 7: 811-23.
- Hellström-Westas L, Westgren U, Rosen I, Svenningsen N. Lidocaine for treatment of severe seizures in newborn infants. *Acta Paediatr Scand* 1988; 77: 79-84.
- Ikonomidou C, Bittigau P, Ishimaru MJ, Koch C, Genz K, Price MT, *et al.* Ethanol-induced apoptotic neurodegeneration and fetal alcohol syndrome. *Science* 2000; 287: 1056-60.
- Ikonomidou C, Bosch F, Miksa M, Bittigau P, Vöckler J, Dikranian K, *et al.* Blockade of NMDA receptors and apoptotic neurodegeneration in the developing brain. *Science* 1999; 283: 70-4.
- Ikonomidou C, Scheer J, Wilhelm T, Juengling F, Titze K, Stöver U, *et al.* Brain morphology alterations following prenatal exposure to antiepileptic drugs. *Eur J Ped Neurol* 2007; 11: 297-301.
- Ikonomidou C, Turski L. Antiepileptic drugs and brain development. *Epilepsy Res* 2010; 88: 11-22.
- Khan O, Chang E, Cipriani C, *et al.* Use of intravenous levetiracetam for management of acute seizures in neonates. *Pediatr Neurol* 2011; 44: 265-9.

- Low E, Boylan GB, Mathieson SR, Murray DM, Korotchikova I, Stevenson NJ, et al. Cooling and seizure burden in term neonates: an observational study. *Arch Dis Child Fetal Neonatal Ed.* 2012; 97: F267-72.
- Liu Y, Shangguan Y, Barks JD, Silverstein FS. Bumetanide augments the neuroprotective efficacy of phenobarbital plus hypothermia in a neonatal hypoxia–ischemia model. *Pediatr Res* 2012; 71: 559-65.
- Lynch BA, Lambeng N, Nocka K, Kensel-Hammes P, Bajjalieh SM, Matagne A, et al. The synaptic vesicle protein SV2A is the binding site for the antiepileptic drug levetiracetam. *Proc Natl Acad Sci USA* 2004; 101: 9861-6.
- Manthey D, Asimiadou S, Stefovska V, Kaindl AM, Fassbender J, Ikonomidou C, Bittigau P. Sulthiame but not levetiracetam exerts neurotoxic effect in the developing rat brain. *Exp Neurol* 2005; 93: 497-503.
- Painter MJ, Scher MS, Stein AD, Armatti S, Wang Z, Gardiner JC, et al. Phenobarbital compared with phenytoin for the treatment of neonatal seizures. *N Engl J Med* 1999; 341: 485-9.
- Painter MJ, Sun Q, Scher MS, Janosky J, Alvin J. Neonates with seizures: what predicts development? *J Child Neurol* 2012; 27: 1022-6.
- Pressler RM, Mangum B. Newly emerging therapies for neonatal seizures. *Semin Fetal Neonatal Med* 2013; 18: 216-23.
- Shany E, Benzaqen O, Watemberg N. Comparison of continuous drip of midazolam or lidocaine in the treatment of intractable neonatal seizures. *J Child Neurol* 2007; 22: 255-9.
- Silverstein FS, Ferriero DM. Off-label use of antiepileptic drugs for the treatment of neonatal seizures. *Pediatr Neurol* 2008; 39: 77-9.
- Slaughter LA, Patel AD, Slaughter JL. Pharmacological treatment of neonatal seizures: a systematic review. *J Child Neurol* 2013 Mar; 28: 351-64.
- Srinivasakumar P, Zempel J, Wallendorf M, Lawrence R, Inder T, Mathur A. Therapeutic hypothermia in neonatal hypoxic ischemic encephalopathy: electrographic seizures and magnetic resonance imaging evidence of injury. *J Pediatr* 2013; 163: 465-70.
- Stefovska V, Uckermann O, Czuczwar M, Smitka M, Czuczwar P, Kis J, et al. Sedative and anticonvulsant drugs suppress postnatal neurogenesis. *Ann Neurol* 2008; 64: 434-45.
- Straiko MM, Young C, Cattano D, Creeley CE, Wang H, Smith DJ, et al. Lithium protects against anesthesia-induced developmental neuroapoptosis. *Anesthesiology* 2009; 110: 862-8.
- Uria-Avellanal C, Marlow N, Rennie JM. Outcome following neonatal seizures. *Semin Fetal Neonatal Med* 2013; 18: 224-32.
- Yacobi S, Ornoy A. Is lithium a real teratogen? What can we conclude from the prospective versus retrospective studies? A review. *Isr J Psychiatry Relat Sci* 2008; 45: 95-106.
- Yon JH, Carter LB, Reiter RJ, Jevtovic-Todorovic V. Melatonin reduces the severity of anesthesia-induced apoptotic neurodegeneration in the developing rat brain. *Neurobiol Dis* 2006 Mar; 21(3): 522-30.
- Zhong J, Yang X, Yao W, Lee W. Lithium protects ethanol-induced neuronal apoptosis. *Biochem Biophys Res Commun* 2006; 350: 905-10.

Neonatal seizures in hypoxic-ischaemic encephalopathy: the impact of therapeutic hypothermia

Evonne Low, Geraldine B. Boylan

Neonatal Brain Research Group, Irish Centre for Fetal and Neonatal Translational Research, Department of Paediatrics and Child Health, University College Cork, Cork, Ireland

Moderate to severe neonatal hypoxic-ischaemic encephalopathy (HIE) affects approximately 1 to 3 per 1,000 live term births and is a major cause of death and long-term neurodisability (Marlow and Budge, 2005; Lawn et al., 2010). Seizures are the hallmark of neurological injury and approximately 45 to 50% of all neonatal seizures are attributable to HIE (Volpe, 2008). However, neonatal seizures continue to present a diagnostic and therapeutic challenge to clinicians worldwide due to their variable clinical expression and poor response to commonly used antiepileptic drugs (AEDs). The adoption of more widespread EEG monitoring in the neonatal intensive care unit over the last 10 years has meant that the true seizure burden of neonates with HIE has been recognized. Previous research has been hampered by the lack of continuous EEG monitoring to characterize and quantify neonatal seizures in this population. In addition, many studies included seizures with varying aetiologies and EEG monitoring was not continuous in the acute phase of injury.

The evidence of benefit for therapeutic hypothermia in HIE is considered sufficient for the widespread implementation of its use in neonatal intensive care units worldwide (NICE guideline 2010; Jacobs et al., 2013; Harris et al., 2014). A meta-analysis of 3 trials which enrolled 767 neonates showed that therapeutic hypothermia reduced the combined rate of death or disability at 18 months (Edwards et al., 2010). More recently, neonates who were treated with therapeutic hypothermia after perinatal asphyxia have shown improved neurocognitive function at 6 to 7 years of age (Azzopardi et al., 2014). Further data are required to clarify whether therapeutic hypothermia is appropriate for severe HIE. Efforts to supplement therapeutic hypothermia with other neuroprotective agents and to extend the neuroprotection window beyond 72 hours may prove useful for this population (Fan and Van Bel, 2010; Faulkner et al., 2011; Aly et al., 2012; Robertson et al., 2013; Herrera EA et al., 2014; Charriaut-Marlangue et al., 2014).

Hypoxic-ischaemic encephalopathy (HIE)

Given that HIE is an evolving process reflecting the evolution of the underlying brain injury (Gunn and Thoresen, 2006), continuous EEG monitoring is essential for assessing cerebral function and for accurate quantification of neonatal seizures. Immediately following the primary hypoxia-ischaemic insult, there is disruption to cerebral oxidative metabolism, cytotoxic oedema develops, excitotoxins accumulate and the EEG is suppressed. Some metabolic recovery is possible over the subsequent 30 to 60 minutes (Tan et al., 1996; Bennet et al., 2007a). A latent phase then follows from about 1 to 6 hours characterized by cerebral hypoperfusion, reduced metabolism and a suppressed EEG. During this period, high energy phosphates return to near normal values (Robertson et al., 2013). However, a secondary injury phase then develops and corresponds to further periods of cytotoxic oedema, accumulation of excitotoxins and hyperperfusion. During this injury phase, there is a failure of cerebral mitochondrial activity (Lorek et al., 1994; Bennet et al., 2006; Wassink et al., 2014) eventually leading to cell death. In moderate to severe brain injury, the background EEG may start to recover during this period and seizures often develop (*Figure 1*). In very severe injury, the EEG can remain suppressed for days and seizures may never emerge.

Seizures and HIE

Seizures are seen in term neonates with significant HIE, usually occurring within the first 24 hours of life (Lynch et al., 2012). In experimental models of HIE, seizures occur either immediately after injury following an asphyxial insult or in a delayed manner 6 to 12 hours after the initial insult when secondary energy failure leads to additional cell death (Scher et al., 2008). Gunn et al. found that if ischaemia lasted 30 minutes or longer, a stereotypic sequence of depressed EEG activity followed by a low frequency epileptiform activity was observed (Gunn et al., 1992). The combination of hypoxia and seizures produces more profound injury in the brain than either factor alone (Wirrell et al., 2001). Seizures add to the hypoxia-ischaemic injury in neonatal animals; the same may be true for neonates (Wirrell et al., 2001; Miller et al., 2002).

In an elegant study by Bjorkman et al. using histology, magnetic resonance imaging and spectroscopy, electrographic seizures in piglets were associated with increased severity of brain injury following an extensive hypoxic-ischaemic insult (Bjorkman et al., 2010).

A recent histological study in the hippocampi of 16 deceased full-term asphyxiated neonates has shown that there were more significant increases in microglial activation and expression of the inflammatory markers, namely interleukin 1β and complement 1q in cases with seizures compared to those without seizures (Schiering et al., 2014). In this study seizures were confirmed with EEG monitoring.

Ideally, accurate identification and quantification of neonatal seizures require continuous multichannel video-EEG monitoring (Boylan and Pressler, 2013). However, continuous video-EEG monitoring is not widely available and as a result, many centres worldwide now use limited two channel aEEG/EEG systems. As long as the limitations of these devices are appreciated, they are still far better than estimating seizure burden using clinical acumen alone (Rennie et al., 2004; Shellhaas et al., 2007; Murray et al., 2008; Malone et al., 2009; Glass et al., 2013).

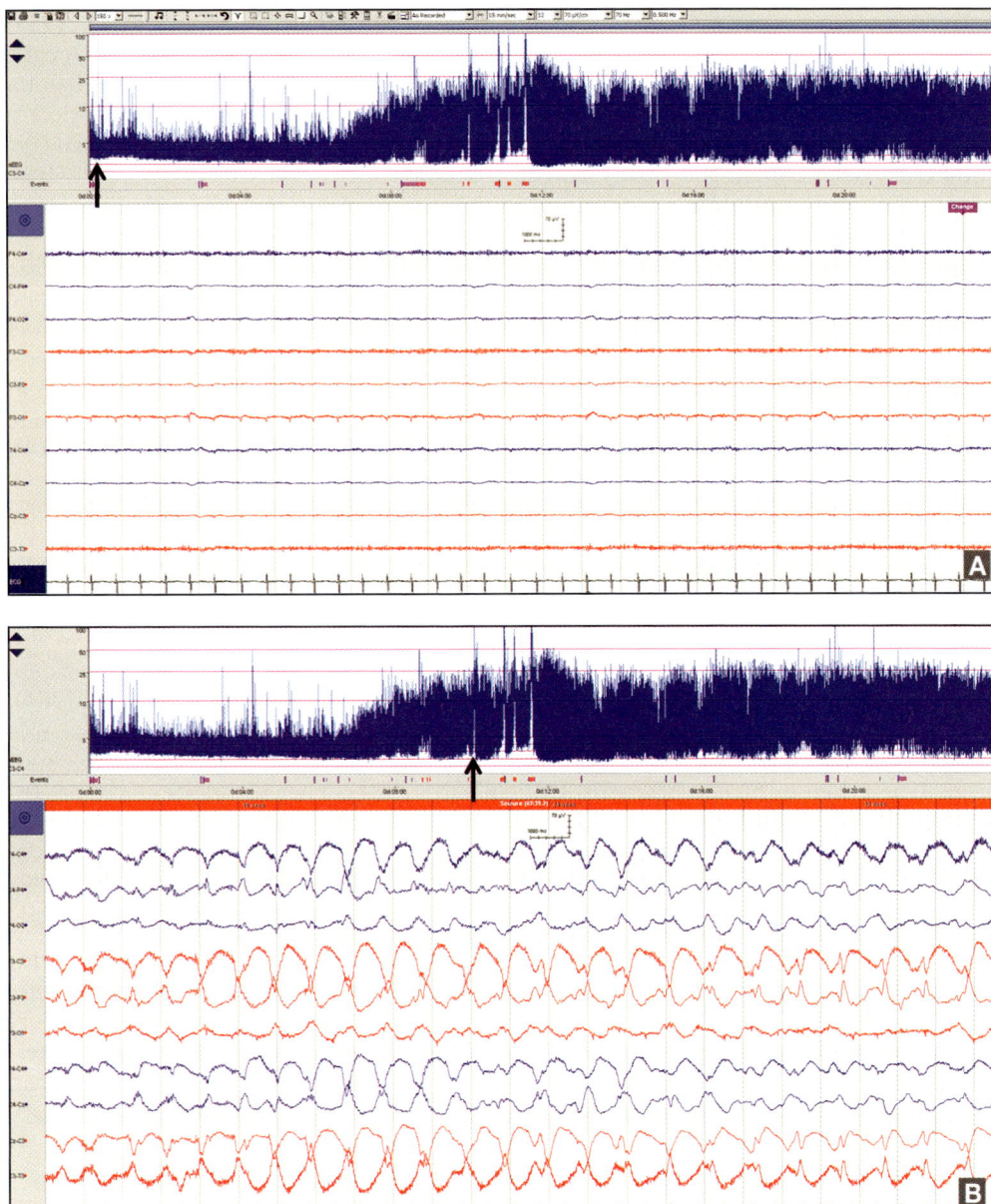

Figure 1. EEG and amplitude-integrated EEG (aEEG) over a 24 hour period from a neonate with poor Apgar scores, cord pH < 7.1 and requiring recuscitation at birth. EEG/aEEG recording commenced when the neonate was three hours old (during the latent phase) while receiving therapeutic hypothermia. Black arrows indicate location of EEG snapshot on aEEG recording.
A: EEG activity was suppressed from the outset and remained suppressed until the neonate was nine hours old.
B: following this period, the EEG began to recover and a burst suppression pattern developed with seizures emerging at 12 hours (probable secondary injury phase) after birth. Seizures responded well to phenobarbitone but a burst suppression background pattern continued.

Seizures occur in moderate and severe HIE only (Sarnat and Sarnat 1976; Levene et al., 1985) and are difficult to control. Studies completed before the widespread use of therapeutic hypothermia show that traditional first and second-line AEDs are often ineffective (Painter et al., 1999; Boylan et al., 2004). There are only a few studies that detail the evolution of electrographic seizure burden in neonates with HIE in the pre-therapeutic hypothermia era (Low et al., 2012; Lynch et al., 2012). Low et al. detailed the extensive electrographic seizure burden of neonates with HIE using continuous video-EEG monitoring; the seizure burden in non-cooled neonates was high and status epilepticus common (*Figure 2a*). Lynch et al. (2012) examined the temporal distribution of seizures in neonates with HIE and found that seizures generally have a short period of high electrographic seizure burden followed by a longer period of low seizure burden, resulting in an accumulation of seizures near the time of seizure onset (a positive skew) (*Figure 2a and b*). Prolonged seizures have been shown to exacerbate pre-existing cerebral damage due to perinatal hypoxic-ischaemia (Yager et al., 2002). Seizures in human neonates with HIE may exacerbate the initial hypoxic-ischaemic injury and require treatment (Miller et al., 2002; Glass et al., 2009; Ancora et al., 2010, Shah et al., 2014). However, this treatment is very difficult to optimize without continuous EEG monitoring.

Hypothermia and HIE

The use of cold as a therapeutic agent has had a long and interesting history in both medicine and surgery (Wang et al., 2006; also refer to the chapter by Ikonomidou in this volume). The concept of hypothermia as a treatment for brain injury is not new; its use as a treatment for perinatal asphyxia was suggested over 65 years ago (Miller et al., 1964). In the 1960s, Miller and Westin studied the physiologic basis for the neuroprotective role of hypothermia as a form of treatment for "asphyxia neonatorum", firstly in newborn animals and then in human newborns (Miller et al., 1964). They demonstrated improved survival without cerebral palsy or mental disability when apnoeic neonates were cooled rapidly after delivery when conventional resuscitation techniques failed. Preliminary studies in adults with coma after resuscitation from out-of-hospital cardiac arrest provided evidence that moderate hypothermia could improve outcomes (Bernard et al., 2002).

Hypothermia delays neuronal depolarisation, decreases the energy requirement for intrinsic cellular support and membrane homeostasis (Nakashima and Todd, 1996; Tooley et al., 2003; Bennet et al., 2007a), reduces cerebral energy metabolism during the primary injury phase, leading to a delay in the progression of primary damage and alleviates post-reperfusion injury. Some studies have shown that cooling markedly delays apoptosis even when it did not completely suppress it (Gunn et al., 2005; Azzopardi et al., 2009a).

Therapeutic hypothermia and neonatal seizures

Several experimental animal studies have demonstrated the effects of hypothermia on seizures (Busto et al., 1989; Globus et al., 1995; Nakashima and Todd, 1996; Tooley et al., 2003; Bennet et al., 2007b). In vitro studies have shown that rapidly cooling the cortex to between 20 and 25°C as quickly as possible after seizure onset resulted in a 90% reduction in seizure burden (Hill et al., 2000). In fetal sheep, hypothermia was associated with a marked reduction in the amplitude of seizures in the first 6 hours after a complete umbilical cord occlusion (Bennet et al., 2007b). In a piglet model of asphyxia, the duration of individual electrographic seizures were reduced in a cooled group when compared to a non-cooled group (Tooley et al., 2003). Hypothermia to 30 or 33°C has been shown to

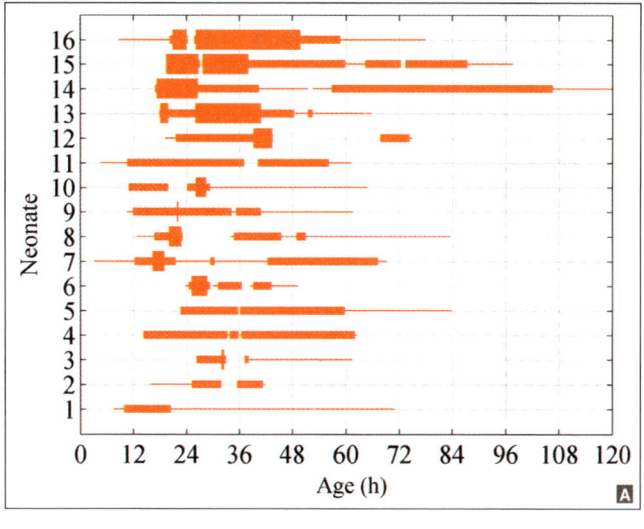
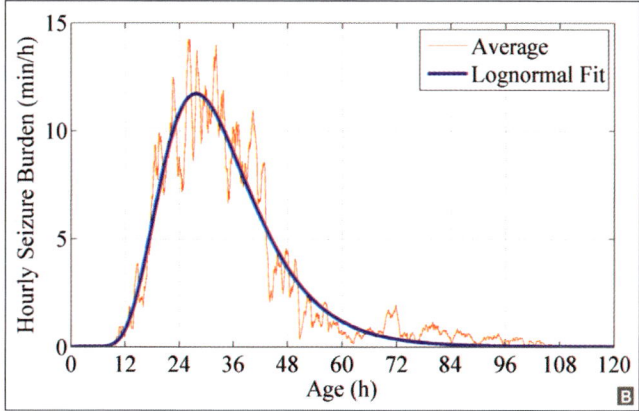

Figure 2. Comparison of the seizure burden between the normothermic and hypothermic neonates with hypoxic-ischaemic encephalopathy (adapted from Low et al., 2012 and Lynch et al., 2012 by Dr Nathan Stevenson).
A and B: at the top (A), a schematic diagram depicting the duration of continuous multichannel EEG monitoring (thin red horizontal lines) in normothermic neonates with electrographic seizures (thick red horizontal lines). The temporal distribution of seizures (at the bottom, B) as quantified using a measure of the hourly seizure in typically shows a large positive skew; such that initial seizures generally have a short period of high electrographic seizure burden followed by a period of reducing seizure burden.

inhibit the release of glutamate in a rat model of cerebral ischaemia (Busto et al., 1989). Other effects of hypothermia such as reduced cytotoxic oedema by reducing amino acid release (Nakashima and Todd, 1996) and inhibition of free oxygen radicals (Globus et al., 1995) may reduce seizure burden. Whether the amplitude, morphology and distribution of electrographic seizures in cooled neonates differ to that of non-cooled neonates will require further investigation.

In our recent study of seizures in neonates with hypothermia, we found that seizure burden was reduced in neonates receiving therapeutic hypothermia compared to a normothermic group [60 *vs* 203 minutes]; and that this was significant in neonates with moderate HIE rather than those with severe HIE (*Figure 2c and d*) (Low et al., 2012). Our findings were

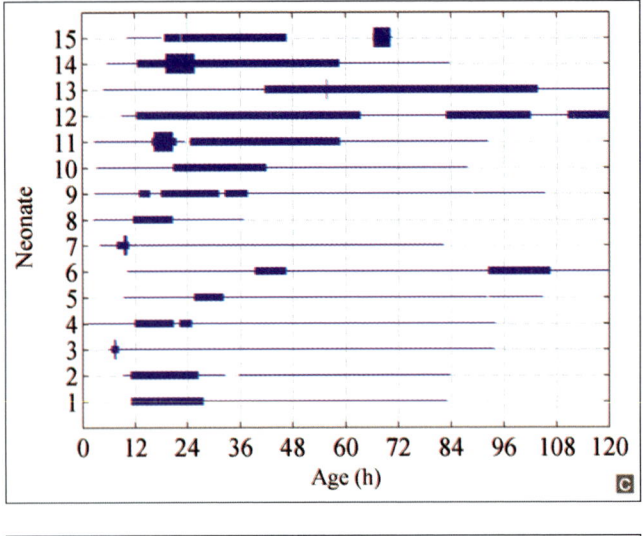

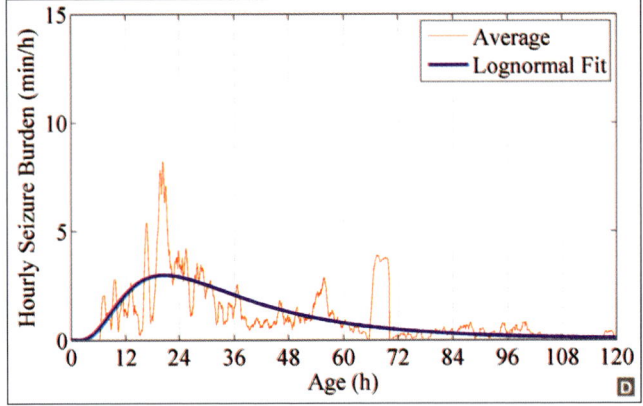

Figure 2 (continued). Comparison of the seizure burden between the normothermic and hypothermic neonates with hypoxic-ischaemic encephalopathy (adapted from Low et al., 2012 and Lynch et al., 2012 by Dr Nathan Stevenson). **C and D:** in the hypothermic group during continuous multichannel EEG monitoring (thin blue horizontal lines), reduced electrographic seizure burden (thick blue horizontal lines) were noted. An altered evolutionary profile, particularly in neonates with moderate rather than in severe hypoxic-ischaemic encephalopathy contributed to this significant reduction in seizure burden in hypothermic neonates. Correspondingly, the hourly seizure burden in this group was also significantly reduced as depicted on the adjacent logarithmic graph.

further confirmed by Srinivasakumar et al. who added MRI findings to their study (Srinivasakumar et al., 2013). In neonates with moderate or severe HIE, we found that electrographic seizure rates were almost identical in non-cooled and cooled cohorts (52% and 48% respectively) (Low et al., 2012). These values are consistent with other studies using multichannel EEG (Rafay et al., 2009; Wusthoff et al., 2011; Nash et al., 2011). However, in 2 of the more recent studies (Wusthoff et al., 2011; Nash et al., 2011), the recorded seizure burden was not quantified and a control cohort (non-cooled) was not available for comparison. In another study, even though seizures were less frequent in a cooled group, this was not significantly different when compared to a non-cooled group (Hamelin et al., 2011).

Status epilepticus

Few studies have reported the occurrence of status epilepticus during cooling. Status epilepticus occurs in neonates with both moderate and severe HIE (Low et al., 2012). In a cooled cohort studied by Srinivasakumar et al., 5 of 19 neonates with status epilepticus were noted to have severe brain injury on MRI (Srinivasakumar et al., 2013). In another cohort of 56 neonates who were cooled, moderate to severe brain injury (detected by MRI at age of 5 days) was more common in neonates with status epilepticus (Glass et al., 2011). A study by Nash et al. also confirmed this finding in 4 of 15 cooled neonates who had status epilepticus and had moderate to severe brain injury (Nash et al., 2011). They concluded that during therapeutic hypothermia, seizures are a risk factor for brain injury, particularly in neonates with status epilepticus. In a study by Wushtoff et al., 23% of neonates undergoing therapeutic hypothermia continued to have status epilepticus (Wusthoff et al., 2011).

Animal studies have advocated the use of therapeutic hypothermia as an adjunct to conventional AEDs to treat status epilepticus (Schmitt et al., 2006). Alternatively, a more effective AED acting as an adjunct to therapeutic hypothermia is much needed to control status epilepticus. Clearly this is an important area for future research, as evidence from small cohort studies shows that neonates undergoing therapeutic hypothermia continue to have periods of status epilepticus which may add further to existing brain injury.

Electroclinical dissociation of seizures

Electroclinical dissociation or electroclinical uncoupling is often described in neonatal seizure studies (Boylan et al., 1999; Zangaladze et al., 2008). When this occurs, the clinical signature accompanying the seizure is abolished and seizures are electrographic only. Many neonates exhibit this phenomenon, particularly those with HIE and it is exacerbated by AED use (Connell et al., 1989; Bye and Flanagan, 1995; Scher et al., 2003). A more detailed overview of this subject is beyond the scope of this particular review, but is discussed in greater detail by Boylan et al. (Boylan et al., 2013).

Electroclinical dissociation is common in neonates treated with therapeutic hypothermia (Yap et al., 2009; Nash et al., 2011; Wusthoff et al., 2011; Glass et al., 2011). Wusthoff et al. report electrographic-only seizures in 47% of neonates treated with therapeutic hypothermia, Nash et al. report 43% and Glass et al. report 57%. Yap et al. monitored a cohort of 20 neonates with selective head cooling (Yap et al., 2009) and monitored seizures with aEEG; they found that 90% of neonates had electrographic-only seizures. The occurrence of electrographic-only seizures in this study is higher than most reports and may reflect the use of specific AED protocols in this population.

Antiepileptic drugs (AEDs) and therapeutic hypothermia

During both the pre and post-therapeutic hypothermia era, phenobarbitone remains the most commonly used first-line AED in most neonatal units worldwide (Bartha et al., 2007; Vento et al., 2010) and has been shown to be effective in treating approximately 50% of neonatal seizures (Painter et al., 1999; Boylan et al., 2002; Booth and Evans, 2004). The reduced efficacy of this GABA-enhancing AED has been linked to altered neuronal chloride transport in the developing brain (Dzhala et al., 2005).

Based on multicentre studies in the United States (Bartha et al., 2007) and in Europe (Vento et al., 2010), there is still no consensus on a standard protocol for the use of AEDs in neonatal seizures. We have previously shown that there was no significant difference between non-cooled and cooled HIE groups with respect to the number, dose and age in hours when first and second-line AEDs were administered (Low et al., 2012). In a rodent study, phenobarbitone was shown to augment the therapeutic effect of cooling (Barks et al., 2010). As an AED, phenobarbitone has the potential to reduce endogenous heat production and thus exaggerate the fall in temperature during active cooling.

It has been known that the half-life of phenobarbitone is significantly increased when neonates are treated with hypothermia (Filippi et al., 2011) and with reduced hepatic metabolism during hypothermia, plasma drug levels will accumulate (Roka et al., 2008). The bioavailability of phenobarbitone in neonates can range from 45 to 500 hours (Takemoto, 2012); it can be variable depending on circumstances (Filippi et al., 2011; van den Broek et al., 2012; Shellhaas et al., 2013) and is different from adults (Marsot et al., 2013). Van den Broek et al. assessed the pharmacokinetics of phenobarbitone in a cohort of 31 neonates ($\geq$ 36 weeks gestation) with HIE who were cooled (van den Broek et al., 2012). The authors advocate the use of up to 40 mg/kg of phenobarbitone in total before proceeding to a second-line AED as plasma levels of phenobarbitone before proceeding to a second-line AED but plasma levels of phenobarbitone should always be checked. Based on a study undertaken before the era of therapeutic hypothermia, phenobarbitone doses higher than 40 mg/kg have been shown to increase neuronal apoptosis (Gilman et al., 1989).

■ Seizures during rewarming following therapeutic hypothermia

Seizures have been reported in the rewarming period following therapeutic hypothermia (Battin et al., 2004; Kendall et al., 2012; Shah et al., 2014). In a rabbit model cooled to a core temperature of 33° C, a decrease in nitric oxide production and hippocampal cell loss were noted during kainate-induced seizures (Takei et al., 2005). During rewarming, there was an increase in nitric oxide production in the hippocampus during seizures. Transient rebound epileptiform activity has previously been observed when hypothermia was discontinued after 72 hours (Gunn et al., 2005). Although rewarming seizures have been anecdotally reported (Battin et al., 2004; Gerrits et al., 2005; Shah et al., 2014), they can continue unabated even after the rewarming period has completed (Kendall et al., 2012). Shah et al. recently showed that in human term neonates, seizures are commonly seen during cooling and a significant second peak of seizures during the rewarming period is not uncommon (Shah et al., 2014). On recommencing therapeutic hypothermia immediately after a period of rewarming, seizures that re-emerge during rewarming can abate without the use of any AED (Kendall et al., 2012).

In our study, seizures were seen in four of 15 cooled neonates when therapeutic hypothermia was discontinued (Low et al., 2012). Two of the 4 cases had a shorter duration of therapeutic hypothermia as a decision was made to redirect in neonatal intensive care. In the remaining 2 neonates, electrographic seizures were observed following discontinuation of therapeutic hypothermia despite the fact that therapeutic hypothermia started at 6 and 9 hours respectively, after birth and continued for 72 hours. The incidence of rewarming seizures remains speculative. Now that EEG monitoring is continuing during the rewarming period, more studies describing the re-emergence of seizures during rewarming may be reported. Although some studies have speculated that rewarming seizures are benign (Battin et al., 2004; Gerrits et al., 2005; Shah et al., 2014), further studies are required to establish their significance.

Therapeutic hypothermia trials and seizures

Neonatal outcome studies have shown that seizures are powerful predictors of death or permanent neurodisability (Pisani et al., 2008; Glass et al., 2009). Previously published neonatal hypothermia trials could not accurately measure seizure burden as their protocols did not include prolonged continuous multichannel EEG monitoring. These studies used clinical (Kwon et al., 2011) and/or aEEG monitoring (Simbruner et al., 2010; Edwards et al., 2010) for seizure recognition. The recently published Neonatal Research Network Whole Body Hypothermia Trial relied on clinical recognition of seizures only (Kwon et al., 2011) and when the authors adjusted for hypothermia and severity of encephalopathy, hypothermia did not appear to have any impact on the frequency of clinical seizures and outcome. However, clinical estimation of seizure burden is notoriously unreliable with the majority of neonatal seizures being subclinical or electrographic only (Murray et al., 2008; Malone et al., 2009).

When available in some participating neonatal institutions in the TOBY trial, the aEEG was used for recruitment and as a monitoring tool during therapeutic hypothermia (Azzopardi et al., 2009b). At recruitment, clinical seizures and seizures detected by aEEG were present in 67% (74/110) and 29% (33/115) of neonates respectively. The trial considered seizures as a complication during therapeutic hypothermia, with a decreasing incidence from day one to four (90% to 23%). Both clinical recognition of seizures and the aEEG are known to both over, and under estimate the true seizure burden (Murray et al., 2008). In addition, the aEEG cannot detect short seizures, seizures that do not generalize and low voltage seizures.

At present, the therapeutic hypothermia registry lead by Azzopardi et al. has not made brain monitoring a prerequisite for cooling (Azzopardi et al., 2007). It was recommended that if possible, some form of cerebral function monitoring should be performed on neonates receiving therapeutic hypothermia either before the induction of cooling or as soon as possible during cooling. We strongly support the view that EEG monitoring is crucial during therapeutic hypothermia and also believe that monitoring should be extended after cooling has been discontinued as seizures may emerge during rewarming.

Unfortunately continuous EEG monitoring is hard to maintain in the neonatal intensive care unit and a specialized team is required for interpretation, which is rarely available. Many centres have now implemented remote monitoring of the EEG by specialized teams but this is expensive and time consuming. A more promising option is in the form of automated seizure detection using specially trained and validated algorithms. Research is ongoing and a number of excellent algorithms have been described for neonates using off-line data analysis. Few to date have been implemented routinely in the neonatal intensive care unit with the notable exception of the BrainZ aEEG monitoring system. One clinical validation trial is currently underway in Europe (ANSeR– Algorithm for Neonatal Seizure Recognition <http://clinicaltrials.gov/show/NCT02160171>) which may provide useful information on the utility of automated seizure detection for term neonates with HIE.

Conclusion

Seizures are common in neonates with HIE who are treated with therapeutic hypothermia. While the number of neonates with seizures is similar in both normothermic and hypothermic groups, the overall seizure burden has reduced during therapeutic hypothermia.

This is particularly evident in neonates with moderate encephalopathy where current therapeutic hypothermia strategies seem to have the greatest benefit. It is not known if this reduced seizure burden contributes to the increased benefit seen following therapeutic hypothermia in moderate encephalopathy, or if it is simply a reflection of reduced neuronal damage during therapeutic hypothermia. Only large multicentre studies using continuous multichannel EEG monitoring in neonates with HIE undergoing therapeutic hypothermia will be able to answer this important question.

This work was supported by a Science Foundation Ireland Research Centre Award (12/RC/2272) and a Wellcome Trust Strategic Translational Award (098983/z/12/z).

References

- Aly H, Mohsen L, Badrawi N, Gabr H, Ali Z, Akmal D. Viability and neural differentiation of mesenchymal stem cells derived from the umbilical cord following perinatal asphyxia. *J Perinatol* 2012; 32: 671-76.
- Ancora G, Soffritti S, Lodi R, *et al*. A combined a-EEG and MR spectroscopy study in term newborns with hypoxic-ischemic encephalopathy. *Brain Dev* 2010; 32: 835-42.
- Azzopardi D, Brocklehurst P, Currie A, Edwards D. UK TOBY Cooling Register Protocol Version 3 [online]. https://www.npeu.ox.ac.uk/tobyregister. 2007.
- Azzopardi DV, Strohm B, Edwards AD, *et al*. Moderate hypothermia to treat perinatal asphyxial encephalopathy. *N Engl J Med* 2009; 361: 1349-58.
- Azzopardi D, Strohm B, Edwards AD, *et al*. Treatment of asphyxiated newborns with moderate hypothermia in routine clinical practice: how cooling is managed in the UK outside a clinical trial. *Arch Dis Child Fetal Neonatal Ed* 2009; 94: F260-64.
- Azzopardi D, Strohm B, Marlow N, *et al*. Effects of hypothermia for perinatal asphyxia on childhood outcomes. *N Engl J Med* 2014; 371: 140-49.
- Barks JD, Liu YQ, Shangguan Y, Silverstein FS. Phenobarbital augments hypothermic neuroprotection. *Pediatr Res* 2010; 67: 532-37.
- Bartha AI, Shen J, Katz KH, *et al*. Neonatal seizures: multicenter variability in current treatment practices. *Pediatr Neurol* 2007; 37: 85-90.
- Battin M, Bennet L, Gunn AJ. Rebound seizures during rewarming. *Pediatrics* 2004; 114: 1369.
- Bennet L, Roelfsema V, Pathipati P, Quaedackers JS, Gunn AJ. Relationship between evolving epileptiform activity and delayed loss of mitochondrial activity after asphyxia measured by near-infrared spectroscopy in preterm fetal sheep. *J Physiol* 2006; 572 (Pt 1): 141-54.
- Bennet L, Roelfsema V, George S, Dean JM, Emerald BS, Gunn AJ. The effect of cerebral hypothermia on white and grey matter injury induced by severe hypoxia in preterm fetal sheep. *J Physiol* 2007; 578 (Pt 2): 491-506.
- Bennet L, Dean JM, Wassink G, Gunn AJ. Differential effects of hypothermia on early and late epileptiform events after severe hypoxia in preterm fetal sheep. *J Neurophysiol* 2007; 97(1): 572-78.
- Bernard SA, Gray TW, Buist MD, *et al*. Treatment of comatose survivors of out-of-hospital cardiac arrest with induced hypothermia. *N Engl J Med* 2002; 346: 557-63.
- Bjorkman ST, Miller SM, Rose SE, Burke C, Colditz PB. Seizures are associated with brain injury severity in a neonatal model of hypoxia-ischemia. *Neuroscience* 2010; 166: 157-67.
- Booth D, Evans DJ. Anticonvulsants for neonates with seizures. *Cochrane Database Syst Rev* 2004: CD004218.

- Boylan GB, Pressler RM, Rennie JM, et al. Outcome of electroclinical, electrographic, and clinical seizures in the newborn infant. *Dev Med Child Neurol* 1999; 41: 819-25.
- Boylan GB, Rennie JM, Pressler RM, Wilson G, Morton M, Binnie CD. Phenobarbitone, neonatal seizures, and video-EEG. *Arch Dis Child Fetal Neonatal Ed* 2002; 86: F165-70.
- Boylan GB, Rennie JM, Chorley G, et al. Second-line anticonvulsant treatment of neonatal seizures: a video-EEG monitoring study. *Neurology* 2004; 62(3): 486-88.
- Boylan GB, Stevenson NJ, Vanhatalo S. Monitoring neonatal seizures. *Semin Fetal Neonatal Med* 2013; 18: 202-8.
- Busto R, Globus MY, Dietrich WD, Martinez E, Valdes I, Ginsberg MD. Effect of mild hypothermia on ischemia-induced release of neurotransmitters and free fatty acids in rat brain. *Stroke* 1989; 20: 904-10.
- Bye A, Flanagan D. Electroencephalograms, clinical observations and the monitoring of neonatal seizures. *J Paediatr Child Health* 1995; 31: 503-7.
- Charriaut-Marlangue C, Nguyen T, Bonnin P, et al. Sildenafil mediates blood-flow redistribution and neuroprotection after neonatal hypoxia-ischemia. *Stroke* 2014; 45: 850-6.
- Connell J, Oozeer R, de VL, Dubowitz LM, Dubowitz V. Clinical and EEG response to anticonvulsants in neonatal seizures. *Arch Dis Child* 1989; 64 (4 Spec No): 459-64.
- Dzhala VI, Talos DM, Sdrulla DA et al. NKCC1 transporter facilitates seizures in the developing brain. *Nat Med* 2005; 11(11): 1205-13.
- Edwards AD, Brocklehurst P, Gunn AJ, et al. Neurological outcomes at 18 months of age after moderate hypothermia for perinatal hypoxic ischaemic encephalopathy: synthesis and meta-analysis of trial data. *BMJ* 2010; 340: c363.
- Fan X, van Bel F. Pharmacological neuroprotection after perinatal asphyxia. *J Matern Fetal Neonatal Med* 2010; 23 (suppl 3): 17-19.
- Faulkner S, Bainbridge A, Kato T, et al. Xenon augmented hypothermia reduces early lactate/N-acetylaspartate and cell death in perinatal asphyxia. *Ann Neurol* 2011; 70: 133-50.
- Filippi L, la MG, Cavallaro G, et al. Phenobarbital for neonatal seizures in hypoxic ischemic encephalopathy: a pharmacokinetic study during whole body hypothermia. *Epilepsia* 2011; 52: 794-801.
- Gerrits LC, Battin MR, Bennet L, Gonzalez H, Gunn AJ. Epileptiform activity during rewarming from moderate cerebral hypothermia in the near-term fetal sheep. *Pediatr Res* 2005; 57: 342-46.
- Gilman JT, Gal P, Duchowny MS, Weaver RL, Ransom JL. Rapid sequential phenobarbital treatment of neonatal seizures. *Pediatrics* 1989; 83: 674-78.
- Glass HC, Glidden D, Jeremy RJ, Barkovich AJ, Ferriero DM, Miller SP. Clinical neonatal seizures are independently associated with outcome in infants at risk for hypoxic-ischemic brain injury. *J Pediatr* 2009; 155: 318-23.
- Glass HC, Nash KB, Bonifacio SL, et al. Seizures and magnetic resonance imaging-detected brain injury in newborns cooled for hypoxic-ischemic encephalopathy. *J Pediatr* 2011; 159: 731-35.
- Glass HC, Wusthoff CJ, Shellhaas RA. Amplitude-integrated electro-encephalography: the child neurologist's perspective. *J Child Neurol* 2013; 28: 1342-50.
- Globus MY, Alonso O, Dietrich WD, Busto R, Ginsberg MD. Glutamate release and free radical production following brain injury: effects of posttraumatic hypothermia. *J Neurochem* 1995; 65: 1704-11.
- Gunn AJ, Parer JT, Mallard EC, Williams CE, Gluckman PD. Cerebral histologic and electrocorticographic changes after asphyxia in fetal sheep. *Pediatr Res* 1992; 31: 486-91.
- Gunn AJ, Battin M, Gluckman PD, Gunn TR, Bennet L. Therapeutic hypothermia: from lab to NICU. *J Perinat Med* 2005; 33: 340-46.
- Gunn AJ, Thoresen M. Hypothermic neuroprotection. *NeuroRx* 2006; 3: 154-69.

- Hamelin S, Delnard N, Cneude F, Debillon T, Vercueil L. Influence of hypothermia on the prognostic value of early EEG in full-term neonates with hypoxic ischemic encephalopathy. *Neurophysiol Clin* 2011; 41: 19-27.
- Harris MN, Carey WA, Ellsworth MA, et al. Perceptions and practices of therapeutic hypothermia in American neonatal intensive care units. *Am J Perinatol* 2014; 31: 15-20.
- Herrera EA, Macchiavello R, Montt C, et al. Melatonin improves cerebrovascular function and decreases oxidative stress in chronically hypoxic lambs. *J Pineal Res* 2014 May 8. [Epub ahead of print].
- Hill MW, Wong M, Amarakone A, Rothman SM. Rapid cooling aborts seizure-like activity in rodent hippocampal-entorhinal slices. *Epilepsia* 2000; 41: 1241-48.
- Jacobs SE, Berg M, Hunt R, Tarnow-Mordi WO, Inder TE, Davis PG. Cooling for newborns with hypoxic ischaemic encephalopathy. *Cochrane Database Syst Rev* 2013; 1: CD003311.
- Kendall GS, Mathieson S, Meek J, Rennie JM. Recooling for rebound seizures after rewarming in neonatal encephalopathy. *Pediatrics* 2012; 130: e451-55.
- Kwon JM, Guillet R, Shankaran, et al. Clinical seizures in neonatal hypoxic-ischemic encephalopathy have no independent impact on neurodevelopmental outcome: secondary analyses of data from the neonatal research network hypothermia trial. *J Child Neurol* 2011; 26: 322-28.
- Lawn JE, Kerber K, Enweronu-Laryea C, Cousens S. 3.6 million neonatal deaths – what is progressing and what is not? *Semin Perinatol* 2010; 34: 371-86.
- Levene ML, Kornberg J, Williams TH. The incidence and severity of post-asphyxial encephalopathy in full-term infants. *Early Hum Dev* 1985; 11: 21-26.
- Lorek A, Takei Y, Cady EB, et al. Delayed ("secondary") cerebral energy failure after acute hypoxia-ischemia in the newborn piglet: continuous 48-hour studies by phosphorus magnetic resonance spectroscopy. *Pediatr Res* 1994; 36: 699-706.
- Low E, Boylan GB, Mathieson SR, et al. Cooling and seizure burden in term neonates: an observational study. *Arch Dis Child Fetal Neonatal Ed* 2012; 97: F267-72.
- Lynch NE, Stevenson NJ, Livingstone V, Murphy BP, Rennie JM, Boylan GB. The temporal evolution of electrographic seizure burden in neonatal hypoxic ischemic encephalopathy. *Epilepsia* 2012; 53: 549-57.
- Malone A, Ryan CA, Fitzgerald A, Burgoyne L, Connolly S, Boylan GB. Interobserver agreement in neonatal seizure identification. *Epilepsia* 2009; 50: 2097-101.
- Marlow N, Budge H. Prevalence, causes, and outcome at 2 years of age of newborn encephalopathy. *Arch Dis Child Fetal Neonatal Ed* 2005; 90: F193-94.
- Marsot A, Brevaut-Malaty V, Vialet R, Boulamery A, Bruguerolle B, Simon N. Pharmacokinetics and absolute bioavailability of phenobarbital in neonates and young infants, a population pharmacokinetic modelling approach. *Fundam Clin Pharmacol* 2014; 28: 465-71.
- Miller JA Jr, Miller FS, Westin B. Hypothermia in the treatment of asphyxia neonatorum. *Biol Neonat* 1964; 6: 148-63.
- Miller SP, Weiss J, Barnwell A, et al. Seizure-associated brain injury in term newborns with perinatal asphyxia. *Neurology* 2002; 58: 542-8.
- Murray DM, Boylan GB, Ali I, Ryan CA, Murphy BP, Connolly S. Defining the gap between electrographic seizure burden, clinical expression and staff recognition of neonatal seizures. *Arch Dis Child Fetal Neonatal Ed* 2008; 93: F187-91.
- Nakashima K, Todd MM. Effects of hypothermia on the rate of excitatory amino acid release after ischemic depolarization. *Stroke* 1996; 27(5): 913-18.
- Nash KB, Bonifacio SL, Glass HC, et al. Video-EEG monitoring in newborns with hypoxic-ischemic encephalopathy treated with hypothermia. *Neurology* 2011; 76: 556-62.
- National Institute for Health and Clinical Excellence (NICE). Controlled cooling to treat newborn babies with brain injury caused by oxygen shortage during birth. Information about NICE procedure guidance. 347; Reference No N2184 [online]. www.nice.org.uk. 2010.

- Painter MJ, Scher MS, Stein AD, et al. Phenobarbital compared with phenytoin for the treatment of neonatal seizures. *N Engl J Med* 1999; 341: 485-89.
- Pisani F, Copioli C, Di GC, Turco E, Sisti L. Neonatal seizures: relation of ictal video-electroencephalography (EEG) findings with neurodevelopmental outcome. *J Child Neurol* 2008; 23: 394-98.
- Rafay MF, Cortez MA, de Veber GA, et al. Predictive value of clinical and EEG features in the diagnosis of stroke and hypoxic ischemic encephalopathy in neonates with seizures. *Stroke* 2009; 40: 2402-07.
- Robertson NJ, Faulkner S, Fleiss B, et al. Melatonin augments hypothermic neuroprotection in a perinatal asphyxia model. *Brain* 2013; 136: 90-105.
- Roka A, Melinda KT, Vasarhelyi B, Machay T, Azzopardi D, Szabo M. Elevated morphine concentrations in neonates treated with morphine and prolonged hypothermia for hypoxic ischemic encephalopathy. *Pediatrics* 2008; 121: e844-49.
- Sarnat HB, Sarnat MS. Neonatal encephalopathy following fetal distress. A clinical and electroencephalographic study. *Arch Neurol* 1976; 33: 696-705.
- Schmitt FC, Buchheim K, Meierkord H, Holtkamp M. Anticonvulsant properties of hypothermia in experimental status epilepticus. *Neurobiol Dis* 2006; 23: 689-96.
- Scher MS, Alvin J, Gaus L, Minnigh B, Painter MJ. Uncoupling of EEG-clinical neonatal seizures after antiepileptic drug use. *Pediatr Neurol* 2003; 28: 277-80.
- Scher MS, Steppe DA, Beggarly M. Timing of neonatal seizures and intrapartum obstetrical factors. *J Child Neurol* 2008; 23: 640-43.
- Schiering IA, de Haan TR, Niermeijer JM, et al. Correlation between clinical and histologic findings in the human neonatal hippocampus after perinatal asphyxia. *J Neuropathol Exp Neurol* 2014; 73: 324-34.
- Shah DK, Wusthoff CJ, Clarke P, et al. Electrographic seizures are associated with brain injury in newborns undergoing therapeutic hypothermia. *Arch Dis Child Fetal Neonatal Ed* 2014; 99: F219-24.
- Shellhaas RA, Soaita AI, Clancy RR. Sensitivity of amplitude-integrated electroencephalography for neonatal seizure detection. *Pediatrics* 2007; 120: 770-7.
- Shellhaas RA, Ng CM, Dillon CH, Barks JD, Bhatt-Mehta V. Population pharmacokinetics of phenobarbital in infants with neonatal encephalopathy treated with therapeutic hypothermia. *Pediatr Crit Care Med* 2013; 14: 194-202.
- Simbruner G, Mittal RA, Rohlmann F, Muche R. Systemic hypothermia after neonatal encephalopathy: outcomes of neo.nEURO.network RCT. *Pediatrics* 2010; 126: e771-78.
- Srinivasakumar P, Zempel J, Wallendorf M, Lawrence R, Inder T, Mathur A. Therapeutic hypothermia in neonatal hypoxic ischemic encephalopathy: electrographic seizures and magnetic resonance imaging evidence of injury. *J Pediatr* 2013; 163: 465-70.
- Takei Y, Sunohara D, Nishikawa Y, et al. Effects of rapid rewarming on cerebral nitric oxide production and cerebral hemodynamics after hypothermia therapy for kainic acid-induced seizures in immature rabbits. *Pediatr Int* 2005; 47: 53-9.
- Takemoto CK, Hodding JH, Kraus DM. *The Pediatric Dosage Handbook, 19th ed*. Hudson, Ohio: Lexi-Comp, Inc, 2012.
- Tan WK, Williams CE, During MJ, et al. Accumulation of cytotoxins during the development of seizures and edema after hypoxic-ischemic injury in late gestation fetal sheep. *Pediatr Res* 1996; 39: 791-7.
- Tooley JR, Satas S, Porter H, Silver IA, Thoresen M. Head cooling with mild systemic hypothermia in anesthetized piglets is neuroprotective. *Ann Neurol* 2003; 53: 65-72.
- van den Broek MP, Groenendaal F, Toet MC, et al. Pharmacokinetics and clinical efficacy of phenobarbital in asphyxiated newborns treated with hypothermia: a thermopharmacological approach. *Clin Pharmacokinet* 2012; 51: 671-9.

- Vento M, de Vries LS, Alberola A *et al*. Approach to seizures in the neonatal period: a European perspective. *Acta Paediatr* 2010; 99(4): 497-501.
- Volpe JJ. *Neurology of the Newborn*. Philadelphia, PA: WB Saunders Company, 2008.
- Wang H, Olivero W, Wang D, Lanzino G. Cold as a therapeutic agent. *Acta Neurochir (Wien)* 2006; 148(5): 565-70.
- Wassink G, Gunn ER, Drury PP, Bennet L, Gunn AJ. The mechanisms and treatment of asphyxial encephalopathy. *Front Neurosci* 2014; 8: 40.
- Wirrell EC, Armstrong EA, Osman LD, Yager JY. Prolonged seizures exacerbate perinatal hypoxic-ischemic brain damage. *Pediatr Res* 2001; 50: 445-54.
- Wusthoff CJ, Dlugos DJ, Gutierrez-Colina A, *et al*. Electrographic seizures during therapeutic hypothermia for neonatal hypoxic-ischemic encephalopathy. *J Child Neurol* 2011; 26: 724-8.
- Yager JY, Armstrong EA, Miyashita H, Wirrell EC. Prolonged neonatal seizures exacerbate hypoxic-ischemic brain damage: correlation with cerebral energy metabolism and excitatory amino acid release. *Dev Neurosci* 2002; 24: 367-81.
- Yap V, Engel M, Takenouchi T, Perlman JM. Seizures are common in term infants undergoing head cooling. *Pediatr Neurol* 2009; 41: 327-31.
- Zangaladze A, Nei M, Liporace JD, Sperling MR. Characteristics and clinical significance of subclinical seizures. *Epilepsia* 2008; 49: 2016-21.

From conventional genetic analysis to next generation sequencing in diagnostics of epilepsies

Johannes R. Lemke

Institute of Human Genetics, University Hospital Leipzig, Germany

Epilepsy is one of the most common neurologic disorders affecting 1 to 3% of the general population during the course of life. It is also one of the most heterogeneous disorders, as it can be the consequence of numerous apparent causes, such as injury, infection, tumour, malformation, metabolic disorders, vascular defects, etc., as well as a myriad of less obvious factors.

Genetic defects account for a significant proportion of epilepsies and a correct genetic diagnosis has implications for several aspects of the disease. It can provide information on the prognosis and the course of the disorder, developmental issues, accompanying medical problems as well as inheritance and recurrence risks. In an increasing number of cases it can even guide antiepileptic therapy.

In the past, the probability of establishing a correct diagnosis very much depended on the individual knowledge and skills of the treating physicians. The recent technical progress in molecular analyses led to the identification of numerous novel genetic entities. It significantly facilitated diagnostic procedures and by that relieves physicians of the obligation of making a precise diagnosis on the basis of (sometimes very unspecific) clinical features alone.

The following paragraphs will give an overview of conventional and novel genetic diagnostic procedures as well as their capabilities and limitations.

■ Conventional genetic diagnostics in epilepsy

Cytogenetic diagnostics

Chromosomal analysis represents the oldest technique to detect genetic defects in patients with intellectual disability (ID) and epilepsy. However, there are very few disorders caused by chromosomal aberrations that can be illustrated by conventional karyotyping with epilepsy as a significant and recurrent feature (*e.g.*, trisomy 21, ring chromosome 20, invdup 15 and few others). These microscopically visible aberrations usually cause syndromic disorders. Isolated forms of epilepsy are usually not associated with large chromosomal aberrations.

Rauch and colleagues described the yield of conventional karyotyping in a cohort of 600 patients with developmental delay or ID with or without epilepsy (Rauch *et al.*, 2006). Among these, they detected 68 cases (11.3%) with aneuploidies, 19 cases (3.2%) with cytogenetically visible segmental losses or gains on chromosomes and 3 cases (0.5%) with apparently balanced *de novo* structural aberrations.

Thus, conventional chromosome analysis can reveal the underlying diagnosis of up to 15% of ID patients. However, this number is specific to ID and cannot easily be adapted to epilepsy alone. Additionally, many of the cases mentioned above could have been diagnosed clinically (55 of the 68 patients had Down syndrome) and the vast majority of chromosome aberrations are also detectable with molecular cytogenetic array techniques. Consequently, Miller and colleagues suggested choosing chromosomal microarray techniques instead of conventional karyotyping as a first-tier clinical diagnostic test for individuals with ID (Miller *et al.*, 2012).

Array diagnostics

Array comparative genomic hybridisation (array CGH) or single nucleotide polymorphism arrays (SNP arrays) allow for a chromosomal analysis at a far higher resolution than classic karyotyping.

Several groups investigated the diagnostic output of array techniques in different spectra of epileptic disorders (*Table I*). In 2011, Kariminejad analysed patients with brain malformations, most of them associated with ID and symptomatic epilepsy and detected rare copy number variants (CNV) in 22.5% of cases (Kariminejad *et al.*, 2011). Striano detected similar rates of rare CNV in epilepsy patients with ID and patients with non-syndromic ID without epilepsy (Striano *et al.*, 2012). Among individuals with various idiopathic, non-lesional epilepsies, Mefford detected rare CNV in 8.9% of cases which is comparable to the detection rate in patients with epileptic encephalopathies (Mefford *et al.*, 2010; 2011). Finally, CNV also play a minor role in idiopathic generalized epilepsy (IGE) (de Kovel *et al.*, 2010).

Thus, especially in patients with epilepsy and additional findings, such as ID or malformations, there is a high probability of identifying the underlying genetic defect with array techniques. In contrast, the diagnostic yield in isolated epilepsy disorders appears to be low.

Table I. Diagnostic yield of array diagnostics in epilepsy disorders

Phenotype	Cohort size	Nr of detected CNV	Detection rate	Reference
Brain malformations	169	38	22.5%	Kariminejad *et al.*, 2011
ID + epilepsy	265	45	17.0%	Striano *et al.*, 2012
Idiopathic epilepsy	517	46	8.9%	Mefford *et al.*, 2010
Epileptic encephalopathy	315	25	7.9%	Mefford *et al.*, 2011
IGE	1,234	22	1.8%	de Kovel *et al.*, 2010

Molecular genetic diagnostics

Direct Sanger sequencing represents the gold standard in molecular genetic diagnostics. Genetic heterogeneity can differ substantially between epilepsy phenotypes and significantly influences the success in detecting disease-causing mutations in an individual disorder. In addition, many phenotypes are overlapping and rather unspecific.

Hundreds of genes have been associated with different forms of epilepsy and with countless phenotypes comprising epileptic seizures as one of their features (Garofalo et al., 2012; Lemke et al., 2012).

SCN1A is the most well-known epilepsy gene to date and poignantly illustrates the benefits and limitations of a Sanger sequencing approach. Mutations in SCN1A encoding the alpha subunit of the voltage-gated sodium channel are associated with several epilepsy phenotypes (pleyotropy) and can be detected in at least 75% of cases with Dravet syndrome (Depienne et al., 2009). Thus, in case of a high clinical suspicion, direct Sanger sequencing is a straightforward approach to confirm the diagnosis. However, in SCN1A-negative Dravet patients, there is a multitude of genes that might alternatively be responsible for the phenotype, such as PCDH19, SCN1B, SCN2A, GABRD, GABRG2, CHD2, GABRA1, STXBP1 and others (Depienne et al., 2012; Suls et al., 2013; Carvill et al., 2014). Some of these genes appear to be extremely rare causes of Dravet syndrome (Kim et al., 2013).

Therefore, direct Sanger sequencing is most appropriate for the genetic screening of phenotypes with little heterogeneity where only a small number of genes need to be analysed. Sanger sequencing is difficult to perform if the phenotype is not specific and hampers a clear clinical diagnosis, or if there are very large or numerous genes involved, each with low individual mutation detection rates.

■ Next generation sequencing (NGS) techniques in epilepsy

Panel diagnostics

Massive parallel sequencing allows for a simultaneous analysis of several genes and loci in a patient in a single approach. Applying this method to genetic testing of a spectrum of heterogeneous disorders, such as epilepsy, overcomes the restrictions of serial Sanger sequencing approaches. Thus, targeted resequencing or panel approaches offer several advantages.

- All genes known to be involved in a phenotypic spectrum are covered by one test.
- Only targeted genes are analysed, preventing incidental findings in diagnostic settings.
- The targeted genes show a better coverage compared to e.g. whole exome sequencing allowing for a more valid conclusion on the presence of sequence alterations (Figure 1). Additionally, for diagnostic purposes, regions with insufficient coverage may be resequenced by conventional methods to provide complete sequence information allowing for exhaustive positive and negative information on sequence alterations.
- In a diagnostic setting, the costs of panel analysis equal the analysis of 2-3 medium-sized genes by Sanger sequencing.
- In several occasions, NGS was able to unravel mutations that had been overlooked using conventional methods.

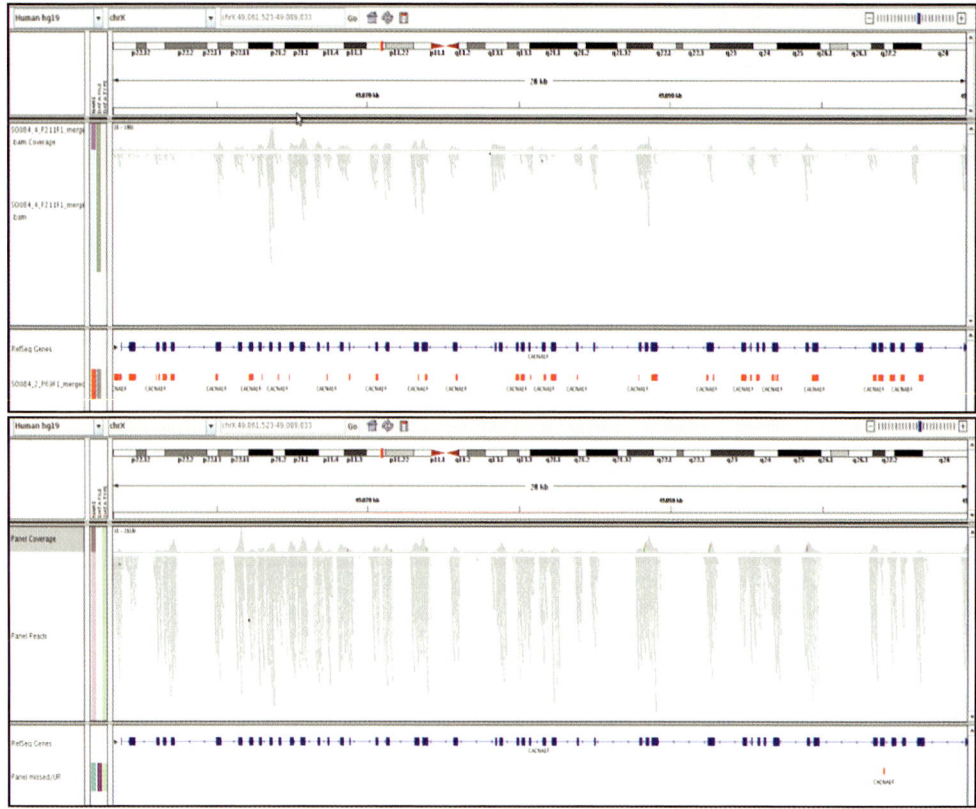

Figure 1 shows a randomly selected gene sequenced with WES (top) and a diagnostic panel (bottom). The coverage (grey peaks) of the panel is significantly higher compared to WES. Regions with a coverage of < 10 reads/base (red bars in bottom line) are widespread in WES and nearly completely abolished in the panel sequence.
(Image provided by Saskia Biskup, CeGaT GmbH, Tübingen, Germany)

Compared to conventional Sanger sequencing, the introduction of panel analysis to genetic diagnostics of epilepsy led to a dramatic gain of information. It was not only possible to analyse all genes of interest at once, but also revealed an alarming number of false negatives in a conventional methods, which is considered to be the gold standard in sequence analysis (Lemke et al., 2012).

NGS is currently still limited in reliably detecting CNV within a gene or a locus. However, even this limitation will most likely be overcome in the near future.

The diagnostic yield depends on the size of the panel and the number of disease-associated genes included, as well as the phenotype of the patients being investigated. Several panel approaches have been published (*Table II*) comprising pure diagnostic approaches (Lemke et al., 2012; Kodera et al., 2013) mixed diagnostic and research approaches (Carvill et al., 2013) and pure research approaches (Klassen et al., 2011). However, the detection rates cannot easily be compared with each other, as there was a different sampling of cohorts as well as different NGS platforms with different stringencies of filter settings of the respective analysis pipelines. Small cohorts (Lemke et al., 2012; Della Mina et al., 2014) may underlie a selection bias towards more severe phenotypes with higher mutation detection rates compared to larger presumably less biased cohorts.

Table II. Diagnostic yield of panel diagnostics in epilepsy disorders

Phenotype	Cohort size	Nr of genes	Nr of detected mutations	Diagnostic yield	Reference
Epilepsy	33	265	16	48.5%	Lemke et al., 2012
Epilepsy	19	67	9	47.3%	Della Mina et al., 2014
Epilepsy	445	265-323	96	21.6%	Lemke, Biskup unpublished data
Epileptic encephalopathy	115	30-50	24	27.8%	
Brain malformations	63	31-43	27	17.0%	
Epileptic encephalopathy	500	65 (including 46 candidates)	52	10.4%	Carvill et al., 2013
Epileptic encephalopathy	53	35	12	22.6%	Kodera et al., 2013

Whole Exome sequencing (WES)

Technically, there is little discrepancy between targeted sequencing of a gene panel and WES. However, regarding the results, there are considerable differences, both in quality and implication.

Diagnostic panels usually cover a few dozen up to a few hundred genes spanning a few hundred up to a few thousand exons, whereas enrichment for WES targets 20,384 genes with 182,726 exons (Agilent Sure Select WES Enrichment, Agilent, Santa Clara, CA, USA). The absolute size of a panel is usually < 1 Mb compared to 51.4 Mb for WES. Thus, sequencing of a panel of genes can be performed with a significantly higher coverage compared to WES (*Figure 1*). Even large panels can be sequenced with a coverage of > 10 reads/base in up to 95% of positions, whereas standard WES often achieves this coverage in only around 70%. However, the sequence quality and coverage constantly improved over the last months and years and a further improvement is to be expected.

In contrast to diagnostic panels that only focus on known relevant genes associated with a certain phenotype, WES reveals genetic alterations anywhere in the exome independent of indication and clinical relevance. Thus, performing WES not only in epilepsy patients might reveal incidental deleterious variants unrelated to the indication for testing. Dorschner and colleagues analysed 1,000 randomly selected exomes of the Exome Variant Server (EVS, NHLBI Exome Sequencing Project, http://evs.gs.washington.edu/EVS/) for pathogenic mutations by comparing variants in 114 disease-associated genes (*e.g.* genes associated with cardiac conduction disease, cancer predisposition, etc.) with described mutations in the Human Gene Mutation Database (HGMD, http://www.hgmd.cf.ac.uk/ac/index.php) (Dorschner et al., 2013). In 23 probands (2.3%), they identified variants that were considered to result in direct medical actions. Thus, before WES is initiated, it must clearly be defined which results are going to be communicated to the respective individual. A retrospective study on 200 WES cases revealed that 16% of adult individuals opt for blinding of incidental findings (Shahmirzadi et al., 2013).

However, in addition to incidental findings, NGS techniques reveal huge amounts of novel variants in known and unknown genes, which significantly complicates the interpretation of results. Additionally, there might be oligogenic findings. Gonzalez and colleagues showed that 17% of 100 diagnostic WES cases harboured mutations in more than one reported gene of either positive or uncertain significance (15% showed aberrations in two genes, 2% showed aberrations in three genes) (Gonzalez et al., 2013).

To minimize interpretational problems, many research studies thus aimed for trio-exome sequencing of index cases together with both parents. This dramatically facilitates the detection of causative *de novo* mutations in dominant as well as compound-heterozygous variants in recessive genes. However, several WES studies revealed approximately 1-2 *de novo* mutations in an individual, sometimes even more. Therefore, the confirmation of a *de novo* origin only is not necessarily sufficient to prove pathogenicity of a genetic variant. Trio-WES in patients with epileptic encephalopathies revealed numerous causative mutations in known epilepsy genes as well as countless putatively causative variants in suspicious genes and variants with currently completely unknown effect. In addition, the NGS sequence results contain regions with poor coverage and even gaps with no coverage at all. Mutations in causative genes might therefore be missed due to insufficient coverage of the region of interest (as shown for patient 520, Lemke et al., 2012).

WES is a very useful tool for analysing patients on a research basis, and it is also one of the most important tools in identifying novel disease-causing genes to date. However, WES in diagnostic settings still remains a very challenging task, especially in cases of single (not trio) exomes without obvious pathogenic mutation detectable at first glance. Evaluation of all unknown variants or resequencing of all underrepresented regions is hardly possible. Nevertheless, databases on coding and splice site variants are rapidly growing and information on many currently unknown variants facilitating interpretation of WES results will certainly be available in the near future.

Surprisingly, WES (*Table III*) appears to not reach the diagnostic yield of various panel approaches (*Table II*). This is in line with the different detection rates of different panels and might similarly be explained by selection bias of cohorts, different platforms and different filter settings rather than by truly methodological issues as *e.g.* underrepresented regions and gaps of coverage.

Table III. Diagnostic yield of exome diagnostics in epilepsy disorders

Phenotype	Cohort size	Likely solved	Diagnostic yield	Reference
Epileptic encephalopathy including:	264	44	16.7%	Epi4K 2013
– infantile spasms	149	18	12.1%	
– Lennox-Gastaut syndrome	115	26	22.6%	
Epileptic encephalopathy	10	7	70.0%	Veeramah et al., 2013

Whole Genome Sequencing (WGS)

WGS usually affords a more comprehensive and uniform coverage compared to targeted NGS approaches, such as WES. This might be a reason why the detection rate (6 out of 32, 19%) of a recent trio-WGS cohort of patients with autism spectrum disorders revealed a higher yield compared to previous studies using trio-WES (Jiang et al., 2013) Several WGS projects in epilepsy disorders are currently ongoing and will show in the near future whether this gain of information holds true for other studies and diseases as well.

However, WGS provides sequence information covering all genomic regions and is not restricted to the coding regions. Little is known on genetic variation in non-coding regulatory regions (promotors, enhancers, silencers, etc.) even of otherwise very well known disease genes. WGS will most probably contribute in elucidating the role of these regions in human disease. Still, WGS is facing similar problems as WES regarding interpretation and validation of rare variants. As available data on genetic variation of non-coding regions is even less, these problems remain immense to date.

Conclusions

The evolution of genetic screening methods of the past years allows for the identification of an increasing number of genetic defects in epilepsy disorders and other heterogeneous diseases.

As described above, array technologies are essential for CNV screening (*Table I*) and cannot yet be easily replaced by NGS techniques. At present time, panel diagnostics appears to yield the highest detection rates in diagnostic settings. However, the diagnostic yield from different studies (*Tables II and III*) cannot be compared directly as there were *i.e.* different modes of analysis and recruitment of patients.

However, with the continuously growing knowledge on genetic variation and creation of clear guidelines on communicating the results to the patient, legal guardians and referring physicians, diagnostic WES might progressively replace panel diagnostics. In contrast, WGS is currently an exclusive scientific screening tool only. Implementation of WGS in diagnostic settings will need far more knowledge on variation of the human reference sequence than currently available.

The knowledge of the underlying genetic defects in human epilepsy disorders will help to elucidate and understand the causative pathomechanisms. Already today, this clearly influences the choice for or against certain antiepileptic drugs (AED) paving the way from empiric AED application towards individual therapies orientating on the actual molecular defect.

Dravet syndrome can serve as an illustrative example (Arzimanoglou, 2009). In the most likely case of a disease-causing mutation in *SCN1A*, epileptologists can select for AED with clear evidence of a beneficial effect in Dravet syndrome. Likewise, there is a list of common standard AED that should be avoided. On the other hand, this list does not necessarily apply to Dravet(-like) patients carrying mutations in *PCDH19*, *CHD2*, etc. Thus, the clinical diagnosis of an epilepsy phenotype without molecular confirmation does not necessarily facilitate therapeutic decisions.

Even if a mutation does not lead to immediate pharmacologic consequences, it may reveal novel targets for individualised therapeutic approaches, such as treatment of epilepsies due to activation of NMDA receptors with memantine or similar NMDA receptor blockers (Lemke *et al.*, 2013; Lemke *et al.*, 2014; Pierson *et al.*, 2014).

Not least, the identification of a causative genetic defect can provide information on prognosis and the individual course of the disorder. It may reveal accompanying medical problems or predispositions to secondary diseases and lead to the initialisation of preventive actions or surveillance. The knowledge of the mode of inheritance helps to counsel patients and their relatives regarding recurrence risks. Finally, a genetic diagnosis can put an end to the search for the underlying aetiology of the individual disorder and the associated stressful (maybe even painful) diagnostic attempts, which may be demanding for the patient as well as the families.

References

- Arzimanoglou A. Dravet syndrome: from electroclinical characteristics tomolecular biology. *Epilepsia* 2009; 50 (suppl 8): 3-9.
- Carvill GL, Heavin SB, Yendle SC, et al. Targeted resequencing in epileptic encephalopathies identifies de novo mutations in CHD2 and SYNGAP1. *Nat Genet* 2013; 45: 825-30.
- Carvill GL, Weckhuysen S, McMahon JM, et al. GABRA1 and STXBP1: novel genetic causes of Dravet syndrome. *Neurology* 2014; 82: 1245-53.
- de Kovel CG, Trucks H, Helbig I, et al. Recurrent microdeletions at 15q11.2 and 16p13.11 predispose to idiopathic generalized epilepsies. *Brain* 2010; 133: 23-32.
- Depienne C, Trouillard O, Saint-Martin C, et al. Spectrum of SCN1A gene mutations associated with Dravet syndrome: analysis of 333 patients. *J Med Genet* 2009; 46: 183-91.
- Depienne C, Gourfinkel-An I, Baulac S, LeGuern E. In: Noebels JL, Avoli M, Rogawski MA, Olsen RW, Delgado-Escueta AV (eds). *Jasper's Basic Mechanisms of the Epilepsies* [Internet]. 4th edition. Bethesda (MD): National Center for Biotechnology Information (US); 2012.
- Dorschner MO, Amendola LM, Turner EH, et al. Actionable, pathogenic incidental findings in 1,000 participants' exomes. *Am J Hum Genet* 2013; 93: 631-40.
- Epi4K Consortium; Epilepsy Phenome/Genome Project. De novo mutations in epileptic encephalopathies. *Nature* 2013; 501: 217-21.
- Garofalo S, Cornacchione M, Di Costanzo A. From genetics to genomics of epilepsy. *Neurol Res Int* 2012; 2012: 876234.
- Gonzalez KD, Shahmirzadi L, Chao E, et al. Annual Meeting of the American Society of Human Genetics, Boston 2013, Poster 1111T.
- Jiang YH, Yuen RK, Jin X, et al. Detection of clinically relevant genetic variants in autism spectrum disorder by whole-genome sequencing. *Am J Hum Genet* 2013; 93: 249-63.
- Kariminejad R, Lind-Thomsen A, Tümer Z, et al. High frequency of rare copy number variants affecting functionally related genes in patients with structural brain malformations. *Hum Mutat* 2011; 32: 1427-35.
- Kim YO, Dibbens L, Marini C, et al. Do mutations in SCN1B cause Dravet syndrome? *Epilepsy Res* 2013; 103: 97-100.
- Klassen T, Davis C, Goldman A, et al. Exome sequencing of ion channel genes reveals complex profiles confounding personal risk assessment in epilepsy. *Cell* 2011; 145: 1036-48.
- Kodera H, Kato M, Nord AS, et al. Targeted capture and sequencing for detection of mutations causing early onset epileptic encephalopathy. *Epilepsia* 2013; 54: 1262-9.
- Lemke JR, Riesch E, Scheurenbrand T, et al. Targeted next generation sequencing as a diagnostic tool in epileptic disorders. *Epilepsia* 2012; 53: 1387-98.
- Lemke JR, Lal D, Reinthaler EM, et al. Mutations in GRIN2A cause idiopathic focal epilepsy with rolandic spikes. *Nat Genet* 2013; 45: 1067-72.
- Lemke JR, Hendrickx R, Geider K, et al. GRIN2B mutations in West syndrome and intellectual disability with focal epilepsy. *Ann Neurol* 2014; 75: 147-54.
- Mefford HC, Muhle H, Ostertag P, et al. Genome-wide copy number variation in epilepsy: novel susceptibility loci in idiopathic generalized and focal epilepsies. *PLoS Genet* 2010; 6: e1000962.
- Mefford HC, Yendle SC, Hsu C, et al. Rare copy number variants are an important cause of epileptic encephalopathies. *Ann Neurol* 2011; 70: 974-85.
- Miller DT, Adam MP, Aradhya S, et al. Consensus statement: chromosomal microarray is a first-tier clinical diagnostic test for individuals with developmental disabilities or congenital anomalies. *Am J Hum Genet* 2010; 86: 749-64.
- Pierson TM, Yuan H, Marsh ED, et al. GRIN2A mutation and early-onset epileptic encephalopathy: personalized therapy with memantine. *Ann Clin Transl Neurol* 2014; 1: 190-8.

- Rauch A, Hoyer J, Guth S, *et al*. Diagnostic yield of various genetic approaches in patients with unexplained developmental delay or mental retardation. *Am J Med Genet A* 2006; 140: 2063-74.
- Shahmirzadi L, Chao EC, Palmaer E, Parra MC, Tang S, Gonzalez KD. Patient decisions for disclosure of secondary findings among the first 200 individuals undergoing clinical diagnostic exome sequencing. *Genet Med* 2014; 16: 395-9.
- Striano P, Coppola A, Paravidino R, *et al*. Clinical significance of rare copy number variations in epilepsy: a case-control survey using microarray-based comparative genomic hybridization. *Arch Neurol* 2012; 69: 322-30.
- Suls A, Jaehn JA, Kecskés A, *et al*. *De novo* loss-of-function mutations in *CHD2* cause a fever-sensitive myoclonic epileptic encephalopathy sharing features with Dravet syndrome. *Am J Hum Genet* 2013; 93: 967-75.
- Veeramah KR, Johnstone L, Karafet TM, *et al*. Exome sequencing reveals new causal mutations in children with epileptic encephalopathies. *Epilepsia* 2013; 54: 1270-81.

Treatable newborn seizures due to inborn errors of metabolism

Jaume Campistol[1], Barbara Plecko[2]

[1] Neurology Department, Hospital Sant Joan de Déu, Universitat de Barcelona, Barcelona, Spain
[2] Division of Neurology, Children's Hospital, University of Zurich, Zurich, Switzerland

---

Neurometabolic diseases comprise a large group of inborn errors of metabolism (IEM) affecting the brain, that have not yet been fully defined (Saudubray, 2012). These diseases are caused by dysfunction of genes that control the intermediary metabolism of carbohydrates, lipids, proteins and vitamins. Accumulating compounds or lack of substrates can provide useful biomarkers in the diagnostic work-up of these rare disorders. Neurometabolic disorders can present with seizures or epilepsy in the newborn period regardless of the metabolic substrate affected (*Table I*). Seizures may be part of a more complex neurologic presentation or be the leading and sometimes only feature of the disease. The physiopathologic mechanisms are often pleomorphic (*Table II*). In general the developing brain is more susceptible to seizures than the adult brain (Arzimanoglou et al., 2004). The age of onset of neurometabolic epilepsy depends on affected pathways and factors linked to the development of the nervous system in a manner that is not always obvious: during the neonatal period, childhood and adolescence, various coordinated gene expression programs are activated and subsequently silenced as the organism grows and matures. Consequently, the effects of a pathogenic gene mutation may remain unnoticed until the mutant gene is activated during a determined stage of development or even in adulthood. For example, the foetal brain preferably consumes products of lipid degradation, including ketone bodies. In neonates, cerebral glucose consumption is still minimal, increasing gradually during infancy and childhood until it reaches up to three times the level of consumption of the newborn. On other occasions, the function of certain defective genes is replaced by others as development progresses, causing reversible or transient clinical symptoms, such as in a special subform of cytochrome c oxidase deficiency that presents with severe hypotonia and weakness, the outcome of which is the restoration of muscle enzyme activity and the normalization of the hypotonia and weakness at a few years of age (Pascual, 2007).

Table I. Inborn Errors of Metabolism (IEM) with seizures in the newborn period or early infancy

Peroxysomal disorders
Non ketotic hyperglycinaemia (NKH)
Molybdenum cofactor deficiency (MOCOD) and Sulfite oxidase deficiency
Urea cycle defects (UCD)
Maple syrup urine disease (MSUD
Organoacidurias (OA)
Pyridoxine dependent epilepsy (PDE)
Pyridoxal 5'-phosphate dependent seizures (PNPO deficiency)
Glut-1 deficiency
Serine deficiency
Menkes disease
Mitochondrial cytopathies

■ Physiopathology

The immaturity of inhibitory systems during early brain development and its dysregulation under metabolic dysfunction play a major role and lower the seizure threshold in neonates. This is explained by the strong expression of inotropic glutamate receptors in general and an expression of receptor subunits that facilitate increased calcium influx (Pascual, 2007). The expression of GABA receptors and GABA glutamate decarboxylase is low in the newborn period. Activation of GABA receptors may be excitatory in the immature brain caused by high intracellular chloride concentrations. There is considerable evidence that alterations in GABA signalling can cause seizures, as well as that seizures can change GABAergic signalling (Rakhade and Jensen, 2009).

Many IEM earlier or later interfere with key functions of brain metabolism such as the transport and utilisation of energy substrates, the production of energy rich phosphates, the metabolic coupling between neurons and astrocytes, the neurotransmitter signalling pathways, the autoregulation of cerebral blood flow and the transport of substrates across the blood brain barrier. In some IEM accumulating compounds may cause direct neurotoxicity and certain triggers as fever or catabolism may precede seizure onset and encephalopathy. In these IEM it is believed that symptoms remain latent until the accumulation of toxic products is sufficient to interfere with cell functions as for example in urea cycle disorders or some organic acidurias. Primary or secondary disturbances in the neurotransmitter pathways with excess of excitation or lack of inhibition in the immature brain can also enhance seizure activity (*Table II*).

Table II. Physiopathology of neonatal seizures in IEM

Reduced energy supply (Glut-1)
Disturbances in neuronal membrane permeability/integrity
Misbalance intra–extracellular ions (OA)
Neurotoxic compounds (UCD, OA, MOCOD)
Neurotransmitters and AA misbalance (PNPO, PDE, NKH, SSADH, GABA)
Molecular transport abnormalities (Menkes)
Polymer accumulation
Neuronal system circuit dysfunction (MOCOD)
Substrate deficiency (Serine)

Table III. Practical approach of IEM disorders with neonatal seizures

1. Detailed medical history, including family pedigree
2. Full physical and neurological examination
3. Extended routine lab: including blood gases, glucose, ammonia, uric acid, lactate and ketones
4. Eventually CSF study: glucose, lactate; storage of 2x1 ml of CSF for later analysis of eg. aminoacids, neurotransmitters, PLP
5. Video EEG and sleep EEG
6. MRI, MRS, neurophysiology
7. Metabolic screening (as targeted as possible)-see Table IV
8. Biochemical analyses in tissues or cell cultures to confirm the metabolic diagnosis, to measure specific enzyme activities and guide genotyping
9. Molecular studies

General approach to the IEM with seizures

Though IEM are rare, they need to be considered as differential diagnoses in the routine work-up, especially in neonatal seizures (*Table III*) (Saudubray, 2012). Unclear etiology and therapy-resistance should always prompt biochemical investigations. A detailed medical history is important, including the family pedigree (*Table IV*), followed by a full physical and neurological examination. The newborn with seizures is an emergency and should immediately be transferred to an intensive care unit where a diagnostic algorithm should be in place. This algorithm will help to exclude the more common causes accounting for about 75% of neonatal seizures, as hypoglycaemia, electrolyte imbalance, hypoxia-ischemia, intracranial haemorrhage, neonatal stroke or CNS infection, followed by an extended urgent routine lab-work to unravel hallmarks of IEM with systemic neonatal decompensation (*Tables IV-V*). If this extended routine lab-work is inconclusive, controlled vitamine trials and selective screening tests have to be performed that may confirm the suspected disease or, at least, serve to place it within a group of metabolic disorders, that has to be investigated further (Pascual et al., 2008; Scriver, 2003; Campistol, 2000). The diagnostic process is not complete until the enzymatic and genetic abnormality causing the disease has been identified.

Table IV. Disease specific metabolites and respective material

Disease	Plasma	Urine	CSF
Urea cycle defects	Ammonia, aminoacids	Orotic acid	
Organic acidurias	Acylcarnitines, aminoacids	Organic acids	
PDE	PA	AASA, PA	(AASA, PA, NT, PLP)
PNPO		Vanil lactate	PLP, NT
ADSL		Purines	
Typical and atypical PKU	Aminoacids	Pterines	(NT)
NKH	Aminoacids		Aminoacids
Serine deficiency	Aminoacids		Aminoacids
MSUD	Aminoacids, acylcarnitines	Organic acids	
Mitochondriopathies	Lactate		Lactate
Glut-1 deficiency	Glucose		Glucose, lactate
Menkes	Copper, ceruloplasmin		
MOCOD	Uric acid	Sulfocisteine	
ISOD		Sulfocisteine	

Table V. Diagnostic suspect of a genetic metabolic encephalopathy with epilepsy

1/ Should be considered mostly with patients (newborn or infant) with unexplained early onset epilepsy poorly responsive to antiepileptic treatment
2/ Seizures are associated with encephalopathy reminiscent of hypoxia – ischaemia (poor feeding, sensory involvement, vomiting, respiratory distress, apnea or unexpected metabolic acidosis)
3/ Seizures are induced by fasting, fever or protein load
4/ Seizures are linked to developmental delay or loss of aquired milestones
5/ Epilepsy begins with a not otherwise explicable status epilepticus
6/ EEG recordings show abnormal background (slowing or burst suppression)
7/ Patients history displays parental consanguinity and or familiar history of unexplained neonatal epilepsy or sudden infant deaths
8/ Refractory seizures in a child under the age of 3 years without an apparent cause

Newborn screening by mass spectrometry is carried out in most high income countries, but programs vary and do not cover for IEM causing neonatal seizures, aside from atypical PKU, biotinidase deficiency, some organic acidurias and some fatty acid oxidation disorders. Some countries mandatorily detect as few as seven inborn errors of metabolism, while it would be possible to detect more than 50 diseases using mass spectrometry, including amino acid disorders. Diagnosing IEM still needs a high degree of clinical suspicion, as there is no particular set of tests that detects all or even most neurometabolic diseases. The most widely used tests can be performed in plasma and urine that should be collected ahead of standardized vitamin trials early in the course of disease. Some IEM will necessitate the analysis of CSF. In this respect thorough sampling and immediate freezing of CSF samples at – 80° helps to avoid the need for repeated spinal taps, as storage at room temperature will not allow later biochemical work-up. *Table IV* lists the IEM causing neonatal seizures and their respective metabolites in body fluids. Confirmatory testing should be done on a genetic level and/or by enzyme assays in appropriate material (fibroblasts, or muscle tissue). Cerebral magnetic resonance imaging (MRI) is a key investigation but in the presence of IEM presenting with neonatal seizures is rarely helpful. The only exception is Molybdenum cofactor deficiency with a diagnostic pattern of brain edema, followed by cystic white matter lesions and brain atrophy.

Proton magnetic resonance spectroscopy (MRS) makes it possible to identify an increasing number of metabolites within the central nervous system by means of a non-invasive *in situ* and *in vivo* procedure and is especially helpful in detecting creatine deficiency syndromes.

In case of a fatal epileptic encephalopathy of unclear etiology, investigations in dried blood spots and fibroblast cultures, which can be obtained during the first 18 hours after death and preserved indefinitely in liquid nitrogen, may be helpful to establish a postmortem diagnosis for further genetic counselling (Marin-Valencia *et al.*, 2010).

■ Seizures and epilepsy in the neonatal period due to IEM with therapeutic options

Of the approximately 750 metabolic diseases that are currently known, some 40%-60% can present with isolated or recurrent convulsive seizures at some point during their course. The cumulative incidence of these disorders is low (1:2,000-3,000 live births), with about 25% of them manifesting during the neonatal period. Early diagnosis has important clinical implications for specific treatment options (Saudubray, 2012).

For IEM manifesting with neonatal metabolic crisis, well established treatment regimens are in place and need the enrolment of a metabolic specialist. Exchange transfusion is effective when it is necessary to eliminate toxic metabolites. Peritoneal dialysis offers a simple alternative but is not as effective as the previous solution or haemodialysis with a much higher clearance.

Longterm treatment for these disorders consists of disease specific, lifelong diets following the principle of substrate reduction thus limiting the flux through the affected metabolic pathway. In an emergency, all the essential nutrients may alternatively be administered parenterally. There are standard diets modified in their protein, carbohydrate or fat content while still satisfying the caloric and essential amino acid requirements for each stage of life. Single disease entities respond to the administration of cofactors or high dose vitamins, that have to be maintained lifelong in the sense of vitamin dependency rather than vitamin deficiency.

Generally, AEDs are not effective in most cases of IEM manifesting with seizures as a hallmark of disease, especially in situations of acute decompensation (Aicardi, 1995). Early and specific treatment can prevent irreversible neurological damage that occurs due to the convulsive seizures and the metabolic derangement and may allow the patient to lead a normal life. In this article we review IEM with seizures or epilepsy of neonatal onset and their specific treatment options.

Defects of vitamin metabolism

Pyridoxine dependent epilepsy (PDE)

This is an autosomal recessive disease characterized by a therapeutic response to pharmacological doses of vitamin B6 (pyridoxine or PLP) and resistance to conventional antiepileptic drugs. For a long time PDE deficiency was assumed to be due to glutamic acid decarboxylase (GAD) deficiency, catalyzing the conversion of glutamate to GABA and requiring vitamin B6 as a cofactor, resulting in decreased GABA concentrations in the brain (Toribe, 2001; Baxter, 1999). Following the description of pipecolic acid as a first biomarker for PDE (Plecko et al., 2000), mutations in the gene encoding for α-aminoadipic semialdehyde (AASA) dehydrogenase (Antiquitin) were identified as the major cause of PDE (Mills et al., 2006; Stockler et al., 2011). α-aminoadipic-semialdehyde dehydrogenase or antiquitin (ATQ) is encoded by the ALDH7A1 or ATQ gene and acts in the catabolism of the essential aminoacid lysine (Mills et al., 2006).

The typical manifestation of PDE is intrauterine or neonatal onset with epileptic spasms, focal myoclonic, tonic or bilateral tonic-clonic seizures within hours or days after birth (Schmitt et al., 2010).

Aside from this, atypical presentations with first manifestation up to three years of age have been described (Gospe, 2010).

The seizures are typically refractory to common anticonvulsants and may progress to status epilepticus. Between episodes the infant can present with hypotonia, sleeplessness, movement disorders suggestive of clinical seizures but without EEG discharges, poor contact, erratic eye movements and myoclonus triggered by acoustic stimuli (Stockler et al., 2011). About one third of the patients show poor adaptation after birth, misleading the clinician to interpret seizures as part of hypoxic ischemic encephalopathy.

In atypical cases, that may account for one third of cases of PDE, onset can be later with West syndrome (Gospe, 2010) or with various seizure types up to the age of 2 years, or with neonatal seizures that may show an initial response to anticonvulsants or to extremely low doses of pyridoxine. About 15% of patients with later proven antiquitin deficiency show an ambiguous response to the first administration of pyridoxine (Mills et al., 2014).

The electroencephalogram (EEG) pattern shows asynchronous bursts of high-voltage generalised epileptiform activity, multifocal discharges, slow spike-wave complexes, burst suppression patterns or hypsarrhythmia in patients with infantile spasms. Neuroimaging can show unspecific findings as hypoplasia of the corpus callosum, cerebellar hypoplasia, cortical atrophy, hydrocephalus, white matter changes and periventricular dysmyelination or intraventricular haemorrhage.

The response to a first dose of intravenous pyridoxine (100 mg) can be quite dramatic (in just a few minutes), with disappearance of seizures and normalisation of the EEG over 24-48 h, but may be accompanied by severe apnea requiring assisted ventilation. In case of ineffectiveness another dose of 100 mg pyridoxine might be given in sequential doses every 5-10 minutes up to a total dose of 500 mg. If intravenous administration is not possible, pyridoxine can be given orally or enterally at equal dose with the same risk of apnea. A delayed response to pyridoxine is possible and treatment should be continued at 30 mg/kg/day in 3 single dosages for at least 3-7 days before concluding that the seizures are not responsive to pyridoxine (Stockler, 2011; Gospe, 2010) or until ATQ deficiency has been excluded by biochemical or genetic testing (Stockler et al., 2011).

In affected patients sudden withdrawal of pyridoxine leads to seizure recurrence, generally within a period of 5-7 days, although in individual cases seizure-free periods up to four weeks have been described. It is recommended, that pyridoxine should be kept lifelong at a dose of 15-30 mg/kg/d with a maximum daily dose around 200-500 mg, divided in 2-3 single dosages. Higher doses may lead to sensory or motor neuropathy. In patients with breakthrough seizures along infections and other stressful situations, transient doubling of the pyridoxine dose is recommended. As only about 25% of PDE patients have normal cognitive outcome despite early seizure control, additional therapeutic strategies have to be developed. Lysine restricted diet has the potential to lower neurotoxic alpha-aminoadipic semialdehyde (AASA) concentrations and has become an additional treatment option for PDE (Karnebeeck et al., 2012; Gallagher et al., 2009; Stockler et al., 2011).

Elevated alpha-aminoadipic semialdehyde (AASA), piperideine-6-carboxylate (P6C) and pipecolic acid (PA) concentrations are found in the CSF, urine or plasma, and serve as reliable biomarkers, while secondary alterations of neurotransmitter metabolism are less consistent (Plecko et al., 2005; Mills, 2006; Struys et al., 2011; Plecko et al., 2007). AASA is also secondarily elevated in molybdenum cofactor deficiency, so that sulfocysteine in urine should be measured simultaneously to avoid a false diagnosis.

AASA in urine and PA in plasma decline upon treatment, but usually remain elevated while on pyridoxine. Other non-specific biochemical disturbances reported are lactic acidosis, hypoglycemia, electrolyte disturbances, hypothyroidism and diabetes insipidus (Mercimek-Mahmutoglu et al., 2012) and may in part improve with pyridoxine treatment. Measurement of the enzyme deficiency in fibroblast homogenates is possible but a difficult laboratory method. The gene ATQ is located on chromosome 5q31. Diagnosis is confirmed by mutation analysis and to date more than 60 different mutations within the 18 exons of the ALDH7A1 gene have been reported. More than half are missense mutations with an altered aminoacid in the protein sequence (Stockler et al., 2011), but large deletions or duplications are not detected by standard sequencing methods. If in the presence of positive biomarkers sequencing does not reveal point mutations, molecular testing for deletions should be performed. Expression studies are helpful in measuring residual enzyme activity of single mutations and are beyond routine.

The outcome of patients with PDE is variable and not as good as the first publications suggested. Some patients have a normal development and remain seizure free on pyridoxine monotherapy, while other patients present incomplete seizure control and marked developmental delay. Some authors therefore distinguish three PDE phenotypes:
- PDE with complete seizure control and normal developmental outcome,
- complete seizure control and developmental delay or autism,
- incomplete seizure control and developmental delay (Scharer et al., 2010).

Due to autosomal recessive inheritance, there is a 25% recurrence risk for subsequent offspring. Intrauterine treatment with 100 mg of pyridoxine should be considered in forthcoming pregnancies, but despite prevention of seizures, is not able to prevent eventual mental retardation (Rankin et al., 2007; Bok et al., 2010). Postpartum confirmation testing has to be done as soon as possible, as high dose pyridoxine treatment might be pro-convulsive in non-affected neonates (Hartmann et al., 2011).

Pyridoxal 5'-phosphate-sensitive seizures or pyridox(am)ine 5'-phosphate oxidase (PNPO) deficiency

Kuo and Wang (2002), Clayton et al. (2003), and Mills et al. (2005) described a small group of newborn infants who presented with therapy-resistant seizures and early infantile epileptic encephalopathy, resulting in death within a few weeks.

The seizures are usually resistant to pyridoxine, but respond to pyridoxal5'-phosphate (PLP), the active vitamin B6 cofactor. Seizures usually cease within 60 minutes from first PLP administration, followed by the onset of hypotonia, respiratory and neurological depression. Again, first administration of PLP can lead to severe apnea so that resuscitation equipment should be at hand. Within a few days the patient returns to normal and the seizures stay controlled, provided the therapy is maintained at 30-50 mg/kg/d administered orally or enterally, divided in four to six single dosages per day. PLP is only available as an oral chemical powder from naturopathic stores and has not been licensed as a drug outside of Asia. PLP should be administered immediately after being dissolved in order to prevent oxidation; monitoring of transaminases is advocated, as one patient has shown liver cirrhosis on longterm use (Mills et al., 2014). The reported cases of PLP dependent seizures are scarce and, except from a few features, have marked overlap with PDE. Patients with PNPO deficiency are frequently born premature and have immediate signs of encephalopathy and seizures, with lactic acidosis and hypoglycaemia. The seizure semiology and EEG findings are indistinguishable from antiquitin deficiency, perhaps with more ocular, facial and other automatisms. Maternal reports of fetal seizures are frequent (more than in the PDE), and a burst suppression pattern EEG is more common than in PDE. In contrast to PDE breakthrough seizures while on PLP are frequently observed and patients may be sensitive to exact intervals of PLP administration throughout the day. If left untreated, the disorder results in death or profound developmental impairment with global brain atrophy and disturbed pattern of myelination (Ruiz et al., 2008). In the early treated patients the outcome is usually much better (Stockler et al., 2011; Porri et al., 2014).

PNPO deficiency lacks a specific biomarker. Raised levels of glycine, threonine and 3-methoxytyrosine, together with a decrease in CSF hydroxyindole acetic acid, and reduction of pyridoxal 5'-phosphate concentrations in CSF are secondary phenomena of cerebral vitamin B6 deficiency and can thus also be found in other conditions. The biomarkers present in Antiquitin deficiency are in the normal range in the PNPO deficient patients. The CSF biochemical profile can mimick that of aromatic L-amino acid decarboxylase deficiency (elevated vanillactate in urine, low concentration of HVA and 5-HIAA, and high concentration of L-dopa, 5-hydroxy-tryptophan and 3-O-methyldopa) (Ormazábal et al., 2008), but single individuals with elevated concentrations of biogenic amines have been described (Porri et al., 2014).

The defect of PLP responsive seizures is located at the pyridox(am)ine 5'-phosphate oxidase, the key-enzyme responsible for converting pyridoxamin 5'-phosphate and pyridoxine into pyridoxal 5'-phosphate (PLP). PLP is the only active vitamin B6 cofactor, acting in more than 140 pyridoxal 5'-phosphate dependent enzymatic reactions, including glutamate oxidation into GABA, lysine degradation and serine formation. Recently a regulatory role of PNPO in PLP recycling and its intracellular transport has been identified, partly explaining why treatment of PNPO deficiency is more difficult than that of PDE. In contrast to Antiquitin deficiency, PNPO deficiency cannot be diagnosed by a specific biomarker. Low PLP in CSF is very suggestive, but has been described in several inborn errors of metabolism (Mills et al., 2005; Footitt et al., 2011). Thus a definite diagnosis can only be established by molecular analysis of the PNPO gene.

The paradigm of exclusive PLP responsiveness has been challenged recently by the description of certain mutations of the PNPO gene, which respond to pyridoxine, but seem to be resistant to PLP (Plecko et al., 2014).

Thus consecutive vitamin trials with pyridoxine, followed by PLP should be a standard procedure in every neonate and biomarkers and genetic testing be performed rigorously.

Other pyridoxine or PLP responsive seizure disorders include neonatal hypophosphatasia (TNSALP deficiency), familial hyperphosphatasia (PIGV deficiency or Mabry syndrome) and hyperprolinemia type 2 (P5CD deficiency) (Plecko, 2013; Stockler et al., 2011; Nunes et al., 2002).

Folinic acid-responsive seizures (FARS)

In 1995 (Hyland et al.) and in 1999 (Torres et al.) described patients with neonatal seizures that were resistant to phenobarbital (PB), and valproic acid (VPA), and some of them also to pyridoxine, but responded to folinic acid (3-5 mg/kg/day) after a variable period of time (3-30 days) (Torres et al., 1999). Despite this, the patients suffered from developmental delay or a fatal course of disease (Nicolai, 2006; Stockler et al., 2011). The analysis of CSF biogenic amines by HPLC showed an unidentified component that was called "peak X" and was used as a disease marker. Recently FARS was identified to be genetically identical to ATQ deficiency, as some patients with "peak X" showed a clear response to pyridoxine and all had positive biomarkers as elevated AASA and PA (Gallagher et al., 2009). The role of folinic acid in PDE is not understood to date, aside from the fact, that peak X is not identical to any biomarker that has so far been recognized with Antiquitin deficiency. In case of a neonate with seizures and an incomplete pyridoxine response, add-on treatment of folinic acid should still be considered (Gospe, 2010; Stockler et al., 2011).

Defects of purine and pyrimidine metabolism

Adenylosuccinate lyase deficiency (ADSL)

This disease usually presents with seizures in the first few days of life or as childhood-onset epilepsy. Although in some patients it is possible to control the seizures, it often develops into an epileptic encephalopathy (Jurecka et al., 2014). It is associated with progressive psychomotor retardation, autistic features and other symptoms due to cerebellar and pyramidal involvement (Castro el al., 2002). This autosomal recessive disease affecting purine metabolism leads to a build-up of succinyl purines: succinylaminoimidazole carboxamide riboside (SAICAr) and succinyladenosine (S-Ado), in the blood, urine and CSF. The gene encoding adenylosuccinate lyase is located on chromosome 22 (22q13.1-q13.2). Treatment with allopurinol, sodium benzoate, purine bases (e.g. adenine), aminoimidazole carboxamide and D-ribose and uridine has had poor results, although in one case D-ribose lead to temporarily improved seizure control (Wolf, 2005; Ciardo et al., 2001).

Amino acidopathies

There are numerous inborn errors of amino acid metabolism that can be accompanied by epileptic seizures in the neonatal period or in the first months of life. The most common, and those that have the greatest impact on the nervous system, are Phenylketonuria (PKU) due to BH4 defects, non-ketotic hyperglycinaemia and serine deficiency (Saudubray, 2012; Wolf et al., 2005).

Atypical Phenylketonuria (PKU) due to BH4 defects

Hyperphenylalaninaemia is usually identified by newborn screening. Further diagnostic work-up includes determination of pterins in urine in order to detect atypical phenylketonuria (PKU). Atypical PKU is due to disorders of tetrahydrobiopterin (BH4) metabolism, the cofactor involved in the hydroxylation of phenylalanine, tyrosine and tryptophane, which are precursors for neurotransmitter synthesis. The defect may lie in the synthesis or in the BH4 recycling process. Affected patients (1% of PKU cases) present with symptoms of neurological impairment due to neurotransmitter deficiency (catecholamines and serotonin). The disorder presents early, with seizures, microcephaly, hypothermia, developmental delay, progressive neurological impairment, breathing difficulties, parkinsonism, myoclonus, chorea, dystonia and pyramidal signs. Refractory epilepsy is common, with infantile spasms or generalised seizures. Dihydropteridine reductase deficiency can be determined by assessing enzyme activity in erythrocytes, fibroblasts and lymphocytes. Treatment is based on dietary protein (phenylalanine) restriction and L-Dopa, 5-hydroxytryptophan and folinic acid supplements (Blau et al., 2011).

Non-ketotic hyperglycinaemia (NKH)

This is caused by a defect in the activity of the glycine degradation system, a multi-enzyme complex present in liver and brain. L-Glycine is an obligatory co-agonist of NMDA receptors; hyperglycinaemia therefore results in overexcitation causing epilepsy and excitotoxicity. The typical history is a mature newborn, presenting with episodes of apnoea, dysautonomia, progressive lethargy and coma within a few days after birth. This is accompanied by segmental and erratic myoclonus which may evolve into epileptic spasms and focal motor seizures resistant to medication. The EEG pattern deteriorates rapidly, with periods of burst-suppression and progression towards hypsarrhythmia after 3 months (Chen et al., 2001). A thin corpus callosum may be a radiologic hint towards the diagnosis. Aside from the neonatal form an atypical presentation with an extrapyramidal movement disorder has been described. NKH is diagnosed by an increased ratio of CSF glycine to plasma > 0.04 with some correlation to phenotype. It is recommended to analyse organic acid levels in urine to exclude "ketotic hyperglycinaemia" (associated with organic aciduria), in which the increase in plasma glycine (normal in CSF) occurs due to inhibition of the hepatic glycine degradation system and the accumulation of toxic organic acids (propionic, methylmalonic and isovaleric aciduria). Recently elevated plasma glycine has been described in a subgroup of mitochondriopathies related to iron-sulfur cluster defects and is accompanied by elevated lactate levels in plasma and CSF. Enzymatic testing for NKH warrants a liver biopsy and has been largely replaced by molecular analysis of the three respective genes involved. Most neonatal forms are caused by P or T protein defects/GCSH or AMT gene (Korman et al., 2006; Kanno et al., 2007; van Hove et al., 2007).

Prenatal diagnosis is possible by molecular analysis in chorionic villi. As glycine is a non-essential aminoacid, dietary restriction is not effective. Sodium benzoate has shown some effect in reducing seizure frequency and glycine levels in plasma but cannot alter the poor longterm prognosis. Strychnine, dextromethorphan (an NMDA receptor antagonist), diazepam, methionine or choline supplements have also been used, but with poor results. The response to AEDs is very limited and VPA must not be used, as it further inhibits glycine metabolism. Transient forms of NKH and a milder course associated with the A802V mutation have been described (Dinopoulos et al., 2011). Thus counselling of parents regarding the prognosis of their affected child should be based on the full genotype.

Serine deficiency

This autosomal recessive disease usually presents with congenital or early onset secondary microcephaly and refractory seizures during the first few months of life, that may evolve into West syndrome. Infants appear unhappy, irritable and hypertonic. More recently a juvenile form with mental decline, absence seizures and behavioural problems has been described (Tabatabaie et al., 2010). Defects have been described in all three steps of serine formation, with a deficiency of the enzyme 3-phosphoglycerate dehydrogenase due to a gene defect PHGDH being the most common. L-serine is an essential component for D-serine and glycine synthesis and as this is an important ligand to NMDA receptors and on the other hand functions as an inhibitory neurotransmitter in the brainstem. In infantile forms cranial MRI can give a clue to diagnosis with significant cerebral atrophy and delayed myelination. Determination of low plasma serine, or -more marked -low CSF serine establish the diagnosis. Patients usually respond favourably to early oral administration of L-serine supplements, 500-700 mg/kg/d, eventually together with glycine (200-300 mg/kg/d) and folinic acid. Intrauterine treatment seems to prevent development of the clinical phenotype (van der Crabben et al., 2013).

Leucinosis or maple syrup urine disease (MSUD)

There is a severe form, which presents during the first week of life with poor feeding, dystonia, generalized seizures and coma, and a burst-suppression EEG pattern. The maple syrup odor is best detectable in organic fluids. Late onset forms typically present with hallucinations and ataxia often triggered by infections or rich protein meals. Patients may present with neutropenia, thrombocytopenia, or pancytopenia. Neuroimaging in the initial stages shows significant cerebral oedema. The symptoms are mainly due to the accumulation of leucine (isoleucine and valine), which at first does not cause changes in the routine laboratory analysis. Metabolic acidosis with an increase in the anion gap, ketonuria, ketoacidosis, moderate hypocalcaemia, hyperlactatemia, and hypo- or hyperglycaemia only arise with the accumulation of 2-oxo-isocaproate, 2-oxoisovalerate and 2-oxomethylvalerate, the break-down products of the three branched chain aminoacids (Scriver et al., 2003; Saudubray, 2012). Diagnosis is based on detecting the characteristic profile as well as L-alloisoleucine in the plasma amino acid and urine organic acid tests. Acute-phase treatment must be aggressive, with peritoneal dialysis or exchange transfusion to rapidly eliminate the accumulated branched-chain amino acids, especially leucine, whilst energy must be supplied in the form of glucose and lipids by a central venous line. Subsequently, patients need a lifelong protein-restricted diet and supplementation with a precursor-free aminoacid mixture.

Organic acidurias

These are biochemical disorders of intermediary metabolism that affect different metabolic pathways of amino acids, fatty acids, ketogenesis, ketolysis, pyruvate, carbohydrates or the Krebs cycle. While some organic acidurias of neonatal onset as propionic aciduria, holocarboxylase synthetase deficiency or isovaleric aciduria cause acute systemic decompensation with severe metabolic acidosis, others as glutaric aciduria or Canavan disease are restricted to the CNS with subacute or chronic brain damage. More than 80 organic acidurias have been reported, and most of them involve the CNS. The variable clinical expression in part, depends on the type of enzyme deficiency, age of onset, accumulated metabolites and triggering factors. In the acute stage, patients present with vomiting, deterioration in their general condition with progressive lethargy and coma, associated with metabolic acidosis with few exceptions for the latter such as glutaric aciduria type I. Myoclonic and other types of seizures are often observed in the acute stage, but as in propionic academia can also occur during the long-term course of disease (Haberlandt et al., 2009). Pancytopenia, metabolic acidosis and ketonuria can appear during decompensation. As the basal ganglia are especially vulnerable to the toxicity of organic acids, symmetric involvement of putamen or globus pallidus should always prompt metabolic investigations. The diagnosis is established by means of quantitative analysis of plasma aminoacids and acylcarnitines as well as urinary organic acid. Again, early diagnosis and treatment are essential to prevent irreversible longterm sequelea. Therefore some of these disorders, as glutaric aciduria type I, have been included in newborn screening programmes of several European countries.

Defects in the urea cycle and related disorders causing hyperammonaemia

Disorders of ureagenesis, due to primary enzymopathies of the urea cycle as well as secondary inhibition by organic acids, bring about hyperammonaemia. The enzyme defects in the urea cycle may be distinguished by their characteristic plasma amino acid profile and the presence or absence of urinary orotic acid (Saudubray, 2012). Age of onset and clinical signs are variable and one third of cases presents in the neonatal period with symptoms of toxic encephalopathy. Initial signs include poor feeding, vomiting, alterations in muscle tone, lethargy, generalised or focal seizures, and, if not treated adequately coma, brain edema and death. Hyperammonemia is an emergency and it is mandatory to stop protein intake and provide adequate caloric supply in order to avoid or limit longterm sequelea such as refractory seizures and neurological deterioration (Campistol, 2000). In argininosuccinic acidaemia a more chronic presentation with trichorrhexis nodosa, irritability, rigidity and refractory seizures is common. Thus plasma ammonia should also be determined in more chronic presentations and needs immediate processing in order to avoid preanalytical errors. The use of valproate should be avoided in this patient group, as it interferes with ammonia detoxification. Phenobarbitone or levetiracetam seem to be safe.

IEM affecting the energetic substrates

Mitochondrial cytopathies

Epilepsy is a frequent manifestation of mitochondrial diseases, illustrating that energy depletion and the accumulation of radicals is lowering the seizure threshold. Some of them manifest during the neonatal period, with seizures being one of the most frequent symptoms. In early onset cases primary lactic acidosis is a leading finding and necessitates the exclusion of secondary lactate elevation due to organic acidurias. Determination of lactate in CSF is especially important and superior to plasma lactate, which can be falsely raised with difficulties in drawing the blood sample. MRI may show bilateral changes of the basal ganglia and in cases of pyruvate dehydrogenase deficiency may show primary malformation of the brainstem. Magnetic resonance spectroscopy (MRS) may reveal elevated lactate peaks. Mitochondriopathies have the unique constellation of Mendelian as well as maternal inheritance through mitochondrial DNA (mtDNA). While some entities as Leigh, MERRF or MELAS syndrome can show well recognizable phenotypes, the majority of mitochondriopathies is of nuclear origin and presents with a more unspecific type of encephalomyopathy. In exceptional cases of recognizable syndromes diagnosis may be confirmed by primary molecular analysis of mtDNA or nuclear DNA, while in most cases with a more unspecific presentation a muscle biopsy and analysis of the oxphos enzymes is still necessary. One exception to this is Alpers disease, or hepatocerebral neurodegeneration, which is caused by autosomal recessive mutations of the POLG1 gene, needed for the replication of mtDNA. Notably in Alpers disease epilepsy that tends to appear in young infants or childhood with myoclonus and ataxia can precede hepatic involvement and may allow suspicion by a specific EEG pattern of unilateral occipital rhythmic high-amplitude delta with superimposed (poly) spikes (RHADS) (Wolf et al., 2009).

In several cases the first manifestation of Alpers disease is status epilepticus, followed by epilepsia partialis continua. Lactic acid levels in plasma and CSF are typically normal and even measurement of oxidative phosphorylation in fresh muscle may be normal. Thus the diagnosis of Alpers disease is by primary genetic testing of the POLG1 gene. Impaired mitochondrial glutamate transport has recently been reported as a cause of early myoclonic encephalopathy (Wolf et al., 2002; Molinari et al., 2004). In all mitochondriopathies the use of sodium valproate should be avoided for the risk of provoking hepatic failure. Some patients may benefit from supplementation of thiamine, riboflavin, L-carnitine or coenzyme Q10 as well as a slowly introduced fat enriched diet (fat to carbohydrates plus protein in gram 1:1 to 3:1).

Glucose transporter type I deficiency

Patients usually appear normal at birth or with some unspecified symptoms as abnormal ocular or generalized movements and present with therapy-resistant focal motor seizures from their first months of life. In addition, especially before meals or at times of fasting patients may exhibit an episodic movement disorder with associated rolling eye movements. About 60% of infants develop acquired microcephaly. Beyond infancy secondary generalization of seizures predominates and more recently Glut-1 deficiency has been described in a cohort of atypical absence epilepsy (Suls et al., 2009). The EEG may be completely normal and preprandial recording should be considered to unravel altered background activity or focal discharges (De Vivo et al., 2002).

Glut-1 deficiency is generally caused by sporadic haploinsufficiency of the blood-brain barrier passive glucose transporter, Glut-1 (SLC2A1 gene), although in milder cases the disease can also be inherited as an autosomal dominant trait (Pascual et al., 2004, 2007). Over 100 different missense mutations have been described so far and about 10% of patients carry deletions, not detected by Sanger sequencing (Leen et al., 2013).

First reports suggested that a CSF/blood glucose ratio < 0.4 confirms the diagnosis, but more recently the use of absolute CSF glucose values below 40 (to 60) mg/dl with respect to age related normal values were considered to be more precise, especially in milder or adult onset cases with paroxysmal exercise induced dyskinesia ± epilepsy (PED, DYT 18). A reduction in glucose uptake by the brain is easily documented by conventional fluordeoxyglucose positron emission tomography (PET), which shows a characteristic pattern of abnormalities. The cranial MRI is usually normal or may show unspecific changes as delayed myelination or brain atrophy. A ketogenic diet (KD) is the only known effective treatment and seizures disappear in the majority of patients (De Vivo et al., 1991; Pascual et al., 2008). The usual recommended ratio of fat to non-fat intake in grams is 3:1, and can be increased to 4:1. Ketosis can be controlled by measurement of urine or blood ketones and patients need to be followed by a dietician with a sick day protocol in place (Klepper et al., 2013).

Menkes disease

The disease can begin in the neonatal period with congenital skull fractures and seizures occurring during the first few months of life. The early phase is dominated by frequent focal clonic seizures with multifocal discharges, that over weeks evolve into infantile spasms with modified hypsarrhythmia (Bahi-Buisson et al., 2006). The diagnosis is suggested by additional typical findings of kinky hair, cutis laxa and bladder diverticles. Menkes disease is caused by mutations in the ATPase 7 gene, an ubiqituous copper transporter encoded on the X-chromosome and located in the trans-Golgi network, that is particularly active in the intestine, from which most of the dietary copper is absorbed (Prasad et al., 2011). Due to impaired copper transport there is malfunction of several copper dependent enzymes as mitochondrial cytochrome c oxidase, lysyl oxidase, superoxide dismutase, dopamine-beta-hydroxylase and tyrosinase (Matsuo et al., 2005), causing elevated plasma lactate due to complex IV deficiency (cytochrome c oxidase), alteration in the molecular bridges of collagen (catalysed by lysyl oxidase) causing hair abnormalities (pili torti, trichorrhexis nodosa, moniletrix and, eventually alopecia), vascular alterations (elongated or toutous vessels and subdural haematoma), and Purkinje cell degeneration in the cerebellum and hypothermia. The serum copper and cerulopasmin are low and the homovanillic acid: vanillylmandelic acid ratio in urine is high. The diagnosis is confirmed by copper uptake studies in fibroblasts or molecular analysis of the ATP7A gene. Early treatment with copper-histidine probably ameliorates some of the symptoms of the disease.

Molybdenum cofactor and Sulfite oxidase deficiency (MOCOD and ISOD)

These two entities have identical clinical presentations and show bilateral myoclonic or tonic-clonic seizures within days after birth that may evolve into status epilepticus. Seventy-five percent of patients were described to have subtle dysmorphic features with elongated face, small nose and puffy cheeks (Johnson et al., 2001). As with many inborn errors of metabolism these seizures are resistant to common anticonvulsants, at least in the initial stage of disease. Many patients show additional signs of encephalopathy, truncal hypotonia and brisk reflexes and may be mistaken for hypoxic ischemic encephalopathy. EEG records show multifocal spike-wave activity or a burst suppression pattern. The MRI may give a clue to diagnosis, revealing generalised brain edema in the early stage, followed by extended cystic changes of the white matter and global brain atrophy. Few patients have shown association with variable primary brain malformation. Beyond infancy a number of ophthalmologic problems has been encountered with both disorders as lense subluxation, optic atrophy or nystagmus. Late onset forms have been described with both disorders and are dominated by movement disorders with seizures being less prominent.

The underlying pathomechanism is directly related to sulfite toxicity, with a neuroexcitatory action on the nervous system. Though molybdenum is a cofactor of xanthin oxidoreductase and aldehyde oxidase as well as sulfite oxidase, it is impairment of the latter enzyme that causes the CNS phenotype in MOCOD as well as in ISOD. Impaired oxidation of xanthin leads to decreased uric acid in plasma in most patients with MOCOD but of course not in those with ISOD. Elevated sulfite in urine occurs in both disorders but commercially available test sticks, have given both, false-negative and false positive results. Thus determination of urinary S-sulfocysteine is the actual gold standard to test for both disorders. Recently elevation of alpha-aminoadipic semialdehyde (AASA), the biomarker for Antiquitin deficiency has been found elevated in patients with MOCOD and ISOD, which is most likely be due to secondary inhibition of AASA dehydrogenase by accumulating sulfite. ISOD as well as MOCOD follow autosomal recessive traits and can be confirmed by respective enzyme studies in cultured fibroblasts. While ISOD is encoded by the SUOX gene, MOCOD can be caused by defects in any of the three genes involved in its synthesis. About 2/3 of MOCOD patients have defects in the MOCS 1 gene, encoding the first precursor (cPMP) in the MoCo biosynthetic pathway and are designated MOCOD type A patients. This prevalent patient group type A may be amenable to intravenous treatment with synthetic cPMP, which should be installed as soon as biochemical results suggest MOCOD, even if genotyping is pending (Veldman et al., 2010). For MOCOD patients type B, harbouring mutations in the MOCS2 gene or single patients harbouring mutations in the GEPH gene, treatment is purely symptomatic. Dextromethorphan, an NMDA receptor antagonist, as well as dietary restriction of sulphur-containing methionine has shown some benefit in single patients as has pyridoxine in those patients with elevated AASA.

Conclusion

There are some forms of neonatal seizures and epilepsies due to inborn errors of metabolism who do not respond to the use of AEDs. In this situation the early start of another type of therapy can prevent neurological deterioration, and seizure control. With specific treatment the patient can lead a normal life without epilepsy and normal development. We reviewed in this chapter the group of metabolic defects that lead to newborn seizures and epilepsy and whose treatment with cofactors is very different from epilepsy management with antiepileptic drugs.

References

- Aicardi J. *Diseases of the nervous system in childhood*. In: Society TS, ed. Clinics in development medicine. London, 1995.
- Arzimanoglou A, Guerrini R, Aicardi J. *Aicardi's Epilepsy in children*. 3rd edition ed. New York: Mac Keith Press, 2004.
- Bahi-Buisson N, Kaminska A, Nabbout R, *et al*. Epilepsy in Menkes disease: analysis of clinical stages. *Epilepsia* 2006; 47: 380-6.
- Baxter P. Epidemiology of pyridoxine dependent and pyridoxine responsive seizures in the UK. *Arch Dis Child* 1999; 81: 431-3.
- Blau N, Hennermann JB, Langenbeck U, Lichter-Konecki U. Diagnosis, classification, and genetics of phenylketonuria and tetrahydrobiopterin (BH4) deficiencies. *Mol Genet Metab* 2011; 104: S2-9.
- Bok LA, Been JV, Struys EA, Jakobs C, Rijper EA, Willemsen MA. Antenatal treatment in two Dutch families with pyridoxine-dependent seizures. *Eur J Pediatr* 2010; 169(3): 297-303.
- Campistol J. Epileptic syndromes in the first year of life and congenital errors of metabolism. *Rev Neurol* 2000; 30 (suppl 1): S60-74.
- Castro M, Pérez Cerdá C, Merinero B. Screening for adenylosuccinate lyase deficiency: clinical, biochemical and molecular findings in four patients. *Neuropediatrics* 2002; 33: 186-9.
- Chen PT, Young C, Lee WT, Wang PJ, Peng SS, Shen YZ. Early epileptic encephalopathy with suppression burst electroencephalographic pattern – an analysis of eight Taiwanese patients. *Brain Dev* 2001; 23: 715-20.
- Ciardo F, Salerno C, Curatolo P. Neurologic aspects of adenylosuccinate lyase deficiency. *J Child Neurol* 2001; 16: 301-8.
- Clayton P, Surtees RAH, De Vile C, Hyland K, Heales SJR. Neonatal epileptic encephalopathy. *Lancet* 2003; 361: 1614.
- De Vivo DC, Leary L, Wang D. Glucose transporter 1 deficiency syndrome and other glycolytic defects. *J Child Neurol* 2002; 17 (suppl 3): 3S15-S25.
- Dinopoulos A, Matsubara Y, Kure S. Atypical variants of nonketotic hyperglycinemia. *Mol Genet Metab* 2005; 86: 61-9.
- Footitt EJ, Heales SJ, Mills PB, Allen GF, Oppenheim M, Clayton PT. Pyridoxal 5'-phosphate in cerebrospinal fluid; factors affecting concentration. *J Inherit Metab Dis* 2011; 34(2): 529-38.
- Gallagher RC, Van Hove JL, Scharer G, Hyland K, Plecko B, Waters PJ, *et al*. Folinic acid responsive seizures are identical to pyridoxine dependent epilepsy. *Ann Neurol* 2009; 65: 550-6.
- Gospe S. Neonatal Vitamin responsive epileptic encephalopathies. *Chang Gung Med J* 2010; 33: 1-12.

- Haberlandt E, Canestini C, Brunner-Krainz M, et al. Epilepsy in patients with propionic acidemia. *Neuropediatrics* 2009; 40: 120-5.
- Hartmann H, Fingerhut M, Jakobs C, Plecko B. Status epilepticus in a neonate treated with pyridoxine because of a familial recurrence risk for antiquitin deficiency: pyridoxine toxicity? *Dev Med Child Neurol* 2011; 53(12): 1150-3.
- Jurecka A, Zikanova M, Jurkiewicz E, Tylki-Szymańska A. Attenuated adenylosuccinate lyase deficiency: a report of one case and a review of the literature. *Neuropediatrics* 2014; 45(1): 50-5.
- Hyland K, Buist NR, Powell BR, et al. Folinic acid responsive seizures: a new syndrome? *J Inherit Metab Dis* 1995; 18: 177-81.
- Johnson JL, Duran M. Molybdenum cofactor deficiency and isolated sulphite oxidase deficiency. In: CR Scriver, AL Beaudet, WS Sly, et al. eds. *The Metabolic and Molecular Bases of Inherited Disease*. New York: McGraw Hill, 2001, pp. 3136-77.
- Kanno J, Hutchin T, Kamada F, Narisawa A, Aoki Y, Matsubara Y, Kure S. Genomic deletion within GLDC is a major cause of non-ketotic hyperglycinaemia. *J Med Genet* 2007; 44(3): e69.
- Klepper J, Leiendecker B. Glut1 deficiency syndrome and novel ketogenic diets. *J Child Neurol* 2013; 28(8): 1045-8.
- Korman SH, Wexler ID, Gutman A, Rolland MO, Kanno J, Kure S. Treatment from birth of nonketotic hyperglycinemia due to a novel GLDC mutation. *Ann Neurol* 2006; 59(2): 411-5.
- Kuo MF, Wang HS. Pyridoxal phosphate-responsive epilepsy with resistance to pyridoxine. *Pediatr Neurol* 2002; 26: 146-7.
- Leen WG, de Wit CJ, Wevers RA, van Engelen BG, Kamsteeg EJ, Klepper J, et al. Child neurology: differential diagnosis of a low CSF glucose in children and young adults. *Neurology* 2013; 10; 81(24): e178-81.
- Marin-Valencia I, Vilaseca MA, Thio M, Garcia Cazorla A, Artuch R, Campistol J. Assesment of the perimortem protocol in neonates for the diagnosis of inborn errors of metabolim. *Eur J Ped Neurol* 2010; 14: 125-30.
- Matsuo M, Tasaki R, Kodama H, Hamasaki Y. Screening for Menkes disease using the urine HVA/VMA ratio. *J Inherit Metab Dis* 2005; 28: 89-93.
- Mercimek-Mahmutoglu S, Horvath GA, Coulter-Mackie M, Nelson T, Waters PJ, Sargent M, et al. Profound neonatal hypoglycemia and lactic acidosis caused by pyridoxine-dependent epilepsy. *Pediatrics* 2012; 129(5): e1368-72.
- Mills PB, Struys E, Jacobs C, Plecko B, Baxter P, Baumgartner M, et al. Mutations in antiquitin in individuals with pyridoxine dependent seizures. *Nat Med* 2006; 12: 307-9.
- Mills PB, Surtees RA, Champion MP, et al. Neonatal epileptic encephalopathy caused by mutations in the PNPO gene encoding pyridox(am)ine 5' phosphate oxidase. *Hum Mol Genet* 2005; 14: 1077-86.
- Mills PB, Camuzeaux SS, Footitt EJ, Mills KA, Gissen P, Fisher L, et al. Epilepsy due to PNPO mutations: genotype, environment and treatment affect presentation and outcome. *Brain*. 2014 Mar 18. [Epub ahead of print].
- Molinari F, Raas-Rothschild A, Rio M, et al. Impaired mitochondrial glutamate transport in autosomal recessive neonatal myoclonic epilepsy. *Am J Hum Genet* 2005; 76: 334-9.
- Nicolai J, van Kranen-Masterbroek VH, Wevers RA, Hurkx WA, Vles JS. Folinic acid responsive seizures initially responsive to pyridoxine. *Ped Neurol* 2006; 34: 164-7.
- Nunes ML, Mugnol F, Bica I, Fiori RM. Pyridoxine-dependent seizures associated with hypophosphatasia in a newborn. *J Child Neurol* 2002; 17: 222-4.
- Ormazábal A, Oppenheim M, Serrano M, Garcia-Cazorla A, Campistol J, Ribes A, et al. Pyridoxal 5' phosphate values in CSF: reference value and diagnosis of PNPO deficiency in pediatric patients. *Mol Genet Metab* 2008; 94: 173-7.
- Pascual JM, Wang D, Lecumberri B, et al. GLUT-1 deficiency and other glucose transporter diseases. *Eur J Endocrinol* 2004; 150: 627-33.

- Pascual JM. *Encephalopathies in Neurology and Clinical Neuroscience*. Philadelphia: Mosby, 2007.
- Pascual J, Campistol J, Gil Nagel A. Epilepsy in inherited metabolic disorders. *The Neurologist*. 2008; 14: S1-11.
- Plecko B, Stöckler-Ispiroglu S, Paschke E, Erwa W, Struys EA, Jakobs C. Pipecolic acid elevation in plasma and cerebrospinal fluid of two patients with pyridoxine dependent epilepsy. *Ann Neurol* 2000; 48(1): 121-5.
- Plecko B, Hikel C, Korenke GC, Schmitt B, Baumgartner M, Baumeister F, et al. Pipecolic acid as a diagnostic marker of pyridoxine dependent epilepsy. *Neuropediatrics* 2005; 36: 200-5.
- Plecko B, Paul K, Paschke E, Stockler-Ipsiroglou S, Struys E, Jacobs C, et al. Biochemical and molecular characterization of 18 patients with pyridoxine dependent epilepsy and mutations of the antiquitin (ALDH7A1) gene. *Hum Mutat* 2007; 28: 19-26.
- Plecko B. Pyridoxine and pyridoxalphosphate-dependent epilepsies. *Handb Clin Neurol* 2013; 113: 1811-7.
- Plecko B, Paul K, Mills P, Clayton P, Paschke E, Maier O, et al. Pyridoxine responsiveness in novel mutations of the PNPO gene. *Neurology* 2014 Mar 21. [Epub ahead of print].
- Porri S, Fluss J, Plecko B, Paschke E, Korff CM, Kern I. Positive outcome following early diagnosis and treatment of pyridoxal-5'-phosphate oxidase deficiency: a case report. *Neuropediatrics* 2014; 45(1): 64-8.
- Prasad AN, Levin S, Rupar CA, Prasad C. Menkes disease and infantile epilepsy. *Brain Dev* 2011; 33: 866-76.
- Rankin PM, Harrison S, Chong WK, Boyd S, Aylett SE. Pyridoxine-dependent seizures: a family phenotype that leads to severe cognitive deficits, regardless of treatment regime. *Dev Med Child Neurol* 2007; 49(4): 300-5.
- Rhakhade SN, Jensen FE. Epileptogenesis in the immature brain: emerging mechanisms. *Rev Neurol* 2009; 5: 380-91.
- Ruiz A, Garcia Villoria J, Ormazabal A, Zschocke J, Fiol M, Navarro Sastre A, et al. A new fatal case of pyridoxamine 5' phosphate oxidase (PNPO) deficiency. *Mol Genet Metab* 2008; 93: 216-8.
- Saudubray JM. *Clinical approach to inborn errors of metabolism in paediatrics*. In: Saudubray JM, van den Berghe G, Walter JH, eds. Inborn metabolic diseases, 5th edition, Chap 1: 3-54, Berlin: Springer, 2012.
- Scharer G, Brocker V, Vasiliou G, Creadon Swindell RC, Gallagher E, et al. The genotypic and phenotypic spectrum of pyridoxine dependent epilepsy due to mutations in ALDH7A1. *J Inherit Met Dis* 2010; 33(5): 571-81.
- Schmitt B, Baumgartner M, Mills PB. Seizures and paroxysmal events: symptoms pointing to the diagnosis of pyridoxine-dependent epilepsy and pyridoxine phosphate oxidase deficiency. *Dev Med Child Neurol* 2010; 52: e133-42.
- Scriver CR, Beaudet AL, Sly L, Valle D. *The metabolic basis of inherited disease*. New York: McGraw Hill, 2003.
- Stockler S, Plecko B, Gospe S, Coulter Mackie M, Connoly M, van Karnebeek C, et al. Pyridoxine dependent epilepsy and antiquitin deficiency. Clinical and molecular characteristics and recommendations for diagnosis, treatment and follow up. *Mol Genet Metab* 2011; 104: 48-60.
- Struys EA, Bok LA, Emal D, Houterman S, Willemsen MA, Jakobs C. The measurement of urinary Δ^1-piperideine-6-carboxylate, the alter ego of α-aminoadipic semialdehyde, in Antiquitin deficiency. *J Inherit Metab Dis* 2012; 35(5): 909-16.
- Suls A, Mullen SA, Weber YG, Verhaert K, Ceulemans B, Guerrini R, et al. Early-onset absence epilepsy caused by mutations in the glucose transporter GLUT1. *Ann Neurol* 2009; 66(3): 415-9.
- Tabatabaie L, Klomp LW, Berger R, de Koning TJ. L-serine synthesis in the central nervous system: a review on serine deficiency disorders. *Mol Genet Metab* 2011; 99: 256-62.
- Toribe Y. High-dose vitamin B(6) treatment in West syndrome. *Brain Dev* 2001; 23: 654-7.

- Torres OA, Miller VS, Buist NM, Hyland K. Folinic acid-responsive neonatal seizures. *J Child Neurol* 1999; 14: 529-32.
- van der Crabben SN, Verhoeven-Duif NM, Brilstra EH, Van Maldergem L, Coskun T, Rubio-Gozalbo E, Berger R, de Koning TJ. An update on serine deficiency disorders. *J Inherit Metab Dis* 2013; 36(4): 613-9.
- Van Hove JL, Vande Kerckhove K, Hennermann JB, Mahieu V, Declercq P, Mertens S, De Becker M, Kishnani PS, Jaeken J. Benzoate treatment and the glycine index in nonketotic hyperglycinaemia. *J Inherit Metab Dis* 2005; 28(5): 651-63.
- Veldman A, Santamaria-Araujo JA, Sollazzo S, *et al*. Successful treatment of molybdenum cofactor deficiency type A with cPMP. *Pediatrics* 2010; 12: e1249-54.
- Wolf B. The neurology of biotinidase deficiency. *Mol Genet Metab* 2011; 104: 27-34.
- Wolf NI, Bast T, Surtees R. Epilepsy in inborn errors of metabolism. *Epileptic Disord* 2005; 7: 67-81.
- Wolf NI, Smeitink JA. Mitochondrial disorders: a proposal for consensus diagnostic criteria in infants and children. *Neurology* 2002; 59: 1402-5.
- Wolf NI, Rahman S, Schmitt B, Taanman JW, Duncan AJ, Harting I, *et al*. Status epilepticus in children with Alpers' disease caused by POLG1 mutations: EEG and MRI features. *Epilepsia* 2009; 50(6): 1596-607.

Determining outcome from neonatal seizures

Francesco Pisani, Carlotta Spagnoli

Child Neuropsychiatry Unit, Neuroscience Department, University of Parma, Italy

In this chapter, we will discuss the main prognostic implications of the occurrence of neonatal seizures, in terms of subsequent mortality and increased risk for neurological sequelae.

We will describe the epidemiology and the clinical characteristics of such neurodevelopmental outcomes and we will then analyse and critically review the most important clinical, electroencephalographic and imaging predictors of unfavourable outcome.

Based on this evidence, we will delineate the thus-far proposed scoring systems for early prognostication following neonatal seizures and resume their predictivity.

Finally, we will conclude by delineating some of the most relevant fields with a potential to significantly impact on outcome in the near future.

■ Description of clinical outcomes and epidemiology

Mortality risk and its trend over the last decades in newborns with neonatal seizures will be analysed and after that we will report on morbidity, mainly focusing on cerebral palsy and intellectual impairment, whereas epilepsy will be treated separately.

Mortality

Mortality after neonatal seizures in hospital-based studies has decreased from approximately 40% reported in studies from the fifties and sixties (Burke, 1954; McInerny and Schubert, 1969; Craig, 1960), even if lower rates, *i.e.* 14% to 26% (Tibbles and Prichard, 1965; Schulte, 1966; Harris and Tizard, 1960) have also been reported in the same period, to more recent figures of 7-16% (Tekgul *et al.*, 2006; Garfinkle and Shevell, 2011a; Ronen, 2007; Scher, 1997). Unsurprisingly, neonatal intensive care unit cohorts in the 80's reported higher figures, especially among preterm infants, with a mortality as high as 57% in the 32-36wGA group and reaching 84% in the group of less than 31wGA, *versus* a 17% mortality in the full-term group (Bergman *et al.*, 1983). Still in the 90's mortality in the NICU was as high as 30% after clinically diagnosed seizures (Brunquell, 2002).

Higher rates of mortality have been associated with EEG-confirmed neonatal seizures in the 1980s ranging from 50% in preterm newborns to 40% in full-term infants (Scher et al., 1993; Scher and Painter, 1989), and have afterwards lowered, even if remain relevant, with a 19% overall mortality, raising to 33.3% in the preterm subgroup, in a neonatal intensive care unit (NICU) based series collecting data in the 5 years between 1999 and 2004 (Pisani et al., 2007).

Comparison between two population-based studies, providing long-term follow-up information, the first one collecting data between 1959 and 1966 (Holden et al., 1982) and the second in the years 1990-1994 (Ronen et al., 2007), show a reduction in mortality from 34.8% in the first to 24% in the latter, mainly attributable to higher mortality in preterm infants (42% versus 16% in the full-term group). It is noteworthy to highlight how the main difference between the two cohorts resides in the much lower proportion of favourable outcomes in the surviving neonates, falling from 70% in the older series to 35% in the more recent one. The correlation between higher mortality rates and lower rates of abnormal outcome was already noted in older studies (Schulte, 1966). This shift from mortality to morbidity, especially in the preterm neonate, represents one of the greatest challenges in current neonatal intensive care. The varying trend in mortality among preterm newborns with neonatal seizures (as derived from studies of the last 40 years) is presented in *Figure 1*.

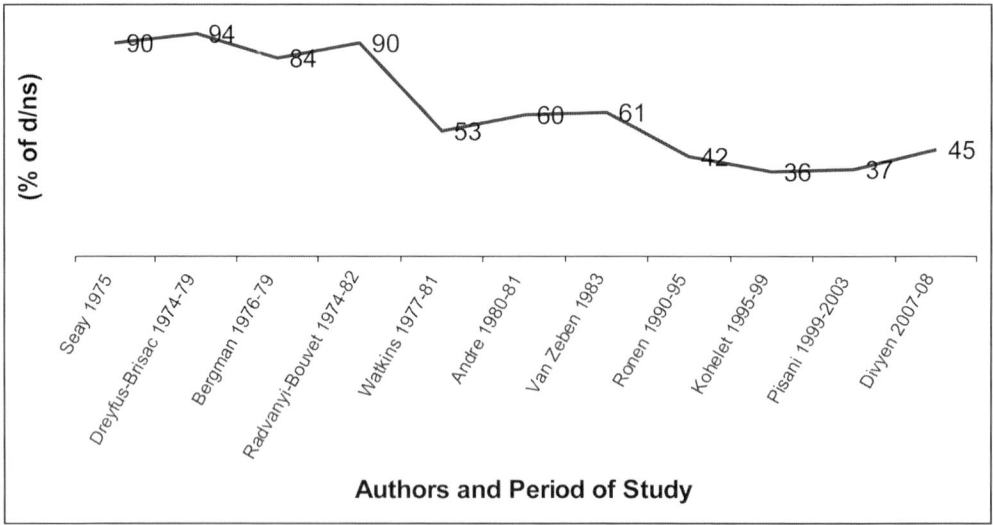

Figure 1. Evolution of the mortality rate in preterm newborns with neonatal seizures.

Morbidity

Following neonatal seizures, the main three neurological outcomes to consider comprise cerebral palsy, global developmental delay/mental retardation and epilepsy, which are often associated in the same patient (Mellits et al., 1982). In a recent hospital-based cohort of both full-term and preterm neonates with EEG-confirmed seizures, 31.7% of patients presented with cerebral palsy, 9.4% isolated and 15.3% associated with both epilepsy and mental retardation (Pisani et al., 2012a). Furthermore, an IQ of less than 70 has been reported in 66.7% of children with motor deficits compared to 11.1% in those without

(Bergman et al., 1983). This association is particularly striking when the outcome epilepsy is considered (Pisani et al., 2012a; Clancy and Legido, 1991; Legido et al., 1991), as the 86.6% of patients with epilepsy also present both learning disability and cerebral palsy.

A smaller proportion of studies have also focused on visual and/or hearing impairment (Bergman et al., 1983), language and microcephaly (Tibbles and Prichard, 1965; Legido et al., 1991). Of note, even in the absence of any major neurological disorders, survivors of neonatal seizures might show minor neuropsychological deficits if re-evaluated in their teenage years: difficulties with spelling, arithmetics and memory, in spite of a normal overall intelligence (Temple et al., 1995).

Cerebral Palsy

The National Collaborative Perinatal Project study reported a rate of 13% of cerebral palsy, which was 30 times higher than the one of newborns without neonatal seizures (Holden et al., 1982), whereas, secondary to a selection-bias towards complex cases, higher rates emerged in survivors from intensive care series (Bergman et al., 1983), with a 31% rate of cerebral palsy and with a wider proportion of affected preterm (59%) as opposed to full-term neonates (41%) (Scher et al., 1993). Nevertheless, when these data are compared to the more recent population-based study, the aforementioned increase in morbidity is apparent, with a rate of 25% of cerebral palsy (17% in full-term neonates and 53% in preterm neonates) (Ronen et al., 2007). When only term babies are considered, the type of motor deficit has been reported as follows: 40% dyskinetic, 16% quadriplegic, 44% hemiplegic (Toet et al., 2005).

Mental Retardation

A second important neurological sequela is represented by learning disability, which prevalence has remained substantially unchanged in the two aforementioned population-based studies, providing a follow-up of 7 to 8 years in the first one and of 10 years in the second: 19% in 1982 versus 20% in 2007, even if this latter study also reports an additional 27% of learning disorders. Selected populations reveal higher rates of intellectual impairment: 42% of preterm neonates and 35% of full-term neonates in a NICU-based population (Scher et al., 1993). For completeness, it can be emphasized that, aside from differences in sampling characteristics and changing epidemiology over time, two additional problems might arise: one regarding the difficulties in comparing studies using different scales to assess the degree of developmental delay and the second regarding the limitation in assessing the IQ in more severely affected patients.

Epilepsy

Although some hospital-based studies have reported percentages as high as 41.4% (Khan et al., 2008) after clinically diagnosed seizures and 56% after EEG-confirmed seizures (Clancy and Legido, 1991), post-neonatal epilepsy has usually been reported to occur in 18-25% of patients (Holden et al., 1982; Dennis, 1978). Recent studies led on mixed cohorts (51.7% full-term with 21.1% preterm ≤ 28 wGA) have confirmed previous results, with a 17.6% overall incidence (Pisani et al., 2012a), whereas a lower rate of 9.4% was reported following aEEG-diagnosed seizures (Toet et al., 2005) (Figure 2). With a mean age of 12.7 months (0.8-41 months) (Clancy and Legido, 1991), an early onset of epilepsy is the rule after neonatal seizures, either already occurring in the neonatal period

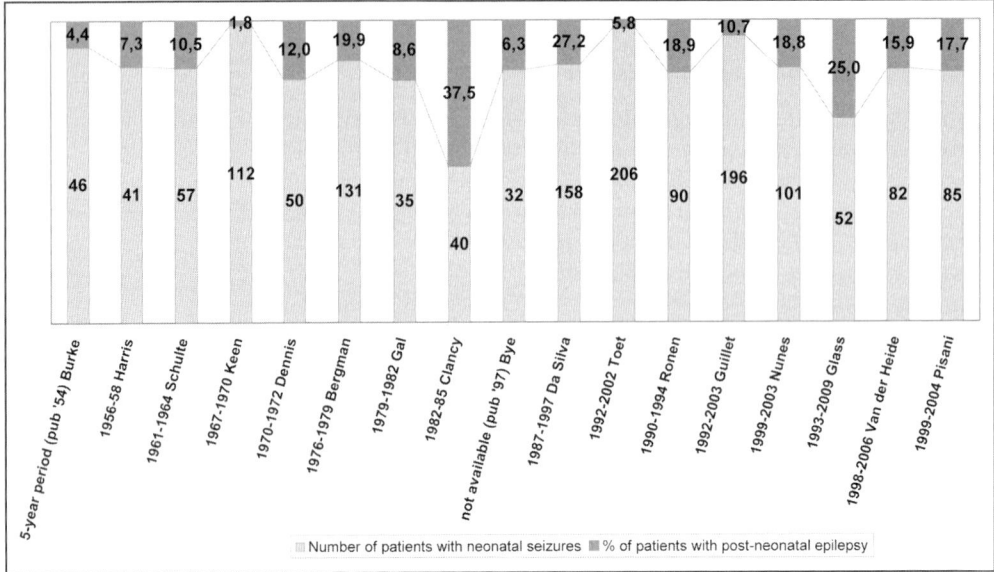

Figure 2. Development of epilepsy after neonatal seizures.

(Bergman et al., 1983; Pisani et al., 2012a) or after a brief latent period, as already noted by Schulte (1966) who observed that it was only between 5 and 20 months that the focal epileptiform discharges recorded in the newborn period were followed by the occurrence of seizures. This observation has remained quite constant from older to more recent studies, with a 50% onset in the first 8 months of life (Bergman et al., 1983), similar to the 58.3% onset within the first year of life, reported after aEEG-diagnosed seizures (Toet et al., 2005).

An only slightly different time distribution is reported by others (Pisani et al., 2012a), with slightly lower rates of onset both after the neonatal period within the first year (13.3%) and after the first year of life (26.6%), compared to 41.6% between 18 months and seven years (Toet et al., 2005).

After neonatal seizures, there is an overrepresentation of severe seizure types (Dennis, 1978), such as infantile spasms, reported in approximately 20-25% of cases (Khan et al., 2008; Pisani et al., 2012a), which seem to be more frequent after perinatal hypoxia, CNS malformation or infection (Watanabe et al., 1982). The occurrence of other syndromes, including EME (8.3%) and EIEE (4.2%) (Khan et al., 2008) is strongly determined by underlying etiology (Watanabe et al., 1982).

Additional seizure types include generalised (possibly partial with secondary generalization) and focal symptomatic seizures (Pisani et al., 2012a; Clancy and Legido, 1991; Khan et al., 2008; Watanabe et al., 1982), which often coexist in the same patient and may generally prove difficult to control (Pisani et al., 2012a; Glass HC et al., 2011). Older studies have also focused on seizure frequency as a measure of postneonatal epilepsy severity, reporting figures of more than one seizure per week in 26.9% of survivors from an intensive care unit (Bergman et al., 1983), and of more than one seizure per month or intractable seizures in 66.7% of a hospital-based series with very high rates of epilepsy (Ortibus et al., 1996).

Predictors of outcome

Factors determining or contributing to prognosis following neonatal seizures can be divided into four different groups:
- clinical variables concerning pre-perinatal history,
- clinical variables concerning brain injury,
- clinical variables concerning seizures characteristics,
- EEG variables.

Clinical variables concerning pre-perinatal history

These comprise factors pertaining to the birthing process and prenatal conditions which could affect outcome: gestational age, birth weight, mode of delivery, Apgar scores, need for resuscitation.

A role for gestational age has been confirmed in many cohorts since earlier studies, with the preterm babies faring significantly worse (Bergman et al., 1983; Holden et al., 1982; Ellison et al., 1981; Andre et al., 1988) and still showing a high mortality (37.1% in very preterm neonates of ≤ 32 wGA) following neonatal seizures (Pisani et al., 2012b). Population-based data reveal strikingly different rates for all reported outcomes: cerebral palsy (53% in preterm *versus* 17% in full-term neonates), epilepsy (40% *vs* 18%) and mental retardation (40% *vs* 14%) (Ronen et al., 2007).

Some authors have used birth weight, sometimes as an alternative to gestational age, advocating a lower error risk (Knauss and Marshall, 1977) and obtained positive results in terms of outcome prediction (Mellits et al., 1982; Ellison et al., 1981; Pisani et al., 2009; Seay and Bray 1977).

Apgar scores, need for resuscitation after 5 minutes (Mellits et al., 1982) and, in some cases, meconium aspiration (Garfinkle and Shevell, 2011b) have been used as perinatal variables mainly representing markers of hypoxic-ischemic injury, implying both an expression of a severity degree and of a specific aetiology (Holden et al., 1982). A correlation between muscle tone at 5 minutes and cerebral palsy was reported, whereas the respiration score was found to correlate with the later development of mental retardation (Holden et al., 1982).

Variables regarding brain injury

The outcome is also significantly related to the aetiology and the severity of the brain injury.

Aetiology of neonatal seizures represents the most important predictor of outcome, as outlined since earlier reports (McInemy and Schubert, 1969; Schulte, 1966; Keen and Lee, 1973). On the more favourable extreme of the spectrum, benign familial neonatal convulsions mainly carry a good prognosis (Ronen et al., 1993) (*Table I*).

Although very rare in current clinical practice, transient metabolic disturbances also carry a good outcome (McInerny and Schubert, 1969) and represent one of the reasons for the higher prevalence of normal survivors in older series. Among metabolic disturbances, only prolonged symptomatic hypoglycaemia might be associated with the development of relevant sequelae (Koivisto et al., 1972). Pyridoxine dependency has been associated with the later development of cognitive deficits, but a relevant role is played by early diagnosis and therapeutic intervention (Baxter, 2001).

Table I. Outcome of neonatal seizures according to etiology

Favourable outcome	Unfavourable outcome
Benign familial neonatal seizures	Meningitis
Transient acquired electrolytes disturbance (sodium, potassium, calcium, magnesium)	Intraventricular haemorrhage (depending on degree)
Isolated subarachnoid haemorrhage	Epileptic encephalopathies
Focal perinatal arterial ischemic stroke	Inborn errors of metabolism
	Congenital brain malformations (depending on underlying diagnosis)
	Prolonged hypoglycaemia
	Pyridoxine dependency

Tekgul *et al.*, 2006; Scher *et al.*, 1993; Legido *et al.*, 1991; Connel *et al.*, 1989; Lombroso 1983 and 1996; Bernes and Kaplan 1994; Klinger *et al.*, 2000.

On the opposite extreme of the spectrum, inborn errors of metabolism and epileptic encephalopathies are associated with a severe prognosis, whereas cortical malformations prognosis is poor (Tekgule *et al.*, 2006) and predicted by the specific diagnosis (Uria-Avellanal *et al.*, 2013).

Nevertheless, the great bulk of cases belong to either hypoxic-ischemic injury or to intraventricular haemorrhage, which imply a significant risk of subsequently altered development or death.

Injury severity, assessed by means of brain imaging, has been consistently linked to the subsequent outcome (Leijser *et al.*, 2006; Ment *et al.*, 2002) and grading systems have been developed for clinical and research aims. It has been repeatedly reported that a severely abnormal cerebral ultrasound scan is an independent predictor of outcome (Ronen *et al.*, 2007; Pisani *et al.*, 2007 and 2009), and this tool has proven very sensitive for detecting aetiologies carrying significant prognostic implications (Vollmer *et al.*, 2003). The presence of a global abnormality on neuroimaging (CT/MRI) has been found to be associated with unfavourable outcome in 100% and with epilepsy in 66% (Ortibus *et al.*, 1996) of the patients. MRI findings in the context of hypoxic-ischemic encephalopathy have been categorised according to the predominant pattern of injury, and these classification systems have been compared with outcomes and proven contributory to more accurate prognostication (Barkovich *et al.*, 1998).

Clinical variables concerning seizure characteristics

These clinical variables are the presence of electrographic seizures, the seizure duration, the response to treatment, the seizure semiology and the postnatal day at onset.

Interestingly, evidence has been gathered for an association between the presence of electrical seizure activity alone and higher rates of mortality and morbidity (Pisani *et al.*, 2012a; Bye *et al.*, 1997), and with the outcomes microcephaly, severe cerebral palsy, and failure to thrive, both in the whole study group and in the subgroup with asphyxia (McBride *et al.*, 2000). The short-term outcome in full-term neonates with hypoxic-ischemic encephalopathy treated for clinical and electrographic seizures or for clinical-only seizures demonstrated a trend towards longer seizure duration in the clinical-only group, and a correlation between seizure severity and MRI findings (van Rooij et al., 2010). Data on the long-term follow-up of patients with electrographic-only seizures *versus* both electrographic and electroclinical seizures are more contradictory, as one study reported the absence of any psychomotor deficits in the first group compared to a 54% prevalence of deficits in the second group (Kurul et al., 2009). Additional data would be required to shed light into this issue, as with the aid of continuous monitoring it is now apparent that electric seizures represent the vast majority of seizure burden in newborns (Murray et al., 2008).

Duration of clinical seizures, which some studies had tried to assess and variably use as prognostic indicator, including prolonged seizure activity, seizures lasting for more than one day, and repetitive seizures (Bergman et al., 1983; Ellison et al., 1981; Andre et al., 1988), has now been substituted by an evaluation of electrographic duration measurements, which will be treated in the paragraph dealing with EEG parameters.

Response to treatment might be another indicator of the outcome. The choice of the best way to measure seizure refractoriness has been dealt differently in various studies. For example, some authors found the need for multiple drugs to treat seizures as the variable correlating with a poor outcome (Ronen et al., 2007; Bergman et al., 1983; Andre et al., 1988) whereas in other instances, the time required to achieve seizure control was also evaluated, finding that no epilepsy developed if neonatal seizures ceased within 48 hours after birth and required no more than two antiepileptic drugs (Toet et al., 2005). Furthermore, in a cohort of neonates requiring at least two antiepileptic drugs, it was demonstrated that the failure to achieve seizure control, rather than the number of administered drugs correlated with an increased risk of poor outcome (van der Heide et al., 2012).

Seizure semiology has been originally studied in an attempt to correlate specific seizure types with prognosis. Although this link was initially confirmed in the setting of clinically diagnosed neonatal seizures, advocating an association between tonic seizures and poor outcome (Bergman et al., 1983; Mizrahi and Kellaway, 1987) and further implications for specific seizure types were reported in an intensive care series, separating subtle and generalised tonic from other seizure types on the basis of a worse prognosis in the former (Brunquell et al., 2002). Other authors have found that clonic seizures with no facial involvement in full-term infants carry a favourable prognosis (Ronen et al., 2007; Boylan et al., 1999), whereas generalized myoclonic seizures in preterm neonates are followed by a high mortality (Ronen et al., 2007). However, even when based on clinical diagnosis, such an association between seizure type and prognosis has not always been confirmed (Tekgul et al., 2007). Furthermore, when a more rigorous diagnosis of neonatal seizures is applied (requiring EEG confirmation), controversial data are collected for focal clonic *versus* non-clonic seizures (Garfinkle and Shevell 2011a; Nagarajan et al., 2012); even the presence of one or more seizure types has failed in consistently predicting outcome when seizure diagnosis is based on EEG (Pisani et al., 2009), in contrast with what was reported in earlier clinically defined series (Brunquell et al., 2002).

Similarly, postnatal day of seizures onset was more relevant in earlier studies (Holden et al., 1982; Mellits et al., 1982), possibly because it reflected different underlying aetiologies (Legido et al., 1991).

Predictors of epilepsy

Taken together, the aforementioned epidemiological data depict a clinical scenario in which epilepsy is interpretable, at least in part, as a marker of severity: patients with epilepsy, in the vast majority of cases, are also affected by cerebral palsy and mental retardation. Such an association has long been recognised, for example it was reported that only the presence of severe sequelae seems to predict seizure recurrence (Gal et al., 1984). Nevertheless, such an explanation, although presumably correct with the current knowledge, is likely to be incomplete, as neonatal seizures could also play an additive or synergistic effect to the one played by brain damage (Legido et al., 1991) and also have an epileptogenic role. In the present discussion, specific risk factors for the development of post-neonatal epilepsy have been subdivided into seizure-related and brain injury-related predictors, although seizure severity cannot be considered completely separated from the underlying brain damage.

When neonatal seizures diagnosis relied on clinical grounds, the number of days with neonatal seizures was found to predict later epilepsy (Holden et al., 1982) and especially when a frequency of more than 10 seizures per hour was present (Clancy and Legido, 1991). More recent studies have demonstrated the presence of neonatal status epilepticus to be highly predictive of the development of epilepsy (Pisani et al., 2007). On the other hand, patients who will later develop epilepsy present with a severely abnormal neurological examination and an abnormal background EEG (Legido et al., 1991), they are more likely to have severely abnormal ultrasound scans (Kato et al., 2010) and diffuse abnormalities in brain imaging (Ortibus et al., 1996). More precisely, children with severe brain injury are more likely to develop epilepsy. Where there is basal ganglia/thalamus predominant injury, epilepsy will be present in 20% of patients (Watanabe et al., 1982).

In patients with hypoxic-ischemic encephalopathy, some tools for prediction of specific seizure types have also been provided, because a severely abnormal background EEG has been associated with the development of myoclonic seizures (Watanabe et al., 1982), and a marked, prolonged depression (for at least 21 days) has been associated with infantile spasms in full-term or near-term newborns (Watanabe et al., 1982; Kato et al., 2010).

EEG variables related to outcome

The main objective while evaluating EEG in newborns is the definition of the background activity, which has proven as one of the most robust predictors of outcome, both in terms of death and later neurological development, whereas the presence of isolated sharp waves is of more limited prognostic value (Rowe et al., 1985). Both degree and duration of recorded abnormalities correlate with outcome (Connel et al., 1989). Of interest, the background activity has also proven more significant for outcome than ictal activity, and, in some studies, than organization of sleep states (Khan et al., 2008).

The detection of normal EEG activity usually bears a favourable outcome (Andre et al., 1988; Connel et al., 1989; Lombroso, 1996; Rowe et al., 1985): in 86% and 70% of cases in two different studies (Rose and Lombroso, 1970; Tibbles and Prichard, 1965). On the other hand, an abnormal EEG is predictive of poor prognosis: when abnormalities are marked (burst-suppression, persistent low voltage or isoelectric, periodic, multifocal) (Rowe et al., 1985; Lombroso, 1983; Rose and Lombroso, 1970) or moderate-severe an unfavourable outcome can be predicted (Legido et al., 1991; Pisani et al., 2008a). This holds particularly true when serial EEGs showing persistent abnormalities are recorded (Connel et al., 1989; Monod et al., 1972; Tharp et al., 1981). In fact, the predictive value of sequential EEGs is stronger than that of a single EEG recording (Khan et al., 2008).

More cautious conclusions should be driven from mildly abnormal background EEG (Tibbles and Prichard, 1965).

Ictal EEG variables are of more limited and controversial value in forecasting outcome. Nevertheless a lot of effort has been put into identifying the more relevant markers, generating a bulk of different cut-offs and measures, often of limited clinical usefulness, either being non-significant or, as already concluded by Connell *et al.*, (1989), providing helpful confirmation to background EEG analysis but not adding to it (*Table II*).

We will only discuss variables shown to be significant or approaching statistical significance in the relative studies.

Table II. Ictal EEG: Evaluated parameters

Related to frequency and topography of ictal discharges (controversial)
• Number of independent electrographic seizure foci
• Seizure discharges characteristics
• Diffusion of discharges
Related to seizure duration and seizure burden
Significant
• Presence of status epilepticus
Controversial
• Ictal Fraction
Insufficient data
• Periodic discharges fraction
• Seizure "severity"
• Seizure slope
Not significant
• Total number of seizures/recording
• Number of seizures/hour(epoch)
• Mean/maximum seizure duration
• Total seizure duration/epoch
• Maximum seizure frequency/day
• Maximum daily seizure duration
• Total EEG seizure duration
• % of each EEG tracing during which any channel shows EEG seizure activity
• Seizure Fraction

Rowe *et al.*, 1985; Legido *et al.*, 1991; Ortibus *et al.*, 1996; Bye *et al.*, 1997; Boylan *et al.*, 1999; Pisani *et al.*, 2007; van Rooij et al 2007; Glass *et al.*, 2011; Nagarajan *et al.*, 2011; Painter *et al.*, 2012.

Number of independent electrographic seizure foci

This parameter has been shown to correlate with outcome at one year of age (Bye *et al.*, 1997). A more recent study has failed to replicate this finding (Nagarajan *et al.*, 2011).

Seizure discharges characteristics

Ictal low frequency focal discharges and localised rhythmic activity have been associated with a worse prognosis, but they tend to occur in the context of an abnormal background (Rowe *et al.*, 1985). Low amplitude discharges are associated with increased mortality and a frequency < 2 Hz of ictal discharges was related with increased morbidity (Nagarajan *et al.*, 2011).

Diffusion of discharges

The contralateral spread of discharges has been related to an adverse outcome (Pisani *et al.*, 2008a), although this result was not reproduced (Nagarajan *et al.*, 2011).

Neonatal status epilepticus

Neonatal status epilepticus is predictive of outcome (Legido et al., 1991) in both full-term and preterm babies and a risk factor for epilepsy in full-term and preterm neonates of less than 29wGA, even when compared with recurrent seizures (Pisani et al., 2007). Its paramount prognostic relevance has been elucidated when, after adjusting for degree of encephalopathy and severity of brain injury, it proved still independently associated with epilepsy (Glass et al., 2011), because this represents a successful attempt to distinguish between an interpretation of status as solely a marker of brain injury severity and the existence of a specific contribution at least to epileptogenesis.

In newborns with hypoxic-ischemic encephalopathy and neonatal status epilepticus, longer duration predicts worse neurodevelopmental outcome and, even if duration of neonatal status epilepticus was not related to outcome in the whole group, it was predictive of outcome in the group with hypoxic-ischemic encephalopathy (van Rooij et al., 2007).

Ictal fraction

The ictal fraction is obtained as the ratio between the total duration of seizures in an EEG and the total duration of the EEG recording per hour. This parameter significantly relates to outcome if longer than 10 minutes (Pisani et al., 2008a). It was designed to provide information independently of absolute EEG duration, so that a wider application in different clinical settings could be possible, providing clear prognostic information and a measure of seizure severity even in case of unavailability of continuous monitoring. However when tested in subsequent studies, a correlation with outcome has not been demonstrated (Nagarajan et al., 2011).

Periodic discharges fraction

This is calculated as the percentage of paroxysmal complexes separated by nearly identical intervals between individual recurrent discharges lasting $\leq$ 10 seconds. It correlates with outcome in univariate analysis (Ortibus et al., 1996).

Severity of individual seizure and seizure slope

Severity of individual seizure is defined as the duration of epileptiform activity in each channel of a standard neonatal montage summed across all channels being active during the seizure, whereas seizure slope is the direction of seizure severity over time prior to treatment.

A mild to moderate seizure severity and a decreasing severity over time are more likely to be associated by a normal or moderately abnormal outcome, whereas if the maximum seizure severity is observed after treatment an adverse outcome is reported to be predictable (Painter et al., 2012).

Number of seizures/hour

This parameter approached significance for the outcome epilepsy and, if less than two seizures per hour were detected in patients with asphyxia, was associated with a favourable outcome in 100% of the patients in a single study (Legido et al., 1991).

Creation and testing of prediction models

In an effort to define prognosis early-on, scoring systems based on readily available clinical variables have been developed. The first one to be proposed (Ellison et al., 1981) was constructed on the basis of the available scientific literature with the aims to identify outcome predictors, to aid treatment decision and to provide a basis for data comparison and to uniform practice between different centres. Data collected in the neonatal period were compared with those pertaining to 3 and 10 months of age. The scored predictive variables in the neonatal period comprised abnormalities on EEG, neurological examination, etiology and type of seizures and birth weight, whereas at 3 months these did not include type of seizures but the presence or absence of seizures since discharge. It was shown that all variables at initial scoring (but seizure duration) predicted mental development, motor function and epilepsy at 10 months and that all scores at 3 months predicted the same outcomes at 10 months, the probability levels being more significant at 3 months of age. Thus, on this basis, the Authors also provided practice guidance for antiepileptic therapy discontinuation. This preliminary study was then validated on a larger cohort (Ellison et al., 1986).

More than 20 years later, a second scoring system was proposed (Pisani et al., 2009) and tested in a cohort of both preterm and full-term infants. In comparison to the previous proposal, it carried some relevant innovations in the choice of scored variables: aside from birth weight, neurological examination and background EEG activity, it included the clinical parameters Apgar score at one minute, efficacy of anticonvulsant therapy and presence or absence of status epilepticus. Moreover, due to its widespread availability on neonatal wards, it also included brain imaging data in the form of ultrasound brain scan findings. The predictive variables, once scored for increasing severity, were then combined to obtain two different outcome prediction models, one excluding and the second including EEG data. Unlike for its predecessor, for this scoring system sensitivity, specificity and positive and negative predictive values (PPV and NPV, respectively) were calculated.

When the cut-off is set at 4, the first prediction model, with a maximum possible total score of 12, has shown a specificity of 85.7%, a specificity of 80.6% (Table III), whereas the second (maximum total score of 13), when a cut-off of 5 is considered, demonstrates a sensitivity of 81.4%, a specificity of 83.3%, a PPV of 90.5% and a NPV of 69.8%, being a better predictor of adverse than of good outcome (Pisani et al., 2009).

A third prediction model has then been proposed, only testing variables and assessing outcome in term infants (Garfinkle and Shevell, 2011c). Based on the evaluation of mode of delivery, time of seizure onset, seizure type, EEG background, and etiology, each categorised to obtain a maximum possible score of 5, it provides the best prognostic reliability when the cut-off is set at 3 (Table III).

Application of these useful tools, relatively simple, in different clinical settings for research aims could enable validation and definition of their reproducibility.

Future perspectives

In the future, the most important factors potentially modifying outcome after neonatal seizures will comprise increased survival of preterm neonates of lower gestational ages and birth weights, possible long-term effects of therapeutic hypothermia on newborns with hypoxic-ischemic encephalopathy, introduction of new antiepileptic drugs with a

Table III. Comparison of the three scoring systems for prognostic assessment after neonatal seizures

Study design	Ellison et al.	Pisani et al.	Garfinkle and Shevell
Subjects (n)	96	106	120
NS diagnosis	clinical	EEG-confirmed	clinical
Included gestational ages	N/A	FT, PT	FT
Follow-up duration	10 mo	2 y	Minimum: 2 y (1 y if normal) Median: 3.5 y if normal and 6 y if abnormal
Analysed outcome	E, MR, motor dysfunction	Favourable/unfavourable (death, CP, E, visual/hearing impairment)	Death, CP, E, GDD
Independent predictors	EEG, neurological examination, etiology, seizure type, BW < or > 1,500 g	BW, 1 min Apgar score, neurological examination, cerebral USS, AEDs efficacy, NSE.	Delivery, time of seizure onset, seizure type, EEG background, etiology
Model fitness	N/A	AUC: 0.917 (95% CI: 0.858-0.975 p < 0.001) Cut-off:4 Se: 85.7%, Sp: 80.6%, PPV: 89.6% NPV: 74.4%	AUC: 0.876 (95% CI: 0.810-0.943 p < 0.001) Cut-off ≥ 3: Se: 81.1%, Sp: 84%, PPV: 84.3%, NPV: 80.8%

AED: antiepileptic drug; AUC: area under the curve; BW: birth-weight; CI: confidence interval; CP: cerebral palsy; E: epilepsy; EEG: electroencephalogram; FT: full-term; g: grams; GDD: global developmental delay; mo: months; MR: mental retardation; (n): number; N/A: not available; NPV: negative predictive value; NS: neonatal seizures; NSE: neonatal status epilepticus; PPV: positive predictive value; PT: preterm; Se: sensitivity; Sp: specificity; USS: ultrasound scan; y: years.

mechanism of action closer to neonatal physiology and possibly used in combination with neuroprotective or antioxidant agents, which could all favour a change in the rate and severity of long-term sequelae. On the other hand, improved monitoring of high-risk newborns could lead to an implementation of prognostication tools, enabling physicians to promptly start the appropriate multidisciplinary follow-up.

Additionally, the medical approach to disability is changing as health-related quality of life measures are increasingly taken into account, with a potential to provide complementary information to be included in outcome evaluation for a better understanding of relevant treatment goals in this complex patients population (Ronen and Rosenbaum, 2013).

References

- Andre M, Matisse N, Vert P, Debruille C. Neonatal seizures-recent aspects. *Neuropediatrics* 1988; 19: 201-7.
- Barkovich AJ, Hajnal BL, Vigneron D, Sola A, Partridge JC, Allen F, et al. Prediction of neuromotor outcome in perinatal asphyxia: evaluation of MR scoring systems. *Am J Neuroradiol* 1988; 19: 143-9.

- Baxter P. Pyridoxine-dependent and pyridoxine-responsive seizures. *Dev Med Child Neurol* 2001; 43: 416-20.
- Bergman I, Painter MJ, Hirsch RP, Crumrine PK, David R. Outcome in neonates with convulsions treated in an intensive care unit. *Ann Neurol* 1983; 14: 642-7.
- Bernes SM, Kaplan AM. Evolution of neonatal seizures. *Pediatr Clin North Am* 1994; 41: 1069-104.
- Boylan GB, Pressler RM, Rennie JM, Morton M, Leow PL, Hughes R, et al. Outcome of electroclinical, electrographic, and clinical seizures in the newborn infant. *Dev Med Child Neurol* 1999; 41: 819-25.
- Brunquell PJ, Glennon CM, DiMario FJ Jr, Lerer T, Eisenfeld L. Prediction of outcome based on clinical seizure type in newborn infants. *J Pediatr* 2002; 140: 707-12.
- Burke JB. The prognostic significance of neonatal seizures. *Arch Dis Child* 1954; 29: 342-5.
- Bye AM, Cunningham CA, Chee KY, Flanagan D. Outcome of neonates with electrographically identified seizures, or at risk of seizures. *Pediatr Neurol* 1997; 16: 225-31.
- Clancy RR, Legido A. Postnatal epilepsy after EEG-confirmed neonatal seizures. *Epilepsia* 1991; 32: 69-76.
- Connell J, Oozeer R, de Vries L, Dubowitz LM, Dubowitz V. Continuous EEG monitoring of neonatal seizures: diagnostic and prognostic considerations. *Arch Dis Child* 1989; 64: 452-8.
- Craig WS. Convulsive movements occurring in the first 10 days of life. *Arch Dis Child* 1960; 35: 336-44.
- Dennis J. Neonatal convulsions: aetiology, late neonatal status and long-term outcome. *Dev Med Child Neurol* 1978; 20: 143-8.
- Ellison PH, Largent JA, Bahr JP. A scoring system to predict outcome following neonatal seizures. *J Pediatr* 1981; 99: 455-9.
- Ellison PH, Horn JL, Franklin S, Jones MG. The results of checking a scoring system for neonatal seizures. *Neuropediatrics* 1986; 17: 152-7.
- Gal P, Sharpless MK, Boer HR. Outcome in neonates with seizures: are chronic anticonvulsants necessary? *Ann Neurol* 1984; 15: 610-1.
- Garfinkle J, Shevell MI. Cerebral palsy, developmental delay, and epilepsy after neonatal seizures. *Pediatr Neurol* 2011a; 44: 88-96.
- Garfinkle J, Shevell MI. Predictors of outcome in term infants with neonatal seizures subsequent to intrapartum asphyxia. *J Child Neurol* 2011b; 26: 453-9.
- Garfinkle J, Shevell MI. Prognostic factors and development of a scoring system for outcome of neonatal seizures in term infants. *Eur J Paediatr Neurol* 2011c; 15: 222-9.
- Glass HC, Hong KJ, Rogers EE, Jeremy RJ, Bonifacio SL, Sullivan JE, et al. Risk factors for epilepsy in children with neonatal encephalopathy. *Pediatr Res* 2011; 70: 535-40.
- Harris R, Tizard JP. The electroencephalogram in neonatal convulsions. *J Pediatr* 1960; 57: 501-20.
- Holden KR, Mellits ED, Freeman JM. Neonatal seizures. I. Correlation of prenatal and perinatal events with outcomes. *Pediatrics* 1982; 70: 165-76.
- Kato T, Okumura A, Hayakawa F, Tsuji T, Hayashi S, Kubota T, et al. Prolonged EEG depression in term and near-term infants with hypoxic ischemic encephalopathy and later development of West syndrome. *Epilepsia* 2010; 51: 2392-6.
- Keen JH, Lee D. Sequelae of neonatal convulsions. Study of 112 infants. *Arch Dis Child* 1973; 48: 542-6.
- Khan RL, Nunes ML, Garcias da Silva LF, da Costa JC. Predictive value of sequential electroencephalogram (EEG) in neonates with seizures and its relation to neurological outcome. *J Child Neurol* 2008; 23: 144-50.

- Klinger G, Chin CN, Beyene J, Perlman M. Predicting the outcome of neonatal bacterial meningitis. *Pediatrics* 2000; 106: 477-82.
- Knauss T, Marshall RE. Seizures in a neonatal intensive care unit. *Dev Med Child Neurol* 1977; 19: 719-28.
- Koivisto M, Blanco-Sequeiros M, Krause U. Neonatal symptomatic and asymptomatic hypoglycaemia: a follow-up study of 151 children. *Dev Med Child Neurol* 1972; 14: 603-14.
- Kurul SH, Sutcuoglu S, Yis U, Duman N, Kumral A, Ozkan H. The relationship of neonatal subclinical electrographic seizures to neurodevelopmental outcome at 1 year of age. *J Matern Fetal Neonatal Med* 2009; 22: 584-8.
- Legido A, Clancy RR, Berman PH. Neurologic outcome after electroencephalographically proven neonatal seizures. *Pediatrics* 1991; 88: 583-96.
- Leijser LM, de Vries LS, Cowan FM. Using cerebral ultrasound effectively in the newborn infant. *Early Hum Dev* 2006; 82: 827-35.
- Lombroso CT. Prognosis in neonatal seizures. *Adv Neurol* 1983; 34: 101-13.
- Lombroso CT. Neonatal seizures: a clinician's overview. *Brain Dev* 1996; 18: 1-28.
- McBride MC, Laroia N, Guillet R. Electrographic seizures in neonates correlate with poor neurodevelopmental outcome. *Neurology* 2000; 55: 506-13.
- McInerny TK, Schubert WK. Prognosis of neonatal seizures. *Am J Dis Child* 1969; 117: 261-4.
- Mellits ED, Holden KR, Freeman JM. Neonatal seizures. II. A multivariate analysis of factors associated with outcome. *Pediatrics* 1982; 70: 177-85.
- Ment LR, Bada HS, Barnes P, Grant PE, Hirtz D, Papile LA, *et al*. Practice parameter: neuroimaging of the neonate: report of the Quality Standards Subcommittee of the American Academy of Neurology and the Practice Committee of the Child Neurology Society. *Neurology* 2002; 58: 1726-38.
- Mizrahi EM, Kellaway P. Characterization and classification of neonatal seizures. *Neurology* 1987; 37: 1837-44.
- Monod N, Pajot N, Guidasci S. The neonatal EEG: statistical studies and prognostic value in full-term and pre-term babies. *Electroencephalogr Clin Neurophysiol* 1972; 32: 529-44.
- Murray DM, Boylan GB, Ali I, Ryan CA, Murphy BP, Connolly S. Defining the gap between electrographic seizure burden, clinical expression and staff recognition of neonatal seizures. *Arch Dis Child Fetal Neonatal Ed* 2008; 93: F187-91.
- Nagarajan L, Ghosh S, Palumbo L. Ictal electroencephalogram in neonatal seizures: characteristics and associations. *Pediatr Neurol* 2011; 45: 11-6.
- Nagarajan L, Ghosh S, Palumbo L. Classification of clinical semiology in epileptic seizures in neonates. *Eur J Paediatr Neurol* 2012; 16: 118-25.
- Ortibus EL, Sum JM, Hahn JS. Predictive value of EEG for outcome and epilepsy following neonatal seizures. *Electroencephalogr Clin Neurophysiol* 1996; 98: 175-85.
- Painter MJ, Sun Q, Scher MS, Janosky J, Alvin J. Neonates with seizures: what predicts development? *J Child Neurol* 2012; 27: 1022-6.
- Pisani F, Cerminara C, Fusco C, Sisti L. Neonatal status epilepticus vs recurrent neonatal seizures: clinical findings and outcome. *Neurology* 2007; 69: 2177-85.
- Pisani F, Copioli C, Di Gioia C, Turco E, Sisti L. Neonatal seizures: relation of ictal video-electroencephalography (EEG) findings with neurodevelopmental outcome. *J Child Neurol* 2008a; 23: 394-8.
- Pisani F, Barilli AL, Sisti L, Bevilacqua G, Seri S. Preterm infants with video-EEG confirmed seizures: outcome at 30 months of age. *Brain Dev* 2008b; 30: 20-30.
- Pisani F, Sisti L, Seri S. A scoring system for early prognostic assessment after neonatal seizures. *Pediatrics* 2009; 124: 580-7.

- Pisani F, Piccolo B, Cantalupo G, Copioli C, Fusco C, Pelosi A, et al. Neonatal seizures and postneonatal epilepsy: a 7-y follow-up study. *Pediatr Res* 2012a; 72: 186-93.
- Pisani F, Copioli C, Turco EC, Sisti L, Cossu G, Seri S. Mortality risk after neonatal seizures in very preterm newborns. *J Child Neurol* 2012b; 27: 1264-9.
- Ronen GM, Rosales TO, Connolly M, Anderson VE, Leppert M. Seizure characteristics in chromosome 20 benign familial neonatal convulsions. *Neurology* 1993; 43: 1355-60.
- Ronen GM, Buckley D, Penney S, Streiner DL. Long-term prognosis in children with neonatal seizures: a population-based study. *Neurology* 2007; 69: 1816-22.
- Ronen GM, Rosenbaum PL. *Concepts and perspectives of "health" and "life quality" outcomes in children and young people with neurological and developmental conditions.* In: Ronen GM, Rosenbaum PL, eds. Life quality outcomes in children and young people with neurological and developmental conditions: concepts, evidence and practice (Chapter 2). Clinics in Developmental Medicine No. 196. London: Mac Keith Press; 2013.
- Rose AL, Lombroso CT. A study of clinical, pathological, and electroencephalographic features in 137 full-term babies with a long-term follow-up. *Pediatrics* 1970; 45: 404-25.
- Rowe JC, Holmes GL, Hafford J, Baboval D, Robinson S, Philipps A, et al. Prognostic value of the electroencephalogram in term and preterm infants following neonatal seizures. *Electroencephalogr Clin Neurophysiol* 1985; 60: 183-96.
- Scher MS, Painter MJ. Controversies concerning neonatal seizures. *Pediatr Clin North Am* 1989; 36: 281-310.
- Scher MS, Aso K, Beggarly ME, Hamid MY, Steppe DA, Painter MJ. Electrographic seizures in preterm and full-term neonates: clinical correlates, associated brain lesions, and risk for neurologic sequelae. *Pediatrics* 1993; 91: 128-34.
- Scher MS. Seizures in the newborn infant. Diagnosis, treatment, and outcome. *Clin Perinatalogy* 1997; 24: 735-72.
- Schulte FJ. Neonatal convulsions and their relation to epilepsy in early childhood. *Dev Med Child Neurol* 1966; 8: 381-92.
- Seay AR, Bray PF. Significance of seizures in infants weighing less than 2,500 grams. *Arch Neurol* 1977; 34: 381-2.
- Tharp BR, Cukier F, Monod N. The prognostic value of the electroencephalogram in premature infants. *Electroencephalogr Clin Neurophysiol* 1981; 51: 219-36.
- Temple CM, Dennis J, Carney R, Sharich J. Neonatal seizures: long-term outcome and cognitive development among "normal" survivors. *Dev Med Child Neurol* 1985; 37: 109-18.
- Tibbles JA, Prichard JS. The prognostic value of the electroencephalogram in neonatal convulsions. *Pediatrics* 1965; 35: 778-86.
- Tekgul H, Gauvreau K, Soul J, Murphy L, Robertson R, Stewart J, et al. The current etiologic profile and neurodevelopmental outcome of seizures in term newborn infants. *Pediatrics* 2006; 117: 1270-80.
- Toet MC, Groenendaal F, Osredkar D, van Huffelen AC, de Vries LS. Postneonatal epilepsy following amplitude-integrated EEG-detected neonatal seizures. *Pediatr Neurol* 2005; 32: 241-7.
- Uria-Avellanal C, Marlow N, Rennie JM. Outcome following neonatal seizures. *Semin Fetal Neonatal Med* 2013; 18: 224-32.
- van Rooij LG, Toet MC, van Huffelen AC, Groenendaal F, Laan W, Zecic A, et al. Effect of treatment of subclinical neonatal seizures detected with aEEG: randomized, controlled trial. *Pediatrics* 2010; 125: 358-66.
- van Rooij LG, de Vries LS, Handryastuti S, Hawani D, Groenendaal F, van Huffelen AC, et al. Neurodevelopmental outcome in term infants with status epilepticus detected with amplitude-integrated electroencephalography. *Pediatrics* 2007; 120: 354-63.

- van der Heide MJ, Roze E, van der Veere CN, Ter Horst HJ, Brouwer OF, Bos AF. Long-term neurological outcome of term-born children treated with two or more anti-epileptic drugs during the neonatal period. *Early Hum Dev* 2012; 88: 33-8.
- Vollmer B, Roth S, Baudin J, Stewart AL, Neville BG, Wyatt JS. Predictors of long-term outcome in very preterm infants: gestational age versus neonatal cranial ultrasound. *Pediatrics* 2003; 112: 1108-14.
- Watanabe K, Kuroyanagi M, Hara K, Miyazaki S. Neonatal seizures and subsequent epilepsy. *Brain Dev* 1982; 4: 341-6.

The epidemiology of infancy onset seizures

Christin Eltze

Great Ormond Street Hospital for Children, UCL Institute of Child Health, London, UK

Epileptic seizures in infancy can present as provoked seizures in close time association with brain insults or injuries (inflicted by trauma, CNS infections, cerebrovascular events, etc.). Such brain insults in early life are a risk factor for epilepsy, defined as a disorder with high risk of recurrent unprovoked seizures, manifesting in later life following variable latency periods. Seizures provoked by fever occur especially frequently in the first year of life (Verity *et al.*, 1985). On a population level the risk of later epilepsy is small (Verity and Golding, 1991). However, in a subgroup of infants febrile seizures may be early manifestations of specific electroclinical syndromes, which will be discussed in more detail in a later chapter (Scheffer *et al.*, this volume, page 205).

Epilepsies with onset in infancy demonstrate great heterogeneity with respect to underlying aetiologies, phenotypes and outcomes. Information in the literature about subgroups, defined either by electroclinical or aetiological features, especially lately by monogenetic disorders, is increasing. Frequently the reported case series originate from hospital or specialist clinic settings and may not be representative of the general population. Considering the advances in development of diagnostic tools especially neuroimaging there is a paucity of recent data describing the entire epilepsy infancy group in a population based setting.

Such data are important to streamline investigation resources for more effective use and to target the group of infants that might benefit most from early therapeutic interventions.

In the following data from a recent population based infancy onset cohort are summarised in the context of data from *childhood epilepsy cohorts* that are composed of infants *and* older children (epilepsy onset 1 month to 16 years).

■ Incidence of newly onset of epilepsy in the first 12 and 24 months of life

The annual incidence estimates of epilepsy onset in childhood in developed countries vary between 38 to 60/100,000 in recent publications (Sillanpaa, 2003; Olafsson *et al.*, 1996; Camfield *et al.*, 1996; Freitag *et al.*, 2001; Olafsson *et al.*, 2005; Larsson and Eeg-Olofsson, 2006). Furthermore it has been well documented that childhood epilepsy onset is most common in the first year of life. Few data are available in the literature with respect to the incidence of epilepsy in children under the age of two years because most epilepsy incidence studies provide age specific data only for the age group less than one year and summarize data in larger age bands (e.g. 1-4 years, 5-9 years, etc.).

The incidence estimates of epilepsy onset in the first year of life in studies conducted in developed countries demonstrate great variability (79-256/100,000/year, see Table I). Some have large confident intervals because of small case numbers (Blom et al., 1978; Olafsson et al., 1996; Freitag et al., 2001). Both geographical and methodological differences including prospective or retrospective study design, ascertainment methods, and case definitions account for the variations of incidence rates. The possibility of case under ascertainment in studies that recruit cases from the populations living in the catchment area of a hospital and/or EEG department using attendance registers as the single source cannot be excluded.

The "North London Epilepsy in Infancy study" is the only study that applied a two-source capture-recapture analysis to adjust ascertainment (Eltze et al., 2013). Infants aged 1 to 24 months with newly diagnosed epilepsy and resident in a defined area of North London (UK) were prospectively notified by hospital and community based paediatricians using direct and indirect notification methods (monthly postal survey, 24 hour telephone hotline). The ascertainment adjusted incidence was 70.1 (95% CI [56.3, 88.5])/100,000 children $< = 2$ years/year, with 76% completeness of ascertainment. Considering the methodological differences that limit comparability this finding is similar to figures that can be derived from two older studies of wider childhood cohorts using single source ascertainment; 81 (95% CI [67, 93])/100,000 children < 2 years/year from a Canadian study (cases identified from regional EEG department) (Camfield et al., 1996), and 61 (95% CI [39, 95])/100,000 children < 2 years/year from the UK 1958 National Child Development Study (screening questionnaires to families enrolled in birth cohort) (Kurtz et al., 1998).

In line with previous investigators the "North London Epilepsy in Infancy study" demonstrated a higher incidence rate of epilepsy in the first year (crude incidence infants < 12 months: 82.1 (95% CI [61.4, 109.8])/100,000/year) compared to the second year of life (infants age 12-24 months: (23.4 (95% CI [13.3, 40.8])/100,000/year), see Figures 1 and 2). The risk presenting with epilepsy in the first 12 months of life was over two times higher compared to second year of life (risk ratio for epilepsy between the "< 12 months" and "12-24 months" groups: 2.33 (95% CI [1.44, 3.76]; $p < 0.005$). These data lend further support to observations in animal models demonstrating increased susceptibility for seizures in the immature brain that result in manifestation of a wide spectrum of pathologies in the first year of life (Haut et al., 2004). The reduced risk in the second year may reflect maturation of inhibitory mechanisms within the neuronal networks that result in an increased seizure threshold.

Little information is available in the literature with respect to the interaction of ethnicity and incidence of epilepsy. Most epilepsy incidence studies were conducted in white European populations or populations with European ancestry whilst studies based in Asia and Africa were looking at relatively homogeneous groups. Some US based studies suggest higher epilepsy prevalence and incidence in the black compared to the white population (Shamansky and Glaser, 1979; Haerer et al., 1986). There is also a suggestion of an age specific relationship between unprovoked seizures and ethnicity. Annegers et al. determined the incidence of epilepsy and unprovoked seizures in members of a multiethnic Health Maintenance Organization using a nested case-control study (Annegers et al., 1999). An

Author, year of publication	Ascertainment period	Country	Case definition	Case ascertainment	Age specific incidence: < 1 year/ 100,000/year, (case numbers)	95% CI
Blom et al., 1978	1973-1974	Sweden	1 or more unprovoked seizures	Retrospective – catchment area approach, using data/records from hospital EEG department, single EEG-service provider in area, follow up of cohort, letter + phone contact	95.7 (3)	32.5-281
Doose et al., 1983	Children born 1957-1966	Germany, Kiel	> 1 unprovoked seizure	Catchment area approach, information obtained retrospectively from hospital records (epilepsy centre)	201.6 (76)	Not available
Verity et al., 1992	Birth cohort one week 1970	United Kingdom	1 or more afebrile seizures	Prospective follow up of birth cohort, screening questionnaire with information subsequently obtained from GP's and hospital records	160 (23)	107-240
Hauser et al., 1993	1935-984	US, Rochester, Minnesota	> 1 unprovoked seizure	Retrospective, information form diagnostic record system	86 (36)	62-119
Braathen et al., 1995	1990-1992	Sweden	> 1 unprovoked seizure	Prospective, catchment area of hospital, epilepsy team	0-2 years: 70 (14)	Not available
Camfield et al., 1996	1977-1985	Canada, Nova Scotia	> 1 unprovoked seizures	Retrospective, catchment area of hospital EEG department	118 (112)	98-143
Olafsson et al., 1996	1993	Iceland	> 1 unprovoked seizure	Retrospective, records of healthcare centres, local hospitals, paediatricians + neurologists contacted	256.5 (4)	99.7-657
Kurtz et al., 1998	Birth cohort one week 1958	United Kingdom	> 1 disturbances of consciousness, not associated with acute fever	Prospective follow up of birth cohort, screening questionnaire with information subsequently obtained from GP's and hospital records	90 (14)	43-38
Freitag et al., 2001	1999	Germany, Heidelberg + Manheim	> 1 unprovoked seizure	Prospective, involving EEG departments, 2 university hospitals and office paediatricians (contacted by letters and phone calls)	146 (5)	47.4-340.1

Table I (continued). Incidence estimates of newly onset epilepsy in the first 1 years of life

Author, year of publication	Ascertainment period	Country	Case definition	Case ascertainment	Age specific incidence: < 1 year / 100,000/year, (case numbers)	95% CI
Olafsson et al., 2005	1995-1999	Iceland	> 1 unprovoked seizure	Prospective, country wide surveillance system – of all healthcare facilities (hospitals, A&E's, EEG departments, radiology departments, etc.)	79.5 (11)	44-132
Durá-Travé et al., 2008	2002-2005	Spain, Navarre	> 1 unprovoked seizure	Prospective, catchment area of children's hospital in (only neuropaediatric department in Navarre area, health care centres and other hospitals in area refer patients with seizures or suspected diagnosis of epilepsy)	95.3 (22)	82.8-107.8
Wirrell et al., 2011	1980-2004	US, Olmsted County, Minnesota	> 1 unprovoked seizures or 1 unprovoked seizures + EEG, neuroimaging or abnormal neurology suggesting enduring predisposition to seizures	Retrospective, search of Rochester Epidemiology Project diagnostic index data base, incidence date – date of diagnosis, data obtained by review of medical files	102.4 (50)	Not available
Eltze et al., 2013	2005-2006	North London, United Kingdom	> 1 unprovoked seizure	Prospective survey of defined geographical area, monthly postal survey and notification by phone/verbal/e-mail, 2 source capture–recapture analysis applied for ascertainment adjustment of case numbers (76% ascertainment)	Crude: 82.1(45) Adjusted: 102.2	Crude: 61.4-109.8 Adjusted: 78.7-132.6
Casetta et al., 2012	1996-2005	Italy, province of Ferrara	> 1 unprovoked seizure	Prospective case registry: hospital based paediatric neurologists + paediatricians (Ferrara university hospital, Lagosanto hospital), outpatients medical records, EEG department, ICD9 code search of hospital discharges, community based paediatricians asked to notify cases	109.4 (23)	69.4-164.1

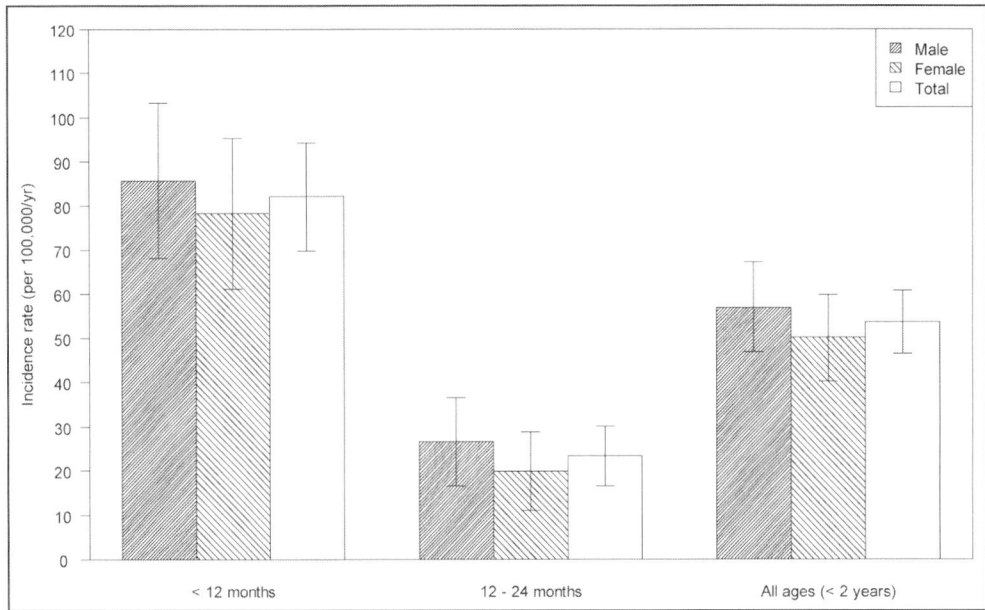

Figure 1. North London Epilepsy in Infancy Study. Age specific incidence rates of epilepsy by sex (bars illustrate 95% CI) (From Eltze et al., 2013, with the kind permission of the journal).

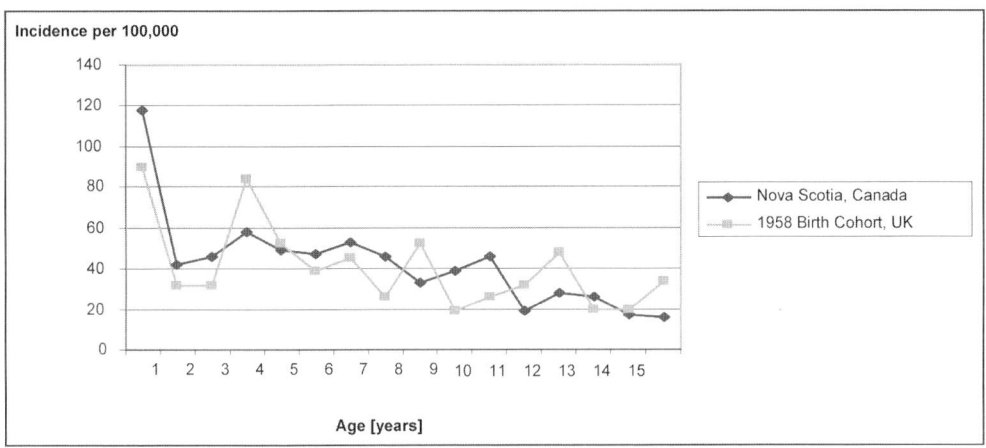

Figure 2. Age specific incidences of childhood epilepsy cohorts based on data from Camfield et al., 1996 and Kurtz et al., 1998.

effect was only demonstrated in young children under the age of 5 years with the risk for first unprovoked seizures being higher for "African-Americans" and "Hispanics" (1.69, 95% CI: 0.73-3.94 and 1.81, 95% CI 0.76-4.32 respectively) compared to the "White" reference group.

The multi-ethnic population of North London provided a setting to investigate the association between ethnicity and infancy onset epilepsy. Data from the "North London Epilepsy in Infancy" incidence cohort showed that Asian infants (including children from

Indian, Pakistani, and Bangladeshi origin) had 3 times higher risk of presenting with epilepsy compared to the "White" group, whilst the risk was not significantly higher in other non-white ethnic groups ("Black" or "Mixed Asian and White") (Eltze et al., 2013).

In a separate study carried out in the same population setting of North London Chin et al. also demonstrated an almost 3 times higher risk of febrile status epilepticus in Asian children compared to the other ethnic groups. The association to epilepsy and ethnicity was less apparent because of the small number of incidence cases related to an underlying diagnosis of epilepsy enrolled in this particular study (NLSTEPSS) (Chin et al., 2006; Chin et al., 2009).

These variations in seizure susceptibility between different ethnic groups are most likely determined by interaction of genetic and environmental factors which require further delineation.

From a global perspective the majority of people with epilepsy live in poor countries (~ 85%) where the reported incidence is higher, 81.7 per 100,000/year in low to middle-income countries compared to 45 in high-income countries (Ngugi et al., 2011; Newton and Garcia, 2012). Although a number of studies from low income countries provide some age specific incidence estimates, data for the first year of life are not specified (Tekle-Haimanot et al., 1997; Mani et al., 1998; Ngugi et al., 2013). The lack of infrastructure especially in rural areas including hospital, clinic registries or regular census data make it difficult to conduct incidence studies and prevalence studies are more practical using survey questionnaires applied by non-medically trained research personnel (Newton and Garcia, 2012). The major difficulty impacting on data collection in infants and very young children is the challenge to differentiate between provoked (febrile or acute CNS infection related seizures) and unprovoked seizures reliably enough to confirm the diagnosis of epilepsy in such settings.

■ How frequently and which electroclinical syndromes are identified?

The most recent proposal for revised terminology and organisation of seizures and epilepsies lists 11 electroclinical syndromes with onset in neonatal period and infancy (*Table II*) (Berg et al., 2010). Many are associated with medication resistant seizures and developmental/cognitive impairments (epileptic encephalopathy) in most patients. A milder course with typically good outcome in the majority of patients can be expected in 4 syndromes.

Information in the literature about the distribution of electroclinical syndromes in a population based setting is limited. One reason is that new infancy onset syndromes have been delineated and added to more recent revisions of the ILAE classification (*i.e.* benign infantile and benign familial infantile epilepsy added in 2001, malignant migrating partial seizures in infancy "considered" in 2001 and added in 2010), which have not been considered in studies applying older classification versions (Engel Jr., 2001; Berg et al., 2010). It is also important to take into account that in prevalence cohorts more severe types of epilepsy associated with higher mortality may be under-represented.

In wider childhood epilepsy cohorts (age 1 month to 15 or 16 years) West syndrome with the typical defining seizure type is most commonly identified (3.7-8%), whilst early infantile epileptic encephalopathy (EIEE) and early myoclonic epileptic encephalopathy (EME) are reported in less than 1% (prevalence studies [Larsson and Eeg-Olofsson, 2006; Oka et al., 2006]), Dravet syndrome (DS) in 1.6 to 2.9% (Dura-Trave et al., 2008; Larsson and

Table II. Electroclinical syndromes – List according to ILAE proposal 2010 (Berg et al., 2010)

Onset in neonatal period	Onset in infancy
Poor outcome in the majority of patients: – Early myoclonic encephalopathy (EME) – Ohtahara syndrome/early infantile epileptic encephalopathy (EIEE)	*Poor outcome in the majority of patients:* – West syndrome – Epilepsy of infancy with migrating focal seizures – Dravet syndrome – Myoclonic encephalopathy in non-progressive disorders
Less severe or benign course in the majority of patients: – Benign familial neonatal epilepsy (BFNE) – Benign neonatal seizures (no traditionally diagnosed as epilepsy)	*Variably severe disease course:* – Febrile seizures *plus* (FS+) – Myoclonic epilepsy in infancy (MEI) *Less severe or benign course in the majority of patients:* – Benign infantile epilepsy – Benign familial infantile epilepsy

Eeg-Olofsson, 2006). The incidence of infantile spasms/West syndrome has been reported by a number of studies between 2.9-4.7 per 10,000 live births (Trevathan et al., 1999; Riikonen and Donner, 1979; Sidenvall and Eeg-Olofsson, 1995). In contrast the incidence for EIEE was estimated in one retrospective study from Japan at 0.1 per 10,000 live births (Hino-Fukuyo et al., 2009). "Epilepsy of infancy with migrating focal seizures" (migrating partial epilepsy in infancy, MPSI) appears to be a particular rare syndrome with an approximated incidence of 0.55/100,000 (McTague et al., 2013). These rare syndromes may, however, be under-reported as some patients may show further evolution to West syndrome/infantile spasms.

A recent study approximated the incidence of mutation positive DS at 1:40,900 live births, based on cases ascertained through the only single genetic laboratory offering genetic analysis for *SCN1A* mutations in the UK during the time of observation (Brunklaus et al., 2012). This figure is likely to be an underestimation because 20-30% of DS cases may be mutation negative and under ascertainment due to failure to request genetic analysis may have occurred especially considering the expanding clinical phenotype.

Few data are available for syndromes with benign or less severe course. Benign familial infantile epilepsy, for example, has been identified in 0.5% of children with new onset epilepsy aged 1 month to 16 years (prevalence cohort, Larsson and Eeg-Olofsson, 2006) and myoclonic epilepsy in infancy in 0.2% and 2.4% of wider new onset childhood epilepsy cohorts (Callenbach et al., 1998; Berg et al., 1999).

Electroclinical syndromes could be identified for 24 (42%) of infants with newly diagnosed epilepsy prospectively enrolled in the North London Epilepsy in Infancy Study (entire cohort n = 57) (Eltze et al. 2013). Clinical, EEG and neuroimaging data were independently rated by two paediatric neurologists with subsequent consensus discussion in cases where discrepancies occurred. The majority had syndromes with poor prognosis associated with epileptic encephalopathy (*Table III*). Syndromes with milder course were recognised in only 5.3% at diagnosis. This supports observations from above quoted studies that self-limiting epilepsies with normal developmental outcome are infrequent in a population based setting.

Table III. North London Epilepsy in Infancy Study: distribution of epilepsy types (Eltze et al., 2013)

Electroclinical syndromes and revised aetiological categories (ILAE Commission Report 2005-2009 [Berg et al. 2010])	N (%)
West syndrome/infantile spasms (7 structural/metabolic, 1 presumed genetic[1], 8 unknown cause)	16 (28%)
Ohtahara syndrome (1 structural/metabolic, 1 unknown cause)	2 (3.5%)
Dravet syndrome (2 genetic: *SCN1A* mutation confirmed)	3 (5.3%)
Benign infantile seizures (non familial)	2 (2.5%)
Myoclonic epilepsy in infancy	1 (1.8%)
Non syndromic epilepsies:	
Structural/metabolic	16 (28%)
Genetic/presumed genetic – Epileptic encephalopathy with KCNQ2 mutation – Monosomy 1p36 – Prader Willi syndrome (15q11-q13 deletion)	3 (5.3%)
Unknown cause and no identifiable electroclinical syndrome	14 (25%)

[1] Chromosomal abnormality – Tetrasomy 15q13-15pter.

In comparison the proportion of recognisable electroclinical syndrome diagnoses in some of the more recent studies of overall childhood epilepsy cohorts varies depending on study design between 28 and 50% (Wirrell et al., 2011; Larsson and Eeg-Olofsson, 2006; Dura-Trave et al., 2008). Prospective design and evaluation of data by paediatric neurologists may have led to the relative high yield of electroclinical syndrome diagnoses in the "North London Epilepsy in Infancy study".

■ What is the distribution of aetiologies in a population based setting?

Advances in neuroimaging and molecular genetics in recent years led to an increase in the identification of underlying causes especially for early onset epilepsies. Clinical syndromic description is thus no longer sufficient to prognosticate on the disease course and decide on the most optimal treatment strategies. The spectrum of aetiologies encountered in infancy is wide and heterogeneous comprising a long list including various types of developmental cortical malformations, chromosomal abnormalities, monogenetic disorders including ion channel gene mutations, metabolic disorders, peri- and post-natally acquired brain lesions.

Data from older mostly hospital or specialist centre based infancy onset epilepsy cohorts suggest that the proportion of confirmed or presumed structural brain pathologies is higher (45-85% of infants with seizure onset in the first year – Matsumoto et al., 1983a; Battaglia et al., 1999; Altunbasak et al., 2007) compared to the overall childhood epilepsy group (18-22%, (Arts, 2003; Berg et al., 1999). However, neuroimaging techniques were limited at the time of the studies and some investigators assumed the presence of structural brain abnormalities based on the history of perinatal complications and developmental impairments. Furthermore it is likely that the infancy onset series originating mostly from specialist settings were biased towards more severe cases.

For the population based "North London Epilepsy in Infancy cohort" magnetic resonance imaging (MRI) data were available for the majority of the enrolled infants (54 [95%] of 57 entire cohort) (Eltze et al., 2013). The yield of MR imaging in this group was high as the independent review of MR images of 51 children by 2 neuroradiologists demonstrated with diagnostically relevant lesions identified in 51%. A similar high proportion of diagnostically relevant abnormalities (57%) were identified in a hospital based cohort of infants presenting with first afebrile seizures from a multi-ethnic inner city population (n = 317, MRI was only performed in 57% of total cohort) (Hsieh et al., 2010).

This is significantly higher than the figure recently reported from a large community based childhood epilepsy cohort (1 months to 16 years, MR data from = 518, 16% aetiologically relevant lesions identified (Berg et al., 2009). The same study reports aetiologically relevant MR findings in infants under the age of 2 years in 25%. These observations support the recommendation in international guidelines to obtain brain MRI imaging in all children with newly onset epilepsy.

In the "North London Epilepsy in Infancy" cohort an underlying aetiology could be determined in 29 (51%) infants enrolled. Developmental and acquired structural brain abnormalities were the commonest identified cause (42%, 24 of 57), whereby developmental brain lesions were most frequent (21%, 12 of 57).

Six children (11%) with monogenetic and chromosomal abnormalities associated with epilepsy were recognised (Table III, Figure 3). At the time of the study, however, the availability of genetic tests including new generation sequencing based technologies to identify monogenetic conditions associated with early onset epileptic encephalopathies was limited. The specific phenotypes of infantile onset epileptic encephalopathy associated with various monogenetic conditions (including *STXBP1, ARX, KCNQ2, SCN2A, PLCB1, KCNT1*) are variable and overlapping (as will be discussed in another chapter). Considering this the proportion of genetic diagnoses in this cohort could have been higher.

However, even in very highly selective populations of infants with epileptic encephalopathy the frequency of specific monogenetic conditions was 10-16% (*i.e., STXB1, CDKL5* in female infants with epileptic encephalopathy) (Deprez et al., 2010; Bahi-Buisson and Bienvenu, 2012). To date the frequency of these conditions in a population based setting is unknown. Although single monogenetic conditions may be rare cumulatively genetic

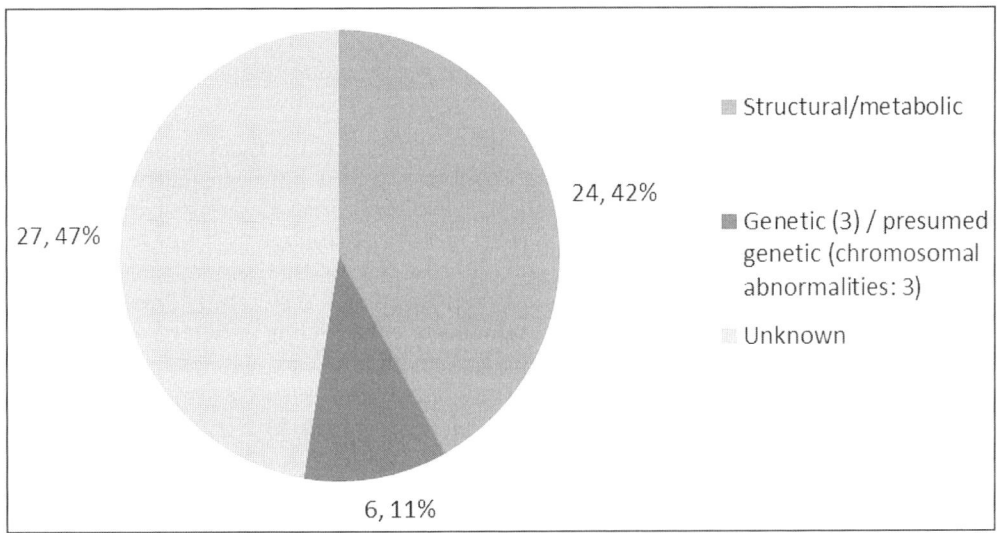

Figure 3. Aetiologies entire cohort (n = 57).

investigations testing multiple candidate genes (using second generation sequencing diagnostic panels of genes) could increase diagnostic yield and reduce the proportion of aetiologically undefined infants.

Electronic data registries to collect data on infants with newly onset epilepsies could provide data about frequency of these genetic epileptic encephalopathies as well as other aetiologies including various types of developmental brain abnormalities.

■ Outcomes

Data from large hospital/specialist centre based series of infants with epilepsy onset in the first 12 to 24 months of age showing persisting seizures in 44-47% suggest a worse outcome compared to overall childhood epilepsy group (Altunbasak et al., 2007; Matsumoto et al., 1983b; Czochanska et al., 1994; Battaglia et al., 1999). However, the follow up periods were shorter compared to those of more recently published childhood epilepsy cohorts (67-70% in 5-year terminal remission, mean follow up 15 and 37 years respectively; Greets et al., 2010; Silanpaa and Schmidt, 2006). One small retrospective population based study of infants with seizure onset in the first 2 years reported 60% (37 of 65) seizure-free and off-antiepileptic medication after a mean follow up of 13 years (range 7.4-19.7 years (Rantala et al., 1999). Presumed or confirmed structural brain abnormalities were in the majority of infancy onset epilepsy series associated with worse outcome.

Neurological impairments are described in a significant proportion of children with infancy onset seizures on follow up (26-67%) in keeping with the higher prevalence of structural brain abnormalities in this group (Chevrie and Aicardi, 1978; Matsumoto et al., 1983b; Czochanska et al., 1994; Datta and Wirrell, 2000; Altunbasak et al., 2007). Forty-six percent of infants enrolled in the "North London Epilepsy in Infancy study" had neurological abnormalities at baseline (Eltze et al., 2013).

The mortality in infancy onset epilepsy is significantly higher (7-11%, Datta and Wirrell, 2000; Matsumoto et al., 1983b; Rantala and Ingalsuo, 1999; Chevrie and Aicardi, 1978; Battaglia et al., 1999) compared to the overall childhood epilepsy group (1.9-3.7%) (Callenbach et al., 2001; Berg et al., 2004a; Camfield et al., 2002). Death in infancy onset epilepsy is similarly as in the overall childhood epilepsy group related to neurologically impairment as well as status epilepticus.

Cognitive impairment on follow up in the infancy onset epilepsy group is more common compared to the overall childhood epilepsy cohort, where it has been recently reported in 26.4% (Berg et al., 2008). In hospital/specialist setting based series of infants with seizure onset in the first 12 to 24 months only 33-42% of children had IQs in normal or borderline range (> 70 or 75), when assessed with standardised assessment tools on follow up (Czochanska et al., 1994; Battaglia et al., 1999; Altunbasak et al., 2007). Various factors were found to be related to poor outcome in these studies including presumed or confirmed structural brain abnormality, seizure onset under 6 months of age, abnormal development at baseline, abnormal neurological examination.

Evaluation of infants with newly onset epilepsy in a population based setting demonstrates that cognitive/developmental impairments are similarly frequent and present already close to diagnosis. Infants enrolled in the "North London Epilepsy in Infancy study" over a 13 months period underwent developmental/cognitive assessment using standardised assessment tools at enrolment and follow up (baseline and 1 year follow up: *Bayley Scales of Infant and Toddler*

Development 3rd edition [Bayley III] (Bayley, 2006a; Bayley, 2006b). Of the 49 infants assessed after a median time interval of 9 weeks (interquartile range 5-15 weeks) following the diagnosis 71% had language composite scores and 63% cognitive composite scores below average, with over half of the infants scoring in the extremely low average (> 2 sd below average). Further analysis was performed to determine predictors of developmental status at presentation.

Principal component analysis was used to generate a single factor from the raw scores of the Baley III and entering this with age at testing into ta multiple regression model with the following factors: "abnormal neurological examination", "presence of interictal discharges on initial EEG", "grossly abnormal EEG background activities", "aetiologically relevant neuroimaging findings", "aetiologically uncertain or incidental neuroimaging findings", "> 20 seizures/seizure clusters prior to developmental assessment" and "developmental status prior to seizure onset". In the final model "presence of interictal discharges on the initial EEG" ($t(32) = -3.1$, $p < 0.01$) and "abnormal neurological examination" ($t(32) = -4.39$, $p < 0.01$) were independently and significantly associated with lower developmental function close to diagnosis with a weaker but not significant effect of "developmental status prior to seizure onset" ($t(32) = 2$, $p = 0.51$; $R^2 = .87$).

Thirty-two of the 49 infants (65%) assessed at enrolment were reassessed at a mean interval of 12.5 months (range 10-18 months).

In order to explore the effect of clinical factors, neuroimaging and EEG findings to the longitudinal change of individual developmental function further analysis was conducted in two steps. The data were reduced using separate principal component analyses for the Bayley III composite scores (language, motor and cognition) at baseline and follow up to generate a single factor: Developmental composite factor at baseline [DCF-0] and follow up [DCF-1]. A repeated measure ANOVA revealed no significant difference between DCF-0 (baseline) and DCF-1 (at follow up). There was also no difference after adjustment for the following factors: "neurological examination", "seizure-free for 6 months", "presence of aetiologically relevant neuroimaging findings", "EEG at enrolment" and "number of AEDs at follow up assessment" (between-group variables) (in preparation for submission).

In the population based "North London Epilepsy in Infancy" cohort the initial developmental status (in the first 3 months after diagnosis) determined the developmental function after short-term follow up. However, small longitudinal changes in developmental function over the relative short observation period may not have become significant due to sample size effects. Small changes in developmental function are likely to be cumulative over time and therefore longer observation periods may be required for longitudinal differences to become significant.

The strong impact of initial developmental status on subsequent progress has also been shown in a larger community based cohort of children with newly onset epilepsy under the age of 3 years (n = 172, 67% under 2 years at onset, complete data sets available for 70% of subjects) (Berg et al., 2004b). Developmental status was assessed in interviews with carers using the Vineland Adaptive Behaviour scales over 3 years. Low baseline scores at baseline were significantly influenced by remote symptomatic aetiology and diagnosis with an epileptic encephalopathy syndrome. After adjustment for aetiology and epileptic encephalopathy syndrome intractable seizures (assessed at 3-year follow up) did not have an effect on baseline Vineland scores. Children without risk factors (no underlying structural brain and not diagnosed with an epileptic encephalopathy at baseline), who had average (normal) adaptive behaviour function at enrolment continued on the same level without deterioration over the 3-year observation period. Whereas children with such risk factors (symptomatic epilepsy, epileptic encephalopathy syndrome, intractable seizures at 3-year follow up) had lower function already at enrolment and demonstrated further decline indicating a failure to acquire skills at an adequate rate.

Although the underlying brain pathology, structural brain abnormality or consequence of molecular genetic defects, is a strong factor that determines cognitive outcome there is also evidence that shorter time lag to start treatment may have an additional impact. This has been especially suggested from studies of children with infantile spasms (Kivity et al., 2004; Hamano et al., 2007; Eisermann et al., 2003; O'Callaghan et al., 2011).

The notion that pharmaco-resistant seizures have an independent negative impact on cognitive outcome especially in those with onset at a very young age is supported by data from children undergoing epilepsy surgery. At pre-surgical evaluation poorer cognitive function was associated with early age of seizure onset and longer duration of epilepsy (Vasconcellos et al., 2001; D'Argenzio et al., 2011).

Furthermore Berg et al. could also show, investigating subjects with seizure onset under 8 years enrolled in the Connecticut childhood epilepsy cohort after 8 to 9 years that cognitive impairment was significantly more frequent in those with pharmaco-resistant seizures and very early seizure onset in infancy compared to those with later seizure onset (Berg et al., 2012).

Concluding remarks

Epilepsy onset in childhood occurs most commonly in the first year of life. The majority of infants present with severe course of epilepsy and developmental/cognitive impairments. The yield of investigations for underlying causes especially structural brain abnormalities and more recently also genetic disorders appears particularly high in this age group compared to epilepsies with later onset in childhood. Clinical presentations are very heterogeneous with age dependent phenotypes that can show evolution from one into another making diagnoses and classifications challenging. The syndromic approach that has guided therapeutic decisions is likely to shift towards a focus on identification of underlying aetiologies. There is a lack of data from resource poor countries that needs to be addressed by future research.

References

- Altunbasak S, Incecik F, Herguner O, Refik BH. Prognosis of patients with seizures occurring in the first 2 years. J Child Neurol 2007; 22: 307-13.
- Annegers JF, Dubinsky S, Coan SP, Newmark ME, Roht L. The incidence of epilepsy and unprovoked seizures in multiethnic, urban health maintenance organizations. Epilepsia 1999; 40: 502-6.
- Arts WF. The dutch study of epilepsy in childhood. In: Jallon P, Berg A, Dulac O, Hauser WA (eds). Prognosis of Epilepsies. Paris: John Libbey Eurotext, 2003, pp. 101-112.
- Bahi-Buisson N, Bienvenu T. CDKL5-related disorders: from clinical description to molecular genetics. Mol Syndromol 2012; 2: 137-52.
- Battaglia D, Rando T, Deodato F, et al. Epileptic disorders with onset in the first year of life: neurological and cognitive outcome. Eur J Paediatr Neurol 1999; 3: 95-103.
- Bayley N. Bayley Scale of Infant and Toddler Development – Third Edition: Techinical Manual. PsychCorp, Hartcourt Assessments, 2006b.

- Bayley N. *Bayley Scales of Infant and Toddler Development – Third Edition: Administration Manual.* 3rd edition. PsychCorp, Harcourt Assessments, 2006a.
- Berg AT, Berkovic SF, Brodie MJ, et al. Revised terminology and concepts for organization of seizures and epilepsies: report of the ILAE Commission on Classification and Terminology, 2005-2009. *Epilepsia* 2010; 51: 676-85.
- Berg AT, Langfitt JT, Testa FM, et al. Global cognitive function in children with epilepsy: A community-based study. *Epilepsia* 2008; 49: 608-14.
- Berg AT, Mathern GW, Bronen RA, et al. Frequency, prognosis and surgical treatment of structural abnormalities seen with magnetic resonance imaging in childhood epilepsy. *Brain* 2009; 132: 2785-97.
- Berg AT, Shinnar S, Levy SR, Testa FM. Newly diagnosed epilepsy in children: presentation at diagnosis. *Epilepsia* 1999; 40: 445-52.
- Berg AT, Shinnar S, Testa FM, Levy SR, Smith SN, Beckerman B. Mortality in childhood-onset epilepsy. *Arch Pediatr Adolesc Med* 2004a; 158: 1147-52.
- Berg AT, Smith SN, Frobish D, et al. Longitudinal assessment of adaptive behavior in infants and young children with newly diagnosed epilepsy: influences of etiology, syndrome, and seizure control. *Pediatrics* 2004b; 114: 645-50.
- Berg AT, Zelko FA, Levy SR, Testa FM. Age at onset of epilepsy, pharmacoresistance, and cognitive outcomes: a prospective cohort study. *Neurology* 2012; 79: 1384-91.
- Blom S, Heijbel J, Bergfors PG. Incidence of epilepsy in children: a follow-up study three years after the first seizure. *Epilepsia* 1978; 19: 343-50.
- Brunklaus A, Ellis R, Reavey E, Forbes GH, Zuberi SM. Prognostic, clinical and demographic features in SCN1A mutation-positive Dravet syndrome. *Brain* 2012; 135: 2329-36.
- Callenbach PM, Geerts AT, Arts WF, et al. Familial occurrence of epilepsy in children with newly diagnosed multiple seizures: Dutch Study of Epilepsy in Childhood. *Epilepsia* 1998; 39: 331-6.
- Callenbach PM, Westendorp RG, Geerts AT, et al. Mortality risk in children with epilepsy: the Dutch study of epilepsy in childhood. *Pediatrics* 1999; 107: 1259-63.
- Camfield CS, Camfield PR, Gordon K, Wirrell E, Dooley JM. Incidence of epilepsy in childhood and adolescence: a population-based study in Nova Scotia from 1977 to 1985. *Epilepsia* 1996; 37: 19-23.
- Camfield CS, Camfield PR, Veugelers PJ. Death in children with epilepsy: a population-based study. *Lancet* 2002; 359: 1891-5.
- Chevrie JJ, Aicardi J. Convulsive disorders in the first year of life: neurological and mental outcome and mortality. *Epilepsia* 1978; 19: 67-74.
- Chin RF, Neville BG, Peckham C, Bedford H, Wade A, Scott RC. Incidence, cause, and short-term outcome of convulsive status epilepticus in childhood: prospective population-based study. *Lancet* 2006; 368: 222-9.
- Chin RF, Neville BG, Peckham C, Wade A, Bedford H, Scott RC. Socioeconomic deprivation independent of ethnicity increases status epilepticus risk. *Epilepsia* 2009; 50: 1022-9.
- Czochanska J, Langner-Tyszka B, Losiowski Z, Schmidt-Sidor B. Children who develop epilepsy in the first year of life: a prospective study. *Dev Med Child Neurol* 1994; 36: 345-50.
- D'Argenzio L, Colonnelli MC, Harrison S, et al. Cognitive outcome after extratemporal epilepsy surgery in childhood. *Epilepsia* 2011; 52: 1966-72.
- Datta AN, Wirrell EC. Prognosis of seizures occurring in the first year. *Pediatr Neurol* 2000; 22: 386-91.
- Deprez L, Weckhuysen S, Holmgren P, et al. Clinical spectrum of early-onset epileptic encephalopathies associated with STXBP1 mutations. *Neurology* 2010; 75: 1159-65.

- Dura-Trave T, Yoldi-Petri ME, Gallinas-Victoriano F. Incidence of epilepsies and epileptic syndromes among children in Navarre, Spain: 2002 through 2005. *J Child Neurol* 2008; 23: 878-82.
- Eisermann MM, DeLaRaillere A, Dellatolas G, et al. Infantile spasms in Down syndrome-effects of delayed anticonvulsive treatment. *Epilepsy Res* 2003; 55: 21-7.
- Eltze CM, Chong WK, Cox T, et al. A population-based study of newly diagnosed epilepsy in infants. *Epilepsia* 2013; 54. 437-45.
- Engel J, Jr. A proposed diagnostic scheme for people with epileptic seizures and with epilepsy: report of the ILAE Task Force on Classification and Terminology. *Epilepsia* 2001; 42: 796-803.
- Freitag CM, May TW, Pfafflin M, Konig S, Rating D. Incidence of epilepsies and epileptic syndromes in children and adolescents: a population-based prospective study in Germany. *Epilepsia* 2001; 42: 979-85.
- Haerer AF, Anderson DW, Schoenberg BS. Prevalence and clinical features of epilepsy in a biracial United States population. *Epilepsia* 1986; 27: 66-75.
- Hamano S, Yoshinari S, Higurashi N, Tanaka M, Minamitani M, Eto Y. Developmental outcomes of cryptogenic West syndrome. *J Pediatr* 2007; 150: 295-9.
- Haut SR, Veliskova J, Moshe SL (2004) Susceptibility of immature and adult brains to seizure effects. *Lancet Neurol* 1998; 3: 608-17.
- Hino-Fukuyo N, Haginoya K, Iinuma K, Uematsu M, Tsuchiya S. Neuroepidemiology of West syndrome and early infantile epileptic encephalopathy in Miyagi Prefecture, Japan. *Epilepsy Res* 2009; 87: 299-301.
- Hsieh DT, Chang T, Tsuchida TN, et al. New-onset afebrile seizures in infants: role of neuroimaging. *Neurology* 2010; 74: 150-6.
- Kivity S, Lerman P, Ariel R, Danziger Y, Mimouni M, Shinnar S. Long-term cognitive outcomes of a cohort of children with cryptogenic infantile spasms treated with high-dose adrenocorticotropic hormone. *Epilepsia* 2004; 45: 255-62.
- Kurtz Z, Tookey P, Ross E. Epilepsy in young people: 23 year follow up of the British national child development study. *BMJ* 1998; 316: 339-42.
- Larsson K, Eeg-Olofsson O. A population based study of epilepsy in children from a Swedish county. *Eur J Paediatr Neurol* 2006; 10: 107-13.
- Mani KS, Rangan G, Srinivas HV, Kalyanasundaram S, Narendran S, Reddy AK. The Yelandur study: a community-based approach to epilepsy in rural South Indi–epidemiological aspects. *Seizure* 1998; 7: 281-8.
- Matsumoto A, Watanabe K, Sugiura M, Negoro T, Takaesu E, Iwase K. Etiologic factors and long-term prognosis of convulsive disorders in the first year of life. *Neuropediatrics* 1983a; 14: 231-4.
- Matsumoto A, Watanabe K, Sugiura M, Negoro T, Takaesu E, Iwase K. Long-term prognosis of convulsive disorders in the first year of life: mental and physical development and seizure persistence. *Epilepsia* 1983b; 24: 321-9.
- McTague A, Appleton R, Avula S, et al. Migrating partial seizures of infancy: expansion of the electroclinical, radiological and pathological disease spectrum. *Brain* 2013; 136: 1578-91.
- Newton CR, Garcia HH. Epilepsy in poor regions of the world. *Lancet* 2012; 380: 1193-201.
- Ngugi AK, Bottomley C, Scott JA, et al. Incidence of convulsive epilepsy in a rural area in Kenya. *Epilepsia* 2013; 54: 1352-9.
- Ngugi AK, Kariuki SM, Bottomley C, Kleinschmidt I, Sander JW, Newton CR. Incidence of epilepsy: a systematic review and meta-analysis. *Neurology* 2011; 77: 1005-12.
- O'Callaghan FJ, Lux AL, Darke K, et al. The effect of lead time to treatment and of age of onset on developmental outcome at 4 years in infantile spasms: evidence from the United Kingdom Infantile Spasms Study. *Epilepsia* 2011; 52: 1359-64.

- Oka E, Ohtsuka Y, Yoshinaga H, Murakami N, Kobayashi K, Ogino T. Prevalence of childhood epilepsy and distribution of epileptic syndromes: a population-based survey in Okayama, Japan. *Epilepsia* 2006; 47: 626-30.
- Olafsson E, Hauser WA, Ludvigsson P, Gudmundsson G. Incidence of epilepsy in rural Iceland: a population-based study. *Epilepsia* 1996; 37: 951-5.
- Olafsson E, Ludvigsson P, Gudmundsson G, Hesdorffer D, Kjartansson O, Hauser WA. Incidence of unprovoked seizures and epilepsy in Iceland and assessment of the epilepsy syndrome classification: a prospective study. *Lancet Neurol* 2005; 4: 627-34.
- Rantala H, Ingalsuo H. Occurrence and outcome of epilepsy in children younger than 2 years. *J Pediatr* 1999; 135: 761-4.
- Riikonen R, Donner M. Incidence and aetiology of infantile spasms from 1960 to 1976: a population study in Finland. *Dev Med Child Neurol* 1979; 21: 333-43.
- Shamansky SL, Glaser GH. Socioeconomic characteristics of childhood seizure disorders in the New Haven area: an epidemiologic study. *Epilepsia* 1979; 20: 457-74.
- Sidenvall R, Eeg-Olofsson O. Epidemiology of infantile spasms in Sweden. *Epilepsia* 1995; 36: 572-4.
- Sillanpaa M. Long-term prognosis in Finnish childhood-onset epilepsy. In: Jallon P, Berg A, Dulac O, Hauser WA (eds). *Prognosis of Epilepsies*. Paris: John Libbey Eurotext, 2003, pp. 127-34.
- Tekle-Haimanot R, Forsgren L, Ekstedt J. Incidence of epilepsy in rural central Ethiopia. *Epilepsia* 1997; 38: 541-6.
- Trevathan E, Murphy CC, Yeargin-Allsopp M. The descriptive epidemiology of infantile spasms among Atlanta children. *Epilepsia* 1999; 40: 748-51.
- Vasconcellos E, Wyllie E, Sullivan S, *et al*. Mental retardation in pediatric candidates for epilepsy surgery: the role of early seizure onset. *Epilepsia* 2001; 42: 268-74.
- Verity CM, Butler NR, Golding J. Febrile convulsions in a national cohort followed up from birth. I--Prevalence and recurrence in the first five years of life. *Br Med J* 1985; 290: 1307-10.
- Verity CM, Golding J. Risk of epilepsy after febrile convulsions: a national cohort study. *BMJ* 1991; 303: 1373-6.
- Wirrell EC, Grossardt BR, Wong-Kisiel LC, Nickels KC. Incidence and classification of new-onset epilepsy and epilepsy syndromes in children in Olmsted County, Minnesota from 1980 to 2004: a population-based study. *Epilepsy Res* 2011; 95: 110-8.

Concept of epileptic encephalopathy: is it relevant?

Federico Vigevano, Nicola Specchio

Department of Neuroscience, Bambino Gesù Children's Hospital, IRCCS, Rome, Italy

Definitions

It is worth saying that most patients with epilepsy do not have a progressive disorder as defined by both seizure worsening and intellectual decline. Indeed, many types of human epilepsies are known that do not progress despite seizure repetition: benign rolandic and occipital epilepsies, absence epilepsies, juvenile myoclonic epilepsy, autosomal dominant nocturnal frontal lobe epilepsy and the majority of lesional epilepsies just to quote the most common ones. Thus, the hypothesis of a progressive worsening induced by epilepsy applies only to limited number of clinical entities particularly to epileptic encephalopathies (EE).

EE are severe conditions, that affect children but also adults, difficult to treat, with variable evolution in terms of seizure remission and cognitive development. The term EE was highlighted by Gastaut when referring to West syndrome and Lennox-Gastaut syndrome (Gastaut *et al.*, 1963). Moreover it was confirmed by Landau and Kleffner who observed patients with aphasia epilepsy related (Landau and Kleffner, 1957).

The modern concept of EE comes from the observation that not only the seizures but also the interictal epileptiform abnormalities need to be considered when dealing with children with these epilepsies.

Dulac (2001) first stressed the idea that both seizures and epileptiform abnormalities might be responsible for the cognitive deterioration. Following this concept, the definition of EE included in the 2001 proposal of the ILAE classification is: Epileptic Encephalopathies are conditions *"in which the epileptiform abnormalities themselves are believed to contribute to progressive disturbance in cerebral function"* (Engel, 2001). This means that not only epileptic seizures, but also severe epileptiform EEG abnormalities contribute to the progressive decline of cerebral functions. In this definition are highlighted three main features that characterize EE: epileptic seizures, EEG abnormalities, cognitive decline. Furthermore the definition was clarified and in 2006 (Engel, 2006) it was added that in EE *"Evidence suggests or supports the notion that there is an epilepsy-dependent neurodevelopmental or neurodegenerative process involved in the evolution of the syndrome (as opposed to an underlying metabolic, degenerative, or encephalitic process)"* and that *"it is important to distinguish between deficits that are due to the cause of the epilepsy, those that are due to pharmacotherapy, and those that are due to the epilepsy itself (EE). Unfortunately, this can be difficult and many EE remain theoretical"* (Engel, 2006).

In the last Report of the ILAE Commission on Classification and Terminology the concept of EE was further clarified: " *Epileptic encephalopathy embodies the notion that the epileptic activity itself may contribute to severe cognitive and behavioural impairments above and beyond what might be expected from the underlying pathology alone (e.g., cortical malformation), and that these can worsen over time. These impairments may be global or more selective and they may occur along a spectrum of severity. Although certain syndromes are often referred to as EE, the encephalopathic effects of seizures and epilepsy may potentially occur in association with any form of epilepsy"* (Berg et al., 2010).

As a consequence of these sentences it is implied that remission of seizures and of epileptiform interictal activity might improve the cognitive development.

The achievement of this definition has required years of debate on severe clinical entities, with onset in pediatric age. Those entities are characterized not only by epileptic seizures, but also by a cognitive deterioration that is strictly related, in terms of period of time and causal effect, to peculiar types of epileptic seizures and EEG patterns.

Epileptic encephalopathy following the current classification

The conditions classified as "epileptic encephalopathy" are listed in *Table I* following the age of onset. We report some of these conditions pointing out the applicability of the concept of EE.

Table I. Epileptic encepahalopathies

Conditions classified as epileptic encephalopathy
Early myoclonic encephalopathy
Early Infantile Epileptic Encephalopathy (Ohtahara syndrome)
West syndrome
Dravet syndrome (Dravet-like syndromes)
Myoclonic status in non-progressive encephalopathies
Lennox-Gastaut syndrome
Landau-Kleffner syndrome
Epilepsy with continuous spike-waves during slow-wave sleep (CSWS or ESES)

Severe neonatal epilepsies with suppression-bursts is a term including the Early Infantile Epileptic Encephalopathy and Early Myoclonic Encephalopathy. In both conditions the electro-clinical pattern is very similar: tonic, myoclonic or focal seizures, with suppression burst on the EEG, and severe delay. The etiology is variable: brain malformations, inborn error of metabolism, genetic abnormalities. Onset is so early that it is not possible to determine if the associated severe cognitive and behavioral impairments are due to both seizures and epileptic abnormalities or to genetic, structural or metabolic brain diseases. In fact the possibilities of clinical improvement with pharmacological or surgical treatment are scarce (Ohtahara et al., 2008; Ohtahara et al., 1976).

Referring to the current definition of EE and considering the severity of structural brain abnormalities, it is very hard to consider the cognitive delay as a consequence of epilepsy and paroxysmal activity.

Dravet syndrome is a severe epilepsy syndrome with onset during the first year of life in apparently normal children. This epileptic entity is due to *a single* etiological factor (SCN1A – interneuron abnormalities) (Martins *et al.*, 2010). It is characterized by a constant electro-clinical pattern, evolving only in terms of intensity and severity, without any possibility of complete resolution. The cognitive impairment, although of variable degree, seems independent from seizure recurrence and EEG abnormalities. It may be considered as a real disease and a specific nosographic entity. Two main studies were performed with the aim of a correlation between seizures, EEG abnormalities and cognitive development. They did not find any significant correlation between the IQ or developmental quotient and the quantitative and qualitative parameters of epilepsy during the first years of life (Ragona *et al.*, 2011, Villeneuve *et al.*, 2014). It is not proven that the cognitive stagnation observed in the first stages of the disease is simply the direct consequence of epilepsy. One hypothesis is that the channelopathy *per se* can play an important role in the pathogenesis of cognitive delay and neurologic abnormalities. (Dravet *et al.*, 2005). This is also supported by the hypothesis that the epileptogenic effects of the SCN1A mutation are mediated by changes in the behavior of inhibitory interneurons in the cortex (Catterall *et al.*, 2010).

West syndrome, Lennox-Gastaut syndrome, and ***Epilepsy with continuous spike-waves during slow-wave sleep (CSWS)*** are conditions in which the EE is clearly the result of a peculiar evolution of epilepsy towards a syndrome specific electro-clinical picture. Cognitive and motor regression is quantifiable and characterized by an evident worsening of the neuropsychological profile if compared to the pre-onset neurocognitive profile. Evolution is variable, ranging from complete remission to very severe conditions, such as drug resistant epilepsy and severe mental retardation.

When referring to West syndrome one might consider that independently from the etiology all patients will experience the same type of seizures and the same EEG pattern during the active phase of the syndrome. Cognitive deterioration appears during this phase, and depending on the etiology might remain stable during this time, or a complete resolution can be observed. The different evolution is related not only to the etiology but also to treatment response, such as to hormonal therapy or early surgical treatment in cases with focal cortical dysplasia.

Epileptic encephalopathy and genetics

The role of genetic mutations as cause of EE is widely discussed. Single genes mutations are already known to be associated with West Syndrome and other early-onset EE, usually with a severe neurodevelopmental compromise and a typical electro-clinical picture (*Table II*).

Many genes cluster in two specific biological pathways: ventral forebrain development and forebrain synapse function. Many of the genes associated with CNVs are involved in the regulatory network that directs ventral forebrain development. Genes in pathways of synaptic function are overrepresented, significantly those involved in GABA-ergic synaptic vesicles transport. Those genes might be responsible of structural abnormalities of the forebrain, and this finding might explain the developments of epileptic spasms, but not entirely the evolution toward an EE (Paciorkowski *et al.*, 2011).

The role of genetics is clearer in conditions such as Tuberous Sclerosis (TS). In TS the risk of developing infantile spasms and the evolution toward an EE is much higher in cases affected by mutations of the TSC2 gene rather than the TSC1 (Dabor *et al.*, 2001).

Table II. Genes involved in epileptic encephalopathies

Gene	Clinical findings
ARX	Lissencephaly, agenesis of the corpus callosum with abnormal genitalia, infantile spasms without brain malformations, syndromic and non-syndromic mental retardation.
CDKL5	Severe global developmental delay, early onset seizures (epileptic spasms, tonic seizures, myoclonias)
FOXG1	Infantile onset of microcephaly, mental retardation, and peculiar jerky movements, lack of speech and motor development and stereotypic movements
GRIN1	Severe mental retardation, Infantile spasms, Lennox-Gastaut syndrome
GRIN2A	Profound global developmental delay and refractory epilepsy characterized by multiple seizure types (partial complex with secondary generalization, tonic, myoclonic, and atypical absence)
MAGI2	Infantile spasms, mental retardation
SLC25A22	Epileptic encephalopathy and no psychomotor acquisition, early myoclonic encephalopathy, migrating partial seizures in infancy
STXBP1	Epileptic spasms, burst-suppression pattern, severe mental retardation

Nevertheless within the spectrum of TSC2 mutations there have been reported differences: the non-terminating mutations located in the central region of the *TSC2* gene (exons 23-33) are associated with a significantly lower risk for IS, and a trend toward a lower prevalence of any type of epilepsy. Therefore not all patients with mutations that have been considered at higher risk for EE present a catastrophic evolution (van Eeghen *et al.*, 2013).

Nonetheless, in many patients, which factors are really major players in the evolution towards EE is still unclear: as for many gene mutations we have to hypothesize the contributing role of other factors, as for structural lesions we might take in consideration possible genetic cofactors

EE are probably related to the malfunction and activation of peculiar networks: ventral forebrain and Gaba-ergic neurons in IS, changes in the behavior of inhibitory interneurons (SCN1A), adhesion molecule (PCDH19), regulated networks in CSWSS, brainstem and thalamus (especially centro-median and anterior thalamus) in LGS.

All structural lesions or genetic mutations, which are responsible for such malfunctions, may provoke EE. However, the triggering factors that may provoke the activation of those systems is not yet known.

▪ Epileptic encephalopathy and the impact on cognition

How epileptiform discharges may impact on cognition is not fully understood. Some hypotheses have been postulated.

Epileptiform discharges can adversely alter neuronal development. Data from animal models of epilepsy suggest that early seizures can provoke structural and physiologic changes in developing neuronal circuits that result in permanent alterations in the balance between neuronal excitation and inhibition, deficit in cognitive function, and increased susceptibility to further seizures (Cilio *et al.*, 2003).

Epileptiform discharges can produce a transient effect on information processing in the brain as it has been shown when studying spikes and slow activity in hypsarrhythmya with EEG coupled with f-MRI. It has been shown that multifocal interictal spikes and high-amplitude slow wave activity within the hypsarrhythmia are associated with the activation of different neuronal networks. Although spikes caused a cortical activation pattern similar to that in focal epilepsies, slow wave activity produced a hypsarrhythmia-specific activation in cortex and subcortical structures such as brainstem, thalamus, and putamen (Siniatchkin et al., 2007).

Epileptiform discharges can produce more long-lasting effects leading to prolonged inhibition of brain areas distant from but connected with epileptic focus. Even if the etiologies of Lennox-Gastaut syndrome (LGS) are diverse, the multiple causes converge into a final common pathway that results in this specific epilepsy phenotype. Significant activation of brainstem and thalamus (especially centro-median and anterior thalamus) associated with epileptiform discharges in patients with LGS have been shown (Siniatchkin et al., 2011).

The therapeutic approach to epileptic encephalopathy

The main goal of the therapeutic approach is to restore the neurological conditions preceding the EE or at least reduce the consequences of this peculiar course of epilepsy.

Medical intervention is expected to achieve a cessation of seizures and a resolution of EEG abnormalities. The treatment of EE is based mainly on the use of specific drugs such as hormonal treatment, Vigabatrin, Stiripentol, Ketogenic diet, Pyridoxine or PLP. Moreover conventional drugs should also be tried, and early surgical treatment in selected cases with a focal lesion (Vigevano et al., 2013). On the basis of the above considerations, it appears that the best results might be reached in those conditions that are truly EE: that is conditions in which cognitive decline is strictly related to the epileptic activity.

Conclusion

Following our debate EE is a dynamic condition not depending on the etiology that may persist over time causing increasingly severe functional effects. It may improve and remit, either spontaneously or with treatment that suppresses the proposed causative epileptic activity.

The term has been used in two ways:
- as a generic classification term for epilepsies with severe cognitive and behavioral outcomes,
- as a pathophysiological process.

We argue that the term is not synonymous with "a severe epileptic syndrome". When a underlying severe brain disorder gives rise to both epilepsy and cognitive and behavioral problems, this entity should not be classified as an epileptic encephalopathy, but rather as an "*encephalopathy with epilepsy*". The crucial difference being that the cognitive and behavioral problems are not a consequence of the epilepsy, but of the underlying cerebral pathology. However, also in "encephalopathy with epilepsy" seizures may aggravate cognitive and behavioral problems and thus treatment of seizures may improve outcomes.

Some disorders, mostly genetically determined, both the epilepsy and the encephalopathy appear to be symptoms of a known or unknown genetic defect and there is no evidence that epileptic activity is primarily responsible for the developmental stagnation. Examples of this include disorders associated with CDKL5, SCN1A, and PCDH19 mutations. However, all spontaneous epileptic phenomena in humans are related to some kind of brain disease (genetic through to structural) and therefore it is likely that all cognitive impairments in children with epilepsy are at least in part a function of etiology.

The concept that deterioration is independent from epilepsy in some conditions was also pointed out by Capovilla who proposed the term of "epileptogenic encephalopathies" when referring to conditions with various etiologies that can produce both deterioration (*per se*) and epilepsy (Capovilla *et al.*, 2013).

Epileptic encephalopathies are dynamic epileptic conditions in which a peculiar evolution related to the activation of specific networks is observed. Although the involvement of cortical and sub-cortical structures is a common finding, those networks seem to be different in various types of EE. We do not yet know which factors may trigger the evolution towards an epileptic encephalopathy.

References

- Berg AT, Berkovic SF, Brodie MJ, Buchhalter J, Cross H, van Emde Boas W, *et al*. Revised terminology and concepts for organization of seizures and epilepsies: Report of the ILAE Commission on Classification and Terminology, 2005-2009. *Epilepsia* 2010; 51: 676-85.
- Capovilla G, Wolf P, Beccaria F, Avanzini G. The history of the concept of epileptic encephalopathy. *Epilepsia* 2013; 54 (suppl 8): 2-5.
- Catterall WA, Kalume F, Oakley JC. NaV1.1 channels and epilepsy. *J Physiol* 2010; 588: 1849-59.
- Cilio MR, Sogawa Y, Cha BH, Liu X, Huang LT, Holmes GL. Long-term effects of status epilepticus in the immature brain are specific for age and model. *Epilepsia* 2003; 44: 518-28.
- Dabora SL, Jozwiak S, Franz DN, Roberts PS, Nieto A, Chung J, Choy YS, *et al*. Mutational analysis in a cohort of 224 tuberous sclerosis patients indicates increased severity of TSC2, compared with TSC1, disease in multiple organs. *Am J Hum Genet* 2001; 68: 64-80.
- Dravet C, Bureau M, Oguni H, Fukuyama Y, Cokar O. Severe myoclonic epilepsy in infancy (Dravet syndrome). In: Roger J, Bureau M, Dravet C, Genton P, Tassinari CA, Wolff P, editors. *Epileptic syndromes in infancy, childhood and adolescence*, 4th ed. France: John Libbey Eurotext; 2005. pp. 89-113.
- Dulac O. Epileptic encephalopathies. *Epilepsia* 2001; 42 (suppl 3): 23-6.
- Eltze C, Chong W, Cox T, *et al*. A population-based study of newly diagnosed epilepsy in infants. *Epilepsia* 2013; 54(3): 437-45.
- Engel J. A proposed diagnostic scheme for people with epileptic seizures and with epilepsy: report of the ILAE Task Force on Classification and Terminology. *Epilepsia* 2001; 42: 1-8.
- Engel J. Report of the ILAE Classification Core Group. *Epilepsia* 2006; 47: 1558-68.
- Gastaut H, Roger J, Ouahchi S, Timsit M, Broughton R. An electroclinical study of generalized epileptic seizures of tonic expression. *Epilepsia* 1963; 4: 15-44.
- Landau WM, Kleffner FR. Syndrome of acquired aphasia with convulsive disorder in children. *Neurology* 1957; 7: 523-30.

- Martin MS, Dutt K, Papale LA, Dubé CM, Dutton SB, de Haan G, Shankar A, Tufik S, Meisler MH, Baram TZ, Goldin AL, Escayg A. Altered function of the SCN1A voltage-gated sodium channel leads to gamma-aminobutyric acid-ergic (GABAergic) interneuron abnormalities. *J Biol Chem* 2010; 285: 9823-34.
- Ohtahara S, Yamatogi Y. Severe encephalopathic epilepsy in early infancy. In: Pellock JM, Bourgeois B, Dodson WE (Eds). *Pediatric epilepsy*. New York: Demos, 2008, pp. 241-7.
- Ohtahara S, Ishida T, Oka E, Inoue H. On the specific age-dependent epileptic syndromes: the early-infantile epileptic encephalopathy with suppression-burst. *No To Hattatsu* 1976; 8: 270-80.
- Paciorkowski AR, Thio LL, Rosenfeld JA, Gajecka M, Gurnett CA, Kulkarni S, Chung WK, *et al*. Copy number variants and infantile spasms: evidence for abnormalities in ventral forebrain development and pathways of synaptic function. *Eur J Hum Genet* 2011; 19: 1238-45.
- Ragona F, Granata T, Dalla Bernardina B, Offredi F, Darra F, Battaglia D, Morbi M, *et al*. Cognitive development in Dravetsyndrome: a retrospective, multicenterstudy of 26 patients. *Epilepsia* 2011; 52: 386-92.
- Siniatchkin M, van Baalen A, Jacobs J, Moeller F, Moehring J, Boor R, Wolff S, Jansen O, Stephani U, *et al*. Different neuronal networks are associated with spikes and slow activity in hypsarrhythmia. *Epilepsia* 2007; 48: 2312-21.
- Siniatchkin M, Coropceanu D, Moeller F, Boor R, Stephani U. EEG-fMRI reveals activation of brainstem and thalamus in patients with Lennox-Gastaut syndrome. *Epilepsia* 2011; 52: 766-74.
- van Eeghen AM, Nellist M, van Eeghen EE, Thiele EA. Central TSC2 missense mutations are associated with a reduced risk of infantile spasms. *Epilepsy Res* 2013; 103: 83-7.
- Vigevano F, Arzimanoglou A, Plouin P, Specchio N. Therapeutic approach to epileptic encephalopathies. *Epilepsia* 2013; 54 (suppl 8): 45-50.
- Villeneuve N, Laguitton V, Viellard M, Lépine A, Chabrol B, Dravet C, Milh M. Cognitive and adaptive evaluation of 21 consecutive patients with Dravet syndrome. *Epilepsy Behav* 2014; 31: 143-8.

The role of EEG in the management of seizures in infancy

Thomas Bast

Epilepsy Center Kork, Kehl, Germany

Without any doubt, EEG plays a major role in both the diagnosis and the classification of epilepsies starting in infancy. The differential diagnosis of paroxysmal clinical events in this age group requires at least documenting a detailed clinical history and the recording of awake and sleep EEG. Ictal video-EEG is the gold standard for the differentiation of either non-epileptic attacks *versus* epileptic seizures, or focal *versus* generalized epileptic seizures. The documentation of classical EEG patterns is essential for the diagnosis of specific electroclinical syndromes. Interictal EEG recordings and the quantification and characterization of seizures by video-EEG are essential in the diagnosis of syndromic and non-syndromic epileptic encephalopathies. Hypsarrhythmia in West syndrome (WS) is a typical example for a pathognomonic EEG pattern influencing therapeutic strategies. This review summarizes the reported data on the crucial diagnostic and therapeutic implications of EEG in epilepsies in infancy.

Differential diagnosis of seizures

Diagnosing epileptic seizures in infants and young children is challenging because symptoms can be subtle, and various forms of non-epileptic paroxysmal events may mimic epileptic seizures (Alam and Lux, 2012). There is a risk of over-interpretation of "interictal" epileptiform activity because epileptic discharges (ED) can be found in about 3% of healthy children (Eeg-Olofson, 1971; Cavazzuti *et al.*, 1980; Okubo *et al.*, 1994). In cases where the diagnosis is not completely certain, video-EEG monitoring with the recording of suspicious attacks is the gold standard. Only 50% of clinical events in neonates were correctly identified as epileptic or non-epileptic when only videos were presented to blinded doctors and other health care professionals (Malone *et al.*, 2009). In this study, clonic seizures were more likely identified as epileptic than subtle seizures. Comparable data with blinded classification based only on semiology is lacking for infants and older children. However, a recent study from Seoul reported non-epileptic events in 143/1,108 (12.9%) children who underwent long-term video-EEG at one centre (Kim *et al.*, 2012). In children under 3 years of age with non-epileptic events, the most common diagnoses were staring, tonic posturing, myoclonus, shuddering, breath holding spells, spasmus nutans, and gastroesophageal reflux. When compared to older children, more with developmental delay (42.9%) were found in the subgroup of patients younger than 6 years of age. This highlights the problem of differentiating abnormal movements from seizures in neurologically impaired infants; 25.3% of the young children had unnecessarily received an antiepileptic treatment. On the other hand, focal seizures with subtle symptoms and automatisms cannot be easily discriminated from the normal behavior of infants (Hamer *et al.*, 1999; Nordli *et al.*, 1997). Video-EEG should be performed in cases of uncertainty.

Even in infants with obvious or proven epileptic seizures, the differentiation between focal onset and generalized seizures is challenging. Focal onset seizures typically present with apparently generalized symptoms. Epileptic spasms and tonic, myoclonic, and hypomotor seizures are the most common seizure types in infants with focal epilepsy (Hamer *et al.*, 1996 and 1999; Fogarasi *et al.*, 2003; Nordli, 2002). Simultaneous ictal video-EEG allows for the differentiation in most of the cases.

■ Diagnosis of electroclinical syndromes

Various epilepsy syndromes start in the neonatal period and in infancy (Berg *et al.*, 2010). Their diagnosis depends mainly on the age of onset, the presence of typical seizure types, and classical EEG patterns. The interictal EEG is typically normal in benign familial neonatal epilepsy, benign (familial) infantile epilepsy, and in the first year after the onset of Dravet syndrome. The absence of EEG abnormalities may be critical for diagnosing these syndromes. Children with glucose-transporter-1 deficiency may present with early onset absences and generalized 2-4/s-spike and waves in the first two years of life, which is an unusual finding in this age group (Suls *et al.*, 2009). Regional or hemispheric alterations of EEG background activity and (multi)focal ED are typical for structural focal epilepsies. However, in infants there is a strong tendency towards propagation and generalization of interictal and ictal epileptiform activity. Many of these patients develop WS.

Classical EEG patterns are hallmarks of the encephalopathic electroclinical syndromes in infancy (*Table I*). Suppression-burst is typical in Ohtahara syndrome (OS) and early myoclonic encephalopathy (EME), with enhancement in sleep in the latter (Wong-Kisiel and Nickels, 2013; Ohtahara and Yamatogi, 2003). While EME is frequently caused by neurometabolic diseases, etiologies of OS are more diverse. These include structural-metabolic causes and genetic defects (*STXBP1* [Saitsu *et al.*, 2008], *ARX* [Kato *et al.*, 2007]). The EEG in malignant migrating partial seizures in infancy (MMPSI) shows almost continual focal seizure patterns. These appear with an independent onset in both hemispheres. The character is confluent, involving non-continuous brain regions with a central and temporal maximum (Wong-Kisiel and Nickels, 2013; Coppola, 2013). Neurometabolic work-up remains negative and, besides some other rare causes, some infants have *KCNT1* mutations (Barcia *et al.*, 2012). The diagnosis of infantile spasms (IS) is based on the combination of epileptic spasms occurring in clusters and hypsarrhythmia in the EEG (Hrachovy and Frost, 2003; Lux and Osborne, 2004). Hypsarrhythmia is mainly characterized by high-voltage slow waves with variable amplitudes (generally > 200 µV). The slowing is combined with ED that arise from many foci with a generally "chaotic" appearance (for review see Hrachovy and Frost, 2013; Lux and Osborne, 2004). There is a lack of synchrony in the EEG. Hypsarrhythmia is usually more pronounced in non-REM sleep, and may disappear in REM. Epileptic spasms may present without hypsarrhythmia, at least for a period of time. The EEG pattern of hypsarrhythmia is more likely present in IS with an early onset. Early in the course of WS, it can be observed more frequently. Various forms of

Table I. Specific EEG patterns in electroclinical syndromes in infancy

Syndrome	Interictal EEG	Ictal EEG
Early infantile epileptic encephalopathy (Ohtahara syndrome)	Suppression-burst (awake, sleep) with high-amplitude (150 to > 350 µV) paroxysms	Desynchronization Generalized or focal epileptic discharges
Early myoclonic encephalopathy	Suppression-burst enhanced in sleep, high-amplitude paroxysms	Desynchronization Variety of paroxysms with focal onset
Malignant migrating partial seizures of infancy	Hemispheric background slowing, multifocal ED (max. temporal, central)	Rhythmic monomorphic alpha/theta discharges in non-continuous brain regions, confluent character, onset from both hemispheres independently
Infantile spasms (West syndrome)	(Modified) hypsarrhythmia. Diffuse, high-amplitude (> 200 µV, even > 500 µV) bilateral slowing. Multifocal epileptic discharges. Electrodecrement. Various forms of modified hypsarrhythmia	Desynchronization and electrodecrement Bilateral epileptic discharges, fast rhythmic patterns

atypical or modified hypsarrhythmia have been described. These include patterns of asymmetry, consistent focal discharges, episodes of voltage attenuation (local, regional, generalized), excessive rapidity or slowing, fragmentation, increased interhemispheric synchronization, increased periodicity, or predominant high-voltage, bilaterally asynchronous slow activity.

The etiologies of IS are diverse, and EEG usually does not allow for a diagnosis of the underlying cause. Persistent asymmetry of the interictal and/or ictal EEG suggests a focal lesion (Wong-Kisiel and Nickels, 2013). Diffuse, high-amplitude fast activity is suggestive for lissencephaly (Gastaut et al., 1987). Aicardi syndrome may present with a "split brain pattern" (Desguerre et al., 2008). *CDKL5* mutation is one of the more common genetic causes of non-structural WS, leading to a typical sequence of clinical and EEG patterns (Bahi-Buisson et al., 2008a and 2008b; Klein et al., 2011). At epilepsy onset from one to 10 weeks, convulsive seizures and a normal interictal EEG are typical. The second stage is characterized by the occurrence of epileptic spasms and hypsarrhythmia. Typically the onset of spasms occurs earlier in *CDKL5* mutations when compared with other etiologies. The period with hypsarrhythmia can be prolonged and may even persist into early childhood. In the third stage of the disease, patients may either become seizure-free, or suffer from tonic and myoclonic seizures that are accompanied by diffuse EEG patterns.

EEG and epilepsy surgery in infancy

In infantile epilepsies, asymmetry of EEG background activity and/or the occurrence of regional interictal ED and seizure patterns may indicate an underlying structural lesion. These findings can be crucial in infants, since some structural lesions cannot be easily detected by MRI in this age group. Focal cortical dysplasia is one of the most important etiologies of pharmacorefractory focal epilepsies. It may be missed by MRI due to an incomplete myelination of the immature brain (Eltze *et al.*, 2005). However, the decision for epilepsy surgery in infants is based on a multimodal approach, and the presence of strictly regional or unilateral EEG abnormalities is not mandatory. In contrast, the preoperative EEG has a low predictive value in children with early brain lesions, including those with hypsarrhythmia (Wyllie *et al.*, 2007). In infants and young children, the presence of non-regional or even bilateral ictal and interictal EEG abnormalities is not correlated with the seizure outcome (Ramantani *et al.*, 2013a and 2013b).

Epileptic encephalopathy

The term "epileptic encephalopathy" was first introduced by Gastaut in 1966 (Gastaut *et al.*, 1966). It reflects the concept that the underlying epileptic activity may contribute to the developmental impairment in children with severe, early onset epilepsy and abundant epileptiform activity. In 2001, Engel defined epileptic encephalopathy as "a condition where the epileptiform abnormalities themselves are believed to contribute to the progressive disturbance of cerebral function" (Engel, 2001). In this concept, epileptic encephalopathies compromised a cluster of electroclinical syndromes including Early Myoclonic Encephalopathy, Ohtahara syndrome, West syndrome, Dravet syndrome, and others. With the latest proposal of the ILAE commission on Classification and Terminology, the concept of epileptic encephalopathy is expanded in the sense, that in every epilepsy "the epileptic activity itself may contribute to severe cognitive and behavioral impairment above and beyond what might be expected from the underlying pathology alone (*e.g.*, cortical malformation), and that this can worsen over time" (Berg *et al.*, 2010). The diagnosis of an epileptic encephalopathy can obviously only be made on the basis of careful clinical observation and (video-) EEG recordings. The latter serves to quantify the burden of clinical and subclinical epileptic activity (for a more detailed discussion on the concept and definition of epileptic encephalopathies also refer to the chapter by Vigevano and Specchio, page 155 in this volume).

Is hypsarrhythmia a kind of non-convulsive status epilepticus?

Some authors strongly believe that the continuous, non-convulsive epileptiform activity contributes to the cognitive deterioration of infants with WS, and that maximal efforts to control hypsarrhythmia should be in order (Dulac, 2001). Others state that hypsarrhythmia may be a surrogate for clinical spasms, and that there is a lack of data supporting the idea of an independent impact of hypsarrhythmia on the long-term cognitive outcome in children with WS (Lux, 2007).

The (cognitive) long-term outcome after WS is mainly determined by the etiology, and most studies failed to differentiate the various factors that possibly influence the outcome. Rener-Primec *et al.* (2006) reported a retrospective study on 48 patients with WS (including 18 cryptogenic cases). The follow-up was three to 13 years. The authors found that the risk of lower mental outcome increased after 3 weeks of hypsarrhythmia. Unfortunately, no details on the statistics leading to this conclusion, *i.e.* the parameters that entered the logistic regression model, were mentioned. The study demonstrates that there is no absolutely strict temporal relation of the disappearance of spasms and the resolution of hypsarrhythmia. Eisermann *et al.* (2003) found that both the treatment lag and the lag to cessation of spasms were correlated with a poor developmental outcome in infants with Down syndrome and IS. Cessation of spasms was defined by the disappearance of clinical seizures in combination with EEG normalization. However, both factors were not differentiated to allow for the analysis of the role of hypsarrhythmia itself. Lux (2007) made the criticism that the effects of different treatment regimens were not mentioned by the authors. Kivity et al. (2004) studied the long-term outcome of infants with cryptogenic infantile spasms after a follow-up of 6 to 21 years. They included 37 patients with infantile spasms of unknown etiology and a normal CT scan. Normal development before onset of spasms, and the absence of other seizure types before and in addition to spasms were further inclusion criteria. A successful treatment with high-dose adrenocorticotropic hormone was started within one month after onset in 22 infants, and all had a normal cognitive outcome. In contrast, the cognitive outcome was normal in only 40% of the 15 infants with a delayed start of the treatment (one to 6.5 months). While the cognitive outcome was good in all 25 infants with normal or only mildly impaired development before the onset of spasms (including four with a delayed start of the therapy), the same applied to only nine of 12 infants with markedly impaired development at onset. Therefore, normal cognitive status at onset and rapid treatment of infantile spasms were associated with a normal long-term outcome. However, the contribution of the duration of hypsarrhythmia was not analyzed. Lux assumed a bias in all the studies because cases with more severe clinical expression may have been diagnosed earlier (Lux, 2007).

Although the effects of ongoing spasms and persisting hypsarrhythmia cannot be discriminated, "the primary objective is to improve the EEG and stop the spasms as soon as possible and to avoid prolonged treatment durations with any form of therapy" (Hrachovy and Frost, 2013).

Can the occurrence of WS in infants at risk be predicted based on EEG?

Patients with neonatal seizures and multicystic periventricular leukomalacia, tuberous sclerosis complex, or malformations of cortical development have a high risk of developing WS. Since a longer lack of treatment is associated with a worse long-term outcome in WS, early or even pre-symptomatic diagnosis would be desirable. The predictive value of EEG changes in neonates is limited, and most studies failed to identify clear markers (Watanabe et al., 1980 and 1982; Ortibus et al., 1996). When combining many clinical variables and patterns of neonatal EEGs, Walther et al. (1987) constructed a model with high sensitivity and specificity regarding later development of WS. However, the complexity of the model seems to reflect the uncertainty of single parameters.

More recently, prolonged suppression of background activity (> 21 days) was identified as a risk factor for later WS in neonates with hypoxic ischemic encephalopathy (Kato et al., 2010).

In a retrospective study, Philippi et al. (2009) assigned repetitively recorded EEGs of infants with later WS to 3 clinical states preceding the onset of spasms. The authors hypothesized that visual inattention is a hallmark of WS (Jambaque et al., 1993; Rando et al., Epilepsia 2004). The visual recognition test (Cohen and Parmelee 1983; Frick and Colombo, 1996) was used to define three clinical states depending on alertness (to objects, caregivers, and noise) and the presence of contact smiling and opticofacial reflex. During a silent period eventually following an initial insult, EEG background activity was normal or only mildly abnormal, and focal and multifocal ED occurred in less than 50% of the time (EEG type 1). During the clinical state of deterioration lasting for several weeks, EEG background activity was definitely abnormal, and bilateral focal and multifocal spikes occurred in 50 to 90% of the time (*EEG type 2*). Finally, EEGs during the last days up to three weeks before the occurrence of spasms showed classical or modified hypsarrhythmia (*EEG type 3*). Based on the gestalt of EEGs, seven blinded reviewers classified numerous recordings and assigned them to one of the three EEG types. The interclass correlation coefficient was 0.73. The median weighted kappa of 0.67 indicated a good interrater reliability. In a third step, all patients that had been investigated at one centre and who were found to have EEGs type 2 were retrospectively analyzed. Eighteen of 22 untreated infants had consecutively developed WS. Only 4 patients did not develop WS. They had been treated with vigabatrin (plus valproate in three) at the time when an EEG type 2 occurred and no spasms were present. Similar findings were reported by Japanese groups. They indicated that bilateral epileptic discharges with a posterior maximum and patterns of rhythmic fast activity may precede the occurrence of IS (Endoh *et al.*, 2007 and 2011).

Consecutive EEG recordings in infants at risk may open up the opportunity for a presymptomatic treatment within the 2 to 6 weeks before spasms would probably occur. However, these data had been retrospectively collected in a few patients, and the EEGs were recorded at variable time points. The idea of a reliable identification of patients who will develop WS must be confirmed by larger and prospective studies.

Conclusion

In combination with clinical features and imaging, EEG plays a major role in the diagnosis and classification of epileptic seizures and electroclinical syndromes in infants. The diagnosis of an epileptic encephalopathy is not possible without EEG. It is still unclear whether or not epileptic EEG activity is a distinct and independent predictor for the cognitive outcome in West syndrome. Repetitively recorded EEGs in infants at risk may help in an early diagnosis of WS, which consequently allows for an early treatment.

The author is grateful to Jim Livingston for editing the manuscript.

References

- Alam S, Lux AL. Epilepsies in infancy. *Arch Dis Child* 2012; 97: 985-92.
- Bahi-Buisson N, Kaminska A, Boddaert N, *et al.* The three stages of epilepsy in patients with CDKL5 mutations. *Epilepsia* 2008; 49: 1027-37.
- Bahi-Buisson N, Nectoux J, Rosas-Vargas H, *et al.* Key clinical features to identify girls with CDKL5 mutations. *Brain* 2008; 131: 2647-61.
- Barcia G, Fleming MR, Deligniere A, *et al.* De novo gain-of-function KCNT1 channel mutations cause malignant migrating partial seizures of infancy. *Nat Genet* 2012; 44: 1255-9.
- Berg AT, Berkovic SF, Brodie MJ, *et al.* Revised terminology and concepts for organization of seizures and epilepsies: report of the ILAE Commission on Classification and Terminology, 2005-2009. *Epilepsia* 2010; 51: 676-85.
- Cavazzuti GB, Cappella L, Nalin A. Longitudinal study of epileptiform EEG patterns in normal children. *Epilepsia* 1980; 21: 43-55.
- Cohen SE, Parmelee A. Prediction of five-year Stanford-Binet scores in preterm infants. *Child Dev* 1983; 54: 1242-53.
- Coppola G. Malignant migrating partial seizures in infancy. *Handb Clin Neurol* 2013; 111: 605-9.

- Desguerre I, Nabbout R, Dulac O. The management of infantile spasms. *Arch Dis Child* 2008; 93: 462-3.
- Dulac O. What is West syndrome? *Brain Dev* 2001; 23: 447-52.
- Eeg-Olofsson O, Petersén I, Selldén U. The development of the electroencephalogram in normal children from the age of 1 through 15 years. Paroxysmal activity. *Neuropadiatrie* 1971; 2: 375-404.
- Eisermann MM, DeLaRaillère A, Dellatolas G, *et al.* Infantile spasms in Down syndrome-effects of delayed anticonvulsive treatment. *Epilepsy Res* 2003; 55: 21-7.
- Eltze CM, Chong WK, Bhate S, *et al.* Taylor-type focal cortical dysplasia in infants: some MRI lesions almost disappear with maturation of myelination. *Epilepsia* 2005; 46: 1988-992.
- Endoh F, Yoshinaga H, Kobayashi K, Ohtsuka Y. Electroencephalographic changes before the onset of symptomatic West syndrome. *Brain Dev* 2007; 29: 630-8.
- Endoh F, Yoshinaga H, Ishizaki Y, *et al.* Abnormal fast activity before the onset of West syndrome. *Neuropediatrics* 2011; 42: 51-4.
- Engel J, Jr. A proposed diagnostic scheme for people with epileptic seizures and with epilepsy: report of the ILAE Task Force on Classification and Terminology. *Epilepsia* 2001; 42: 796-803.
- Fogarasi A, Boesebeck F, Tuxhorn I. A detailed analysis of symptomatic posterior cortex seizure semiology in children younger than seven years. *Epilepsia* 2003; 44: 89-96.
- Frick JE, Colombo J. Individual differences in infants visual attention: recognition of degraded visual forms by four-month-olds. *Child Dev* 1996; 67: 188-204.
- Gastaut H, Roger J, Soulayrol R, *et al.* Epileptic encephalopathy of children with diffuse slow spikes and waves (alias "petit mal variant") or Lennox syndrome. *Ann Pediatr* (Paris) 1966; 13: 489-99.
- Gastaut H, Pinsard N, Raybaud C, Aicardi J, Zifkin B. Lissencephaly (agyria-pachygyria): clinical findings and serial EEG studies. *Dev Med Child Neurol* 1987; 29: 167-80.
- Hamer HM, Wyllie E, Luders HO, Kotagal P, Acharya J. Symptomatology of epileptic seizures in the first three years of life. *Epilepsia* 1999; 40: 837-44.
- Hrachovy RA, Frost JD Jr. Infantile epileptic encephalopathy with hypsarrhythmia (infantile spasms/West syndrome). *J Clin Neurophysiol* 2003; 20: 408-25.
- Hrachovy RA, Frost JD Jr. Infantile spasms. *Handb Clin Neurol* 2013; 111: 611-8.
- Jambaque I, Chiron C, Dulac, Raynaud C, Syrota P. Visual inattention in West syndrome: a neuropsychological and neurofunctional imaging study. *Epilepsia* 1993; 34: 692-700.
- Kato M, Saitoh S, Kamei A, *et al.* A longer polyalanine expansion mutation in the *ARX* gene causes early infantile epileptic encephalopathy with suppression-burst pattern (Ohtahara syndrome). *Am J Hum Genet* 2007; 81: 361-6.
- Kato T, Okumura A, Hayakawa F, *et al.* Prolonged EEG depression in term and near-term infants with hypoxic ischemic encephalopathy and later development of West syndrome. *Epilepsia* 2010; 51: 2392-6.
- Kim SH, Kim H, Lim BC, *et al.* Paroxysmal nonepileptic events in pediatric patients confirmed by long-term video-EEG monitoring–Single tertiary center review of 143 patients. *Epilepsy Behav* 2012; 24: 336-40.
- Kivity S, Lerman P, Ariel R, *et al.* Long-term cognitive outcomes of a cohort of children with cryptogenic infantile spasms treated with high-dose adrenocorticotropic hormone. *Epilepsia* 2004; 45: 255-62.
- Klein KM, Yendle SC, Harvey AS, *et al.* A distinctive seizure type in patients with *CDKL5* mutations: Hypermotor-tonic-spasms sequence. *Neurology* 2011; 76: 1436-8.
- Lux AL, Osborne JP. A proposal for case definitions and outcome measures in studies of infantile spasms and West syndrome: consensus statement of West Delphi group. *Epilepsia* 2004; 45: 1416-28.

- Lux AL. Is hypsarrhythmia a form of non-convulsive status epilepticus in infants? *Acta Neurol Scand* 2007; 186 (suppl): 37-44.
- Malone A, Ryan CA, Fitzgerald A, et al. Interobserver agreement in neonatal seizure identification. *Epilepsia* 2009; 50: 2097-101.
- Nordli DR Jr, Kuroda MM, Hirsch LJ. The ontogeny of partial seizures in infants and young children. *Epilepsia* 2001; 42: 986-90.
- Nordli DR Jr. Infantile seizures and epilepsy syndromes. *Epilepsia* 2002; 43 (suppl 3): 11-6.
- Ohtahara S, Yamatogi Y. Epileptic encephalopathies in early infancy with suppression-burst. *J Clin Neurophysiol* 2003; 20: 398-407.
- Okubo Y, Matsuura M, Asai T, et al. Epileptiform EEG discharges in healthy children: prevalence, emotional and behavioral correlates, and genetic influences. *Epilepsia* 1994; 35: 832-41.
- Ortibus EL, Sum JM, Hanh JS. Predictive value of EEG for outcome and epilepsy following neonatal seizures. *Electroencephalogr Clin Neurophysiol* 1996; 98: 175-85.
- Philippi H, Wohlrab G, Bettendorf U, et al. Electroencephalographic evolution of hypsarrhythmia: toward an early treatment option. *Epilepsia* 2008; 49: 1859-64.
- Ramantani G, Kadish NE, Brandt A, et al. Seizure control and developmental trajectories after-hemispherotomy for refractory epilepsy in childhood and adolescence. *Epilepsia* 2013; 54: 1046-55.
- Ramantani G, Kadish NE, Strobl K, et al. Seizure and cognitive outcomes of epilepsy surgery in infancy and early childhood. *Eur J Paediatr Neurol* 2013; 17: 498-506.
- Randò T, Bancale A, Baranello G, et al. Visual function in infants with West syndrome: correlation with EEG patterns. *Epilepsia* 2004; 45: 781-6.
- Rener-Primec Z, Stare J, Neubauer D. The risk of lower mental outcome in infantile spasms increases after three weeks of hypsarrhythmia duration. *Epilepsia* 2006; 47: 2202-5.
- Saitsu H, Kato M, Mizuguchi T, et al. De novo mutations in the gene encoding STXBP1 (MUNC18-1) cause early infantile epileptic encephalopathy. *Nat Genet* 2008; 40: 782-8.
- Suls A, Mullen SA, Weber YG, et al. Early-onset absence epilepsy caused by mutations in the glucose transporter GLUT1. *Ann Neurol* 2009; 66: 415-9.
- Walther B, Schmitt T, Reitter B. Identification of infants at risk for infantile spasms by neonatal polygraphy. *Brain Dev* 1987; 9: 377-90.
- Watanabe K, Miyazaki S, Hara K, Hakamada S. Behavioral state cycles, background EEGs and prognosis of newborns with perinatal hypoxia. *Electroencephalogr Clin Neurophysiol* 1980; 49: 618-25.
- Watanabe K, Kuroyanagi, Hara K, Miyazyki S. Neonatal seizures and subsequent epilepsy. *Brain Dev* 1982; 4: 341-46.
- Wong-Kisiel LC, Nickels K. Electroencephalogram of age-dependent epileptic encephalopathies in infancy and early childhood. *Epilepsy Res Treat* 2013: 743203.
- Wyllie E, Lachhwani DK, Gupta A, et al. Successful surgery for epilepsy due to early brain lesions despite generalized EEG findings. *Neurology* 2007; 69: 389-97.

Optimizing imaging in aiding management

William Davis Gaillard, Matthew Whitehead, Jonathan Murnick

Center for Neuroscience and the Division of Neuroradiology, Children's National Medical Center, George Washington University School of Medicine and Health Sciences, Washington DC, USA

The aims of imaging in the event of recent onset seizures or newly recognized epilepsy are to establish etiology, to help classify the seizure disorder, to inform acute and long term treatment, and to help provide prognosis (Gaillard *et al.*, 2009). In refractory epilepsy imaging is performed to identify patients who are (or may not) be surgical candidates – primarily by seeking to identify a focal abnormality that, when found and removed, is generally considered associated with a good or excellent surgical outcome. Imaging is also performed to establish etiology, if not previously determined, and identify reasons for failure of medical management. Truly normal imaging, including in children with focal seizures, should raise the possibility of a genetic cause, or perhaps (in older infants) an immune aetiology. Because of the high yield of imaging in infants with new onset seizures/epilepsy (see below) MRI is viewed as optimal care in the evaluation of infants with new onset seizures/epilepsy (Gaillard, 2009). MRI may also be performed to assess impact of therapy (as in tumors) or to assess the ill effects of treatment, as in infants on high does vigabatrin therapy (Pearl, 2009). Imaging with fMRI, DTI, PET, SPECT is reserved for children with medically refractory epilepsy, or a catastrophic epilepsy, who are being evaluated for epilepsy surgery.

There are several possible categories of image findings:
- normal MRI (which may not be normal, see below),
- incidental and findings not clinically relevant (arachnoid cysts, chiari I, etc.),
- non-specific and likely not relevant (*e.g.* mild atrophy, ventriculomegally, delayed myelination) that do not indicate etiology but hint at an injured brain,
- abnormal findings of uncertain significance such as focal encephalomalacia/gliosis, abnormal and relevant for etiology and prognosis.

Of the relevant findings:
- some will require urgent intervention (hematoma, acute hydrocephalus),
- others may identify a subacute process that has therapeutic or prognostic implications (brain tumor, leukodystrophy, inborn error of metabolism),
- others identify a focal (static) abnormality that offers the possibility of elective (*e.g.* surgical) intervention (FCD, MTS),
- some will confirm a suspected static lesion (*e.g.* porencephaly, residual of IVH, arterial stroke).

Some findings will suggest other lines of evaluation and counseling, for example findings suggestive of a metabolic disease/inborn error of metabolism or genetic cause that may also direct treatment, or indicate particularly poor prognosis. Finally, high quality imaging can often provide insights into the timing and mechanisms of injury.

The studies that are abnormal and significant can be viewed as acquired or not (congenital, developmental); and can also be viewed as focal, multifocal, or generalized. Of those acquired, infectious, hypoxic ischaemic encephalopathy (HIE), trauma, neoplasm, and seizure induced changes are the most relevant. Generalized or bilateral multifocal abnormalities (HIE, generalized MCD e.g. lissencephaly, metabolic, congenital infection; TS) are more likely to be associated with poor long term developmental outcomes, and, with the possible exception of TS, not amenable to surgical intervention. The identification of solitary focal abnormalities (Vascular (stroke, AVM, angiomatosis), mesial temporal sclerosis (MTS), developmental tumor, focal cortical dysplasia (FCD) is germane as one aim for imaging is to identify epilepsy that is amenable to surgery. Some abnormalities will also suggest medical management is unlikely to be effective (lissencephaly, hemimegalencephaly).

A limitation common to imaging studies is the lack of control data with regard to clinical imaging sequences for much of this age range (Gaillard et al., 2011).Substantial control data are more readily available for neonates (who will readily sleep in the scanner) and for children three years and older (Katzman et al., 1999). It is not feasible to obtain extensive control data in this age due to the unacceptable need for sedation. However, several studies that have laboriously acquired normal infant (1-24 mo) data, usually by waiting for children to fall asleep in the scanner, are beginning to appear in the literature. These include normal anatomical MRI (Altaye, 2008; Sanchez, 2012; Akiyama, 2103), DTI atlases and white matter tract development (Geng, 2012; Sadeghi, 2013), and structural (DTI) and functional (BOLD) connectivity (Tymofiyeva, 2013; Damaraju, 2013). These data have not been applied to epilepsy populations; rather, most are directed at recovery from neonatal injury and autism. It is not possible to obtain control data for PET and SPECT studies due to radiation exposure, but pseudo control data are available for limited populations for FDG-PET (Chugani, 1987; Kinnala, 1996; Van Bogaert, 1998) and Xenon (CBF) SPECT (Chiron, 1992). These later studies show the rapid increase in glucose consumption and CBF in these early years that presumably reflects synapse formation.

There are very few prospective imaging studies involving children with new onset, or newly recognized, seizures/epilepsy with standardized protocols involving CT or MRI in infants (one – twenty four months). No studies satisfy American Academy of Neurology (http://tools.aan.com/globals/axon/assets/9023.pdf) requirements for Class I data. There are two Class I epidemiologic studies that include imaging. Imaging, however, was not a primary aim of these studies thus relegating the image aspects of the study to lower class (Berg et al., 2000; Shinnar et al., 2001). There are two prospective observational Class II studies focused on infants, one in infants with a first unprovoked seizure (Hsieh et al., 2010), and one in infants with new onset epilepsy (Eltze et al., 2013). These two infant studies establish the substantial yield of abnormal findings in this population, relevant findings seen in 33-45%, and confirm superiority of MRI over CT. Furthermore acute abnormalities can be identified in nearly 10% of infants with new onset afebrile seizures that may change management. MRI will show abnormalities not seen on CT, and that are pertinent in half of these infants. Both series identify malformations of cortical development as the most common finding. There is one Class III study that evaluated CT in children with new onset afebrile seizures that also found substantial yield of identifying focal abnormalities using CT when seizures were focal and children were younger than 33 months (Sharma et al., 2003). As primary generalized epilepsies are rare in this age (Shinnar et al., 1994; Hsieh et al., 2010) the yield of imaging is high and is supported by ILAE and AAN guidelines for imaging patients with focal findings as optimal evaluation of new onset seizures in this age range (Hirtz et al., 2000; Gaillard et al., 2009). These above studies may underestimate the identification of relevant abnormalities. There are reports (Class IV) that imaging abnormalities with MRI may disappear or appear with maturation of white matter that help define or obscure malformations of cortical development (Sankar et al., 1995; Eltze et al., 2005; Takanashi & Barkovich, 2003). There are no data regarding the utility of higher magnetic fields for infants. There are limited data to suggest in older populations, primarily in adults, that 3T MRI may improve identification and delimitation of relevant abnormalities such as FCD and MTS (Knake, 2005; Strandberg, 2008; Zijlmans, 2009; Craven 2012; Winston, 2013). There are no published data at 7T for the epilepsy populations.

Structural and functional imaging are advocated in the evaluation of infants and children for medically refractory surgery because of the impression that the resection of focal abnormalities is associated with good surgical outcomes. Long term longitudinal outcome in patients with MCD however is 40% (Hamiwka, 2005); outcome may be optimized if there is removal of the epileptiogenic zone based on ECOG and imaging (Krsek, 2009; Perry, 2010). The ability to identify and remove abnormal tissue is thus important for surgical success. There are no Class I or Class II studies evaluating the utility of MRI for evaluating children for epilepsy surgery in the infant age range. However, reason dictates that MRI will have a higher yield in refractory patients than in new onset seizure patients, especially as MCD and developmental tumors are the most common entities for surgical management in this age group (Harvey et al., 2008).

Although there is no current consensus regarding specific MR pulse sequence prescription in the evaluation of infantile seizures, a collection of T1, T2, and diffusion weighted images in varying planes are most often utilized. Age-dependent progression of myelination causes an ever-changing MR contrast resolution in the infantile period, complicating MR pulse sequence decisions. The most difficult age to image is approximately 8-14 months. The reason for this has to do with the process of myelination (Yakovlev, 1967) that occurs from posterior to anterior, caudal to rostral, and from medial to lateral brain regions (Almli, 2007). Myelin, depending on its maturity, exhibits changing signal intensity on T1 and T2 weighted images.

For identification of malformations of cortical development (MCD), particularly subtle FCD, it is critical to image the gray-white junction throughout the cerebral hemispheres as clearly as possible. Maximum sensitivity for FCD is achieved by viewing this interface with the highest spatial resolution and highest tissue contrast achievable. Some of the factors affecting spatial resolution are discussed below. In the first two years of life, tissue contrast between the cortical gray matter and subcortical white matter is greatly dependent on the stage of myelination. On T1WI, unmyelinated white matter is hypointense compared to gray matter. As myelin matures in the first year of life, the T1WI signal in white matter increases, becoming isointense to gray matter, and ultimately hyperintense. For T2WI, unmyelinated white matter is hyperintense to gray matter. As myelin matures there is a relative reduction in T2 signal; it becomes isointense and subsequently hypointense to gray matter.

In the neonate, the subcortical white matter is nearly entirely unmyelinated and the gray-white junction can be well evaluated on both T1WI and T2WI. As myelination progresses, the white matter T1 signal increases sooner than the T2 signal decreases. By about 6 months of age, subcortical white matter is nearly isointense to gray matter over large segments of the cerebral hemispheres on T1WI, and the tissue contrast needed to detect FCD is lost. However, subcortical white matter remains hypointense to gray matter on T2WI, so the T2WI are the preferred sequences for detecting FCD at this age.

As myelination continues to progress, the subcortical white matter becomes more nearly isointense to gray matter on T2WI, as well. For this reason, the ages of approximately 8-14 months offer the lowest sensitivity for FCD, as tissue contrast at the gray-white interface is relatively poor on both T1WI and T2WI. At this age, MR spectroscopy and FDG-PET may be especially helpful (Caruso, 2013; Chugani, 1996) (see below). By about 16 months, the white matter has become T1 hyperintense throughout most of the brain, and T1WI is the most sensitive sequence for FCD. At this age, only the anterior frontal and anterior temporal lobes remain difficult to evaluate, as these are the last regions to complete myelination. By 24 months, the myelination has progressed to essentially an adult appearance on MRI, and both T2WI and T1WI show good gray-white contrast throughout the brain.

In infants, small brain size is an obstacle to optimal signal to noise ratios and spatial resolution, parameters of utmost importance in the search for epileptogenic disease processes. Assuming a constant image matrix, decreasing the field of view to accommodate for head size will decrease the signal to noise ratio. The matrix size can then be decreased, however, spatial resolution will be sacrificed. Increasing the number of excitations improves the signal to noise ratio (at the cost of time), as does decreasing the receiver bandwidth (also at the cost of time).

The following sequences are recommended for **children younger than age two years** (Gaillard, 2009): high resolution sagittal, axial, coronal T2 weighted (or 3D); 3D T1 weighted, T2 FLAIR, and oblique coronal high resolution T2 weighted perpendicular to the hippocampal formation. Specific protocols for ages in this range are detailed below.

For FCD, thin slice acquisition is important. Classical imaging markers of type II FCD include cortical thickening, blurring of grey-white margin, and increased signal, thus the need for high resolution/small voxel size acquisition. Adjunctive sequences may include perfusion images (*e.g.* arterial spin labelling (ASL) and magnetization transfer T1WI.

ASL perfusion is a technique that depicts cerebral perfusion (mL/100 g tissue/min) by magnetically tagging arterial blood in the neck (Deibler, 2008). Cortical hyperperfusion is present in the ictal phase; hypoperfusion which may be visible in epileptogenic regions in the interictal state (Deibler, 2008; Pendse, 2010) is an unreliable method for identifying the epileptogenic zone.

Magnetization transfer T1WI has been shown to be of utility for detection of cortical tubers and cortical dysplasia, especially in patients with incomplete brain myelination (Kadom, 2010). Magnetization transfer T1WI images appear to be of greater use and reliability on 1.5 rather than 3T scanners.

Macroscopically normal brain structure as viewed on MR does not exclude underlying structural and/or functional pathology. In patients with metabolic disease, MRS may be the only abnormal sequence. In this arena, MRS can be useful in the evaluation of both partial and generalized seizure disorders (Caruso, 2013). Multivoxel MRS can assist with lesion localization/lateralization in patients both with and without temporal lobe epilepsy, evaluate extent of disease, and assess related metabolic derangements which may indicate the seizure origin or be a consequence thereof (Miller, 2013; Fountas, 2012). Spectroscopy may compliment morphologic information in patients with Rasmussen's encephalitis and tuberous sclerosis (Matthews, 1990; Yapici, 2005). If a structural lesion is discovered, single voxel MRS may help reveal its nature, whether neoplastic, inflammatory, infectious, ischemic, or metabolic.

Tables I and II provide parameters and sequences used at one institution where two separate predesigned MR protocols are tailored for patients less than and greater than one year of age (*Tables I and II*). The choice of sequences and sequence parameters vary according to field strength and scanner model, in addition to individual site preferences and experience. Field of view must be adjusted for head size. For 3D images, field of view and matrix size are typically scaled down in synchrony for patients less than one year to maintain a constant signal to noise ratio. T2-weighted sequences represent the foundation of the first year of life protocol, including coronal 3D T2 CUBE (reformatted into axial, coronal, sagittal planes), axial and sagittal fast recovery fast spin echo (FRFSE) T2, sagittal T2 FLAIR CUBE images (reformatted into axial, coronal, and sagittal planes), and coronal fat sat fast FRFSE T2WI of the entire brain as well as coronal oblique high resolution FRFSE T2WI perpendicular to the long axis of the hippocampal formations. Additional sequences include 3D sagittal T1WI (reformatted into axial, coronal, and sagittal planes), axial SWAN, axial ASL, axial DTI with 25 directions of encoding (highest quality research DTI may use up to 60 directions, primarily for tractography, but requires more time), and single voxel MR spectroscopy (SV MRS) with voxel placed on the left basal ganglia (TE = 288). We include the MRS sequence for patients under 12 months of age, since seizure is more likely to represent an initial presentation of a metabolic disorder in this age group than in older children. Axial T1 weighted magnetization transfer images are acquired if the patient weights 12 kg or more, as SAR deposition can be an issue.

In patients older than one year, a similar pulse sequence set is acquired with the following omissions: sagittal T2, coronal T2 CUBE, and MRS. The 3D sequence orthogonal plane reformats are displayed at 2mm contiguous slice thickness, trading some spatial resolution for signal to noise ratio enhancement. If possible, seizure patients should undergo scans on a 3T MR (Discovery MP750, General Electric, Milwaukee, WI) with a 32-channel head coil, especially if focal seizures are known or suspected. A smaller head coil is often necessary in patients under three months (8 channel). Neonates are typically imaged without sedation, just after feeding. Infants often require general anesthesia for diagnostic image acquisition as even subtle motion artifact can severely plaque image quality. Generally, the total imaging time varies from 25-40 minutes.

The yield of the MRI study may be maximized if the interpreting neuroradiologist (or other reader) is aware of any localizing information. In particular he or she should be informed of any localizing findings from EEG. The seizure characteristics are also important information that should be shared, particularly when the EEG is negative or nonspecific. The reader can then concentrate the search for subtle focal abnormalities in the region of the suspected seizure focus.

While imaging with MRI may be optimal for any infant with epilepsy, imaging resources may be scarce. CT provides helpful information and may change management, especially in urgent settings, but may be falsely reassuring when "normal" (Hsieh *et al.*, 2009) and also conveys radiation exposure to immature brains especially when expertise is lacking

Table I. Sample 3T brain MR protocol and imaging parameters for children < 1 year. Differences from > 1 year protocol are highlighted in bold

Sequence	Plane	TR	TE	TI	FA	Nex	ETL	FOV	ST	SS	Matrix	BW
T2 FRFSE	axial	3500	100	0	90	2	14	18×16	2	2.2	320×224	×25
T2 FRFSE	**sagittal**	**3500**	**100**	**0**	**90**	**1**	**21**	**18×16**	**2**	**2**	**320×224**	**25**
T2 CUBE	**coronal**	**2500**	**82**	**0**	**90**	**1**	**100**	**18×18**	**1**	**1**	**256×256**	**50**
T2 FRFSE fat sat	coronal	3500	100	0	90	1	21	20×17	3.5	3.5	288×288	31.2
T2 FRFSE hippocampi	coronal oblique	3000	100	0	90	3	28	16×14	3	3	384×288	31.2
T2 FLAIR CUBE	sagittal	6000	130	1847	90	1	140	21×20	1.2	0.6	224×224	31.2
DTI	axial	10000	82	0	90	1	1	22×22	3	3	128×128	250
T1 FSPGR	sagittal	8	3	450	12	1	1	18×16	1	0.5	224×224	31.2
ASL	axial	4400	11	1025	111	3	1	24×24	3	3	512×8	62.5
MT	axial	500	10	0	90	1	1	18×18	5	6	320×192	62.5
SWAN	axial	39	24	0	15	0.69	6	18×16	3	1.5	320×224	62.5
MRS	**NA**	**1500**	**288**	**0**	**90**	**8**	**1**	**2×2×2**	**na**	**na**	**na**	**na**

FRFSE: fast recovery fast spin echo; ASL: arterial spin labeling; DTI: diffusion tensor images; FSPGR: fast spoiled gradient echo; SWAN: susceptibility weighted angiography; MT: magnetization transfer spin echo T1; MRS: magnetic resonance spectroscopy; TR: repetition time (ms); TE: echo time (ms); TI: inversion time (ms); FA: flip angle; Nex: #excitations; ETL: echo train length; FOV: field of view (cm); ST: slice thickness (mm); SS: slice spacing (mm); BW: bandwidth (kHz).

Table II. Sample 3T brain MR protocol and imaging parameters for children > 1 year. Differences from < 1 year seizure protocol are highlighted in bold

Sequence	Plane	TR	TE	TI	FA	Nex	ETL	FOV	ST	SS	Matrix	BW
T2 FRFSE	axial	3500	100	0	90	2	25	20×17	2	2.2	**320×320**	31.2
T2 FRFSE fat sat	coronal	3500	100	0	90	1	21	20×17	3.5	3.5	288×288	31.2
T2 FRFSE hippocampi	coronal oblique	3000	100	0	90	3	**23**	**16×16**	3	3	384×288	31.2
T2 FLAIR CUBE	sagittal	6000	130	1847	90	1	140	22×21	1.4	0.7	**256×256**	31.2
DTI	axial	10000	82	0	90	1	1	24×24	3	3	128×128	250
T1 FSPGR	sagittal	8	3	450	12	1	1	**22×22**	1	0.5	**265×256**	31.2
ASL	axial	4400	11	1025	111	3	1	24×24	3	3	512×8	62.5
MT	axial	500	10	0	90	1	1	**20×17**	5	7	320×192	62.5
SWAN	axial	39	24	0	15	0.69	6	20×20	3	1.5	320×224	62.5

FRSE: fast recovery fast spin echo; ASL: arterial spin labeling; DTI: diffusion tensor images; FSPGR: fast spoiled gradient echo; MT: magnetization transfer spin echo T1; SWAN: susceptibility weighted angiography; MRS: magnetic resonance spectroscopy; TR: repetition time (ms); TE: echo time (ms); TI: inversion time (ms); FA: flip angle; Nex: #excitations;ETL: echo train length; FOV: field of view (cm); ST: slice thickness (mm); SS: slice spacing (mm); BW: bandwidth (kHz).

(Brenner et al., 2001). MRI in this age range often requires sedation (except in young infants who may be able to be scanned when asleep), and are most informative when interpreted by those skilled in reading infant MRI. Thus, there are circumstances when imaging may not be practical. In this setting imaging may be reserved for those who:
- require evaluation for neurological and neurosurgical emergencies (status epilepticus, increased ICP, etc.),
- do not respond to medications (there is a theoretical risk that brain tumors or vascular malformations may not identified with this strategy),
- reserved only for those considered for epilepsy surgery assuming resources are available for such consideration. If seizures persist then repeat imaging may be necessary when brain maturation allows identification of developmental abnormalities (Gaillard, et al., 2009).

Early detection and intervention are thought to result in improved outcomes, for seizure control, cognition, and socialization, especially for the catastrophic epilepsies that often have a structural etiology (MCD, FCD, Stroke, TS) and risks for surgery are low (Devlin, 2003; Jonas, 2005; Pulsifer, 2004; Smith, 2004; Elliott, 2008). When MRI is thought to be normal functional imaging with PET and SPECT is conducted to identify the epileptogenic zone. As with MRI there are no Class I or II studies examining utility of functional imaging with PET or SPECT in infants for epilepsy surgery. It is thought that the utility of ^{18}FDG-PET in this age group in part derives from an ability to identify the functional expression of focal developmental abnormalities that may not be apparent on structural imaging studies due to immaturity of myelination (Chugani, 1990; Chugani, 1996, 2013). For these reasons FDG-PET may provide higher yield than in older MRI "negative" patients. Epileptogenic cortex, including MCD/FCD, often are hypometabolic thus exhibit decreased FDG-uptake in the interictal state. The area of hypometabolism may be more widespread than the epileptogenic zone but is invariably ipsilateral to the epilepsy focus (except in TS, see below). Focal FDG-PET abnormalities, especially when co-registered with MRI, may result in re-review of MRI that identifies a structural abnormality (usually FCD, I or II) (Salamon, 2008; Chassoux, 2012). When MRI remains normal underlying pathology usually shows either type I or type II FCD. Bilateral abnormalities on FDG-PET are associated with poor outcomes from surgery (Chugani, 1996, 2012; Moosa, 2012). ^{11}C AMT PET is a precursor of serotonin and also the excitatory quinolinic and kynurenic amino acids. FCD may exhibit increased uptake of AMT and thus be identified (Juhász, 2003). In children with facilitated spasms or focal epilepsy and TS, tubers are hypometabolic. However, AMT PET may exhibit focal increased uptake in approximately 50% of patients and when found are thought to be helpful in identifying the epileptogenic tuber (Chugani, 2013). While children with a (history) of facilitated spasms may have focal FDG-PET abnormalities that helps identify the seizure focus and identify candidates who may benefit from surgery (Chugani, 1990, 1996), patients with active infantile spasms may exhibit unstable FDG-PET findings. In this setting persistently focal abnormalities may be helpful (Metsahonkala, 2002).

Ictal SPECT, and more importantly ictal subtraction SPECT (where ictal and interictal studies are normalized, placed in common space and the interictal image is subtracted from the ictal study then co-registered with a high resolution MRI) are also reported to be helpful in identifying or confirming the epileptogenic zone in infants and helping to guide surgery in the few published class III and IV studies (Véra, 1999; Kaminska, 2003; Hartley, 2002). This has been reported with either of the CBF SPECT ligands (ECD, HMPAO). Ictal subtraction SPECT is a little less reliable than FDG-PET for lateralization of the seizure focus due to propagation effects, as certainty of findings reflects rapidity of administering the ligand in relation to seizure onset. As with PET, SPECT has also been used in children with TS and spasms to help identify the epileptogenic tuber (Koh, 1999; Kakisaka, 2009; Aboian, 2011). Interictal cerebral blood flow based studies such as SPECT, ^{15}O water PET, and ASL-MRI are unreliable for localizing and lateralizing the seizure focus.

Imaging may also be used to identify regions to spare during surgery, when avoidable. Traditionally, the main concerns are to identify primary motor and sensory cortex (*e.g.* motor, vision). While it may be possible to identify receptive language cortex resection of language cortex in children before two years is associated with excellent recovery and re-organization. DTI may be used to identify the optic radiations and the descending motor fibers (Gentz, 2012). fMRI, may be challenging in neonates and the very young as the BOLD effect may be paradoxical due to altered hemoglobin binding and concentration especially if there is persistent fetal hemoglobin. Infants are not sufficiently cognizant to execute performance based tasks, thus all tasks are passive and performed while asleep or under (light) sedation. Some investigators have used listening to a mothers voice with reverse speech control to isolate temporal speech areas (Dehaene-Lambertz, 2002, 2006), though most use stories or auditory clues without control and identify primary auditor cortex, or flashing checkerboards to identify primary visual cortex. Passive movement of the foot or hand can identify motor and sensory cortex. (Deep) Anesthesia abolishes the BOLD response but light sedation does not (Altman, 2001; Bernal, 2012; Barba, 2012).

Conclusion

There is no substitute for (early) high quality MRI with an age appropriate epilepsy protocol interpreted by those skilled in reading infant MRI. When focal epilepsy is known or suspected, information regarding the presumed epileptogenic zone should be readily available to the neuroradiologist or other reader at the time of interpretation for improved diagnostic yield. Imaging yield is optimum if obtained before 6-8 months, and if normal may need to be repeated, with optimal resolution not occurring until 24 months or more following myelination maturation. When MRI is normal, and seizures remain refractory, FDG PET, and in some circumstances AMT–PET, may be helpful aids in identifying the epileptogenic zone, as is Ictal (subtraction) SPECT. Truly MRI negative studies may also suggest under appreciated genetic (or immune) causes.

References

- Aboian MS, Wong-Kisiel LC, Rank M, Wetjen NM, Wirrell EC, Witte RJ. SISCOM in children with tuberous sclerosis complex-related epilepsy. *Pediatr Neurol* 2011 Aug; 45(2): 83-8; doi: 10.1016/j. pediatrneurol. 2011. 05. 001.
- Akiyama LF, Richards TR, Imada T, Dager SR, Wroblewski L, Kuhl PK. Age-specific average head template for typically developing 6-month-old infants. *PLoS One* 2013 Sep 12; 8(9): e73821.
- Almli CR, Rivkin MJ, McKinstry RC; Brain Development Cooperative Group. The NIH MRI study of normal brain development (Objective-2): newborns, infants, toddlers, and preschoolers. *Neuroimage* 2007 Mar; 35(1): 308-25.

- Altaye M, Holland SK, Wilke M, Gaser C. Infantbrain probability templates for MRI segmentation and normalization. *Neuroimage* 2008 Dec; 43(4): 721-30; doi: 10. 1016/j. neuroimage. 2008. 07. 060. Epub 2008 Aug 13.
- Altman NR, Bernal B. Brain activation in sedated children: auditory and visual functional MR imaging. *Radiology* 2001 Oct; 221(1): 56-63.
- Barba C, Montanaro D, Frijia F, Giordano F, Blümcke I, Genitori L, et al. Focal cortical dysplasia type IIb in the rolandic cortex: functional reorganization after early surgery documented by passive task functional MRI. *Epilepsia* 2012 Aug; 53(8): e141-5; doi: 10. 1111/j. 1528-1167. 2012. 03524. x. Epub 2012 Jun 12.
- Berg AT, Testa FM, Levy SR, Shinnar S. Neuroimaging in children with newly diagnosed epilepsy: a community-based study. *Pediatrics* 2000; 106(3): 527-32.
- Bernal B, Grossman S, Gonzalez R, Altman N. FMRI under sedation: what is the best choice in children? *J Clin Med Res* 2012 Dec; 4(6): 363-70.
- Brenner D, Elliston C, Hall E, Berdon W. Estimated risks of radiation-induced fatal cancer from pediatric CT. *AJR Am J Roentgenol* 2001; 176: 289-96.
- Caruso P, Johnson J, Thibert R, Rapalino O, Rincon S, Ratai EM. The use of magnetic resonance spectroscopy in the evaluation of epilepsy. *Neuroimaging Clin N Am* 2013; 23(3): 407-24.
- Chassoux F, Landré E, Mellerio C, Turak B, Mann MW, Daumas-Duport C, Chiron C, Devaux B. Type II focal cortical dysplasia: electroclinical phenotype and surgical outcome related to imaging. *Epilepsia* 2012; 53(2): 349-58.
- Chiron C, Raynaud C, Mazière B, Zilbovicius M, Laflamme L, Masure MC, et al. Changes in regional cerebral blood flow during brain maturation in children and adolescents. *J Nucl Med* 1992 May; 33(5): 696-703.
- Chugani HT, Conti JR. Etiologic classification of infantile spasms in 140 cases: role of positron emission tomography. *J Child Neurol* 1996; 11: 44-8.
- Chugani HT, Luat AF, Kumar A, Govindan R, Pawlik K, Asano E. α-[11C]-Methyl-l-tryptophan–PET in 191 patients with tuberous sclerosis complex. *Neurology* 2013; 81(7): 674-80.
- Chugani HT, Phelps ME, Mazziotta JC. Positron emission tomography study of human brain functional development. *Ann Neurol* 1987 Oct; 22(4): 487-97.
- Chugani HT, Shields WD, Shewmon DA, Olson DM, Phelps ME, Peacock WJ. Infantile spasms: I. PET identifies focal cortical dysgenesis in cryptogenic cases for surgical treatment. *Ann Neurol* 1990; 27: 406-13.
- Craven IJ, Griffiths PD, Bhattacharyya D, Grunewald RA, Hodgson T, Connolly DJ, et al. 3. 0 T MRI of 2000 consecutive patients with localisation-related epilepsy. *Br J Radiol* 2012 Sep; 85(1017): 1236-42.
- Daghistani R, Widjaja E. Role of MRI in patient selection for surgical treatment of intractable epilepsy in infancy. *Brain Dev* 2013; 35: 697-705.
- Damaraju E, Caprihan A, Lowe JR, Allen EA, Calhoun VD, Phillips JP. Functional connectivity in the developing brain: A longitudinal study from 4 to 9 months of age. *Neuroimage* 2013 Aug 27; 84C: 169-80.
- Dehaene-Lambertz G, Dehaene S, Hertz-Pannier L. Functional neuroimaging of speech perception in infants. *Science* 2002 Dec 6; 298(5600): 2013-5.
- Dehaene-Lambertz G, Hertz-Pannier L, Dubois J, Mériaux S, Roche A, Sigman M, et al. Functional organization of perisylvian activation during presentation of sentences in preverbal infants. *Proc Natl Acad Sci USA* 2006 Sep 19; 103(38): 14240-5.
- Deibler AR, Pollock JM, Kraft RA, Tan H, Burdette JH, Maldjian JA. Arterial spin-labeling in routine clinical practice, part 2: hypoperfusion patterns. *Am J Neuroradiol* 2008; 29(7): 1235-41.
- Deibler AR, Pollock JM, Kraft RA, Tan H, Burdette JH, Maldjian JA. Arterial spin-labeling in routine clinical practice, part 3: hyperperfusion patterns. *Am J Neuroradiol* 2008; 29(8): 1428-35.

- Devlin AM, Cross JH, Harkness W, Chong WK, Harding B, Vargha-Khadem F, et al. Clinical outcomes of hemispherectomy for epilepsy in childhood and adolescence. *Brain* 2003 Mar; 126 (Pt 3): 556-66.
- Elliott IM, Lach L, Kadis DS, Smith ML. Psychosocial outcomes in children two years after epilepsysurgery: has anything changed? *Epilepsia* 2008 Apr; 49(4): 634-41; doi: 10. 1111/j. 1528-1167. 2007. 01498. x. Epub 2007 Dec 28.
- Eltze CM, Chong WK, Bhate S, Harding B, Neville BG, Cross JH. Taylor-type focal cortical dysplasia in infants: some MRI lesions almost disappear with maturation of myelination. *Epilepsia* 2005; 46: 1988-92.
- Eltze CM, Chong WK, Cox T, Whitney A, Cortina-Borja M, Chin RF, Scott RC, Cross JH. A population-based study of newly diagnosed epilepsy in infants. *Epilepsia* 2013; 54: 437-45.
- Fountas KN, Tsougos I, Gotsis ED, Giannakodimos S, Smith JR, Kapsalaki EZ. Temporal pole proton preoperative magnetic resonance spectroscopy in patients undergoing surgery for mesial temporal sclerosis. *Neurosurg Focus* 2012; 32(3): E3.
- Gaillard WD, Chiron C, Cross JH, Harvey AS, Kuzniecky R, Hertz-Pannie L, et al. Guidelines for imaging infants and children with recent-onset epilepsy. *Epilepsia* 2009; 50: 2147-53.
- Gaillard WD, Cross JH, S Duncan JS, Stephan H, Theodore WH. Epilepsy imaging study guideline criteria: commentary on diagnostic testing study guidelines & practice parameters. *Epilepsia* 2011; 52: 1750-6.
- Geng X, Gouttard S, Sharma A, Gu H, Styner M, Lin W, et al. Quantitative tract-based white matter development from birth to age 2 years. *Neuroimage* 2012 Jul 2; 61(3): 542-57.
- Hamiwka L, Jayakar P, Resnick T, Morrison G, Ragheb J, Dean P, et al. Surgery for epilepsy due to cortical malformations: ten-year follow-up. *Epilepsia* 2005 Apr; 46(4): 556-60.
- Hartley LM, Gordon I, Harkness W, Harding B, Neville BG, Cross JH. Correlation of SPECT with pathology and seizure outcome in children undergoing epilepsysurgery. *Dev Med Child Neurol* 2002 Oct; 44(10): 676-80.
- Harvey AS, Cross JH, Shinnar S, Mathern BW; ILAE Pediatric Epilepsy Surgery Survey Taskforce. Defining the spectrum of international practice in pediatric epilepsy surgery patients. *Epilepsia* 2008; 49: 146-55.
- Hirtz D, Ashwal S, Berg A, Bettis D, Camfield C, Camfield P, et al. Practice parameter: evaluating a first nonfebrile seizure in children: report of the quality standards subcommittee of the American Academy of Neurology, The Child Neurology Society, and The American Epilepsy Society. *Neurology* 2000; 55: 616-23.
- Hsieh DT, Taeun Chang T, Tsuchida TN, Vezina LG, Vanderver A, Siedel J, et al. New onset afebrile seizures in infants: Presenting characteristics. *Neurology* 2010; 74: 150-6.
- Jonas R, Asarnow RF, LoPresti C, Yudovin S, Koh S, Wu JY, Sankar R, Shields WD, Vinters HV, Mathern GW. Surgery for symptomatic infant-onset epileptic encephalopathy with and without infantile spasms. *Neurology* 2005 Feb 22; 64(4): 746-50.
- Jonas R, Nguyen S, Hu B, Asarnow RF, LoPresti C, Curtiss S, et al. Cerebral hemispherectomy: hospital course, seizure, developmental, language, and motor outcomes. *Neurology* 2004 May 25; 62(10): 1712-21.
- Juhász C, Chugani DC, Muzik O, Shah A, Asano E, Mangner TJ, et al. Alpha-methyl-L-tryptophan PET detects epileptogenic cortex in children with intractable epilepsy. *Neurology* 2003 Mar 25; 60(6): 960-8.
- Kadom N, Trofimova A, Vezina GL. Utility of magnetization transfer T1 Imaging in children with seizures. *J Neuroradiol* 2010; 37(1): 60-3.
- Kakisaka Y, Haginoya K, Ishitobi M, Togashi N, Kitamura T, Wakusawa K, et al. Utility of subtraction ictalSPECT images in detecting focal leading activity and understanding the pathophysiology of spasms in patients with West syndrome. *Epilepsy Res* 2009 Feb; 83(2-3): 177-83.

- Kaminska A, Chiron C, Ville D, Dellatolas G, Hollo A, Cieuta C, et al. IctalSPECT in children with epilepsy: comparison with intracranial EEG and relation to postsurgical outcome. *Brain* 2003 Jan; 126(Pt 1): 248-60.
- Katzman GL, Dagher AP, Patronas NJ. Incidental findings on brain magnetic resonance imaging from 1000 asymptomatic volunteers. *JAMA* 1999; 282: 36-9.
- Kinnala A, Suhonen-Polvi H, Äärimaa T, Kero P, Korvenranta H, Ruotsalainen U, et al. Cerebral metabolic rate for glucose during the first six months of life: an FDG positron emission tomography study. *Arch Dis Child Fetal Neonatal Ed.* 1996 May; 74(3): F153-7.
- Knake S, Triantafyllou C, Wald LL, Wiggins G, Kirk GP, Larsson PG, et al. 3T phased array MRI improves the presurgical evaluation in focal epilepsies: a prospective study. *Neurology* 2005 Oct 11; 65(7): 1026-31.
- Koh S, Jayakar P, Resnick T, Alvarez L, Liit RE, Duchowny M. The localizing value of ictalSPECT in children with tuberous sclerosis complex and refractory partial epilepsy. *Epileptic Disord* 1999 Mar; 1(1): 41-6.
- Krsek P, Kudr M, Jahodova A, Komarek V, Maton B, Malone S, et al. Localizing value of ictal SPECT is comparable to MRI and EEG in children with focal cortical dysplasia. *Epilepsia* 2013 Feb; 54(2): 351-8; doi: 10. 1111/epi. 12059. Epub 2013 Jan 7.
- Krsek P, Maton B, Jayakar P, Dean P, Korman B, Rey G, et al. Incomplete resection of focal cortical dysplasia is the main predictor of poor postsurgical outcome. *Neurology* 2009 Jan 20; 72(3): 217-23; doi: 10. 1212/01. wnl. 0000334365. 22854. d3. Epub 2008 Nov 12.
- Li W, Wait SD, Ogg RJ, Scoggins MA, Zou P, Wheless J, et al. Functional magnetic resonance imaging of the visual cortex performed in children under sedation to assist in presurgical planning. *J Neurosurg Pediatr* 2013 May; 11(5): 543-6.
- Matthews PM, Andermann F, Arnold DL. A proton magnetic resonance study of focal epilepsy in humans. *Neurology* 1990; 40(6): 985-9.
- Metsähonkala L, Gaily E, Rantala H, Salmi E, Valanne L, Äärimaa T, et al. Focal and global cortical hypometabolism in patients with newly diagnosed infantile spasms. *Neurology* 2002; 58(11): 1646-51.
- Miller E, Widjaja E. Magnetic resonance spectroscopy in epilepsy from MR Spectroscopy of Pediatric Brain Disorders. In: Bluml S and Panigrahy A, editors. *MR spectroscopy of pediatric brain disorders*. New York: Springer, 2013.
- Moosa AN, Gupta A, Jehi L, Marashly A, Cosmo G, Lachhwani D, et al. Longitudinal seizure outcome and prognostic predictors after hemispherectomy in 170 children. *Neurology* 2013; 80(3): 253-60.
- Pearl PL, Vezina LG, McCarter R, Molloy-Wells E, Trzcinski S, Saneto RP, et al. Cerebral MRI abnormalities associated with vigabatrintherapy. *Epilepsia* 2009; 50: 184-94.
- Pendse N, Wissmeyer M, Altrichter S, Vargas M, Delavelle J, Viallon M, Federspiel A, Seeck M, Schaller K, Lövblad KO. Interictal arterial spin-labeling MRI perfusion in intractable epilepsy. *J Neuroradiol* 2010; 37(1): 60-3.
- Perry MS, Dunoyer C, Dean P, Bhatia S, Bavariya A, Ragheb J, et al. Predictors of seizure freedom after incomplete resection in children. *Neurology* 2010 Oct 19; 75(16): 1448-53; doi: 10. 1212/WNL. 0b013e3181f88114.
- Pulsifer MB, Brandt J, Salorio CF, Vining EP, Carson BS, Freeman JM. The cognitive outcome of hemispherectomy in 71 children. *Epilepsia* 2004 Mar; 45(3): 243-54.
- Sadeghi N, Prastawa M, Fletcher PT, Wolff J, Gilmore JH, Gerig G. Regional characterization of longitudinal DT-MRI to study white matter maturation of the early developing brain. *Neuroimage* 2013 Mar; 68: 236-47.
- Salamon N, Kung J, Shaw SJ, Koo J, Koh S, Wu JY, et al. FDG-PET/MRI coregistration improves detection of cortical dysplasia in patients with epilepsy. *Neurology* 2008; 71(20): 1594-601.

- Sanchez CE, Richards JE, Almli CR. Neurodevelopmental MRI brain templates for children from 2 weeks to 4 years of age. *Dev Psychobiol* 2012 Jan; 54(1): 77-91.
- Sankar R, Curran JG, Kevill JW, Rintahaka PJ, Shewmon DA, Vinters HV. Microscopic cortical dysplasia in infantile spasms: evolution of white matter abnormalities. *Am J Neuroradiol* 1995; 16: 1265-72.
- Shandal V, Veenstra AL, Behen M, Sundaram S, Chugani H. Long-term outcome in children with intractable epilepsy showing bilateral diffuse cortical glucose hypometabolism pattern on positron emission tomography. *J Child Neurol* 2012 Jan; 27(1): 39-45.
- Sharma S, Riviello JJ, Harper MB, Baskin MN. The role of emergent neuroimaging in children with new-onset afebrile seizures. *Pediatrics* 2003; 111: 1-5.
- Shinnar S, Kang H, Berg AT, Goldensohn ES, Hauser WA, Moshé SL. EG abnormalities in children with a first unprovoked seizure. *Epilepsia* 1994; 35: 471-6.
- Shinnar S, O'Dell C, Mitnick R, Berg AT, Moshe SL. Neuroimaging abnormalities in children with an apparent first unprovoked seizure. *Epilepsy Res* 2001; 43: 261-9.
- Smith ML, Elliott IM, Lach L. Cognitive, psychosocial, and family function one year after pediatric epilepsysurgery. *Epilepsia* 2004 Jun; 45(6): 650-60.
- Strandberg M, Larsson EM, Backman S, Källén K. Pre-surgical epilepsy evaluation using 3TMRI. Do surface coils provide additional information? *Epileptic Disord* 2008 Jun; 10(2): 83-92; doi: 10.1684/epd. 2008. 0194.
- Takanashi J, Barkovich AJ. The changing MR imaging appearance of polymicrogyria: a consequence of myelination. *Am J Neuroradiol* 2003; 24: 788-93.
- Tymofiyeva O, Hess CP, Ziv E, Lee PN, Glass HC, Ferriero DM, *et al*. DTI-based template-free cortical connectome study of brain maturation. *PLoS One* 2013 May 13; 8(5): e63310.
- Van Bogaert P, Wikler D, Damhaut P, Szliwowski HB, Goldman S. Regional changes in glucose metabolism during brain development from the age of 6 years. *Neuroimage* 1998 Jul; 8(1): 62-8.
- Véra P, Kaminska A, Cieuta C, Hollo A, Stiévenart JL, Gardin I, *et al*. Use of subtraction ictal SPECT co-registered to MRI for optimizing the localization of seizure foci in children. *J Nucl Med* 1999 May; 40(5): 786-92.
- Winston GP, Micallef C, Kendell BE, Bartlett PA, Williams EJ, Burdett JL, *et al*. The value of repeat neuroimaging for epilepsy at a tertiary referral centre: 16 years of experience. *Epilepsy Res* 2013 Aug; 105(3): 349-55; doi: 10. 1016/j. eplepsyres. 2013. 02. 022. Epub 2013 Mar 26.
- Yakovlev PI, Lecours AR. The myelogenetic cycles of regional maturation of the brain. In: Minkowski A, editor. *Regional Development of the Brain in Early Life*. Oxford: Blackwell Scientific Publications, 1967.
- Yapici Z, Dincer A, Mefkure E. Proton spectroscopic findings in children with epilepsy owing to tuberous sclerosis complex. *J Child Neurol* 2005; 20(6): 517-22.
- Zijlmans M, de Kort GA, Witkamp TD, Huiskamp GM, Seppenwoolde JH, van Huffelen AC, *et al*. 3T versus 1. 5T phased-array MRI in the presurgical work-up of patients with partial epilepsy of uncertain focus. *J MagnResonImaging* 2009 Aug; 30(2): 256-62; doi: 10. 1002/jmri. 21811.

"Benign" epilepsies in infants: are they always benign?

Julitta de Bellescize[1], Nicola Specchio[2], Alexis Arzimanoglou[1]

[1] Epilepsy, Sleep and Pediatric Neurophysiology Department (ESEFNP), University Hospitals of Lyon (HCL), Lyon, France
[2] Department of Neuroscience, Bambino Gesù Children's Hospital, IRCCS, Rome, Italy

---

Until recently, nearly all "idiopathic" focal and generalized epilepsies were labelled as "*benign*". For some of the syndromes the term was also introduced as part of the name, in opposition to "severe", "catastrophic" or progressive epileptic disorders with uncertain prognosis or outcome. The overall accepted, but rather confusing and quasi-synonymous use of the terms "benign" and "idiopathic" reflected, in a way, progresses in the etiological workup of epilepsies. The terminological problem was partially created by benign childhood epilepsy with centro-temporal spikes (BECTS) and some related entities with focal seizures, with inconsistent onset and without morphological causes. They were obviously categorically different from lesional focal epilepsies but their nosological place was unclear. The solution was to create an umbrella class of "localization-related epilepsies" for all syndromes with focal seizures. This was meant as an interim solution until the matter would be better understood (Wolf *et al.*, 2014). In the absence of identifiable underlying factors these syndromes were defined on the basis of the seizure semiology, related EEG traits and the hypothesis of a genetic predisposition. Despite their various clinical presentations, the qualification "benign" introduced in the ILAE classifications of 1985 and 1989, referred to their common natural history with specific age related seizure onset, self-limited course and excellent evolution in adulthood.

In 2001, a "benign epilepsy syndrome" was defined as an entity characterized by epileptic seizures that are easily treated, or require no treatment, that remits without sequelae. In 2001 the ILAE commission on Classification and Terminology recognized as benign three epileptic syndromes in infancy (Engel, 2001): two focal epilepsy syndromes, with onset during the first year of life – benign infantile seizures (BIS) and benign familial infantile seizures (BFIS) – and benign myoclonic epilepsy of infancy (BMEI), which is the earliest form of generalized idiopathic epilepsy.

In the updated 2006 ILAE Task Force report on syndromes (Engel, 2006) it was suggested to combine benign familial and sporadic infantile seizures to a single entity with regard to their similar phenotype except for the familial occurrence. Moreover the qualification "benign" was removed from benign myoclonic epilepsy of infancy with the simple footnote "because this is not benign in some infants". The argument commonly used is that the label "benign" should be reserved to those conditions for which a good prognosis can be predicted from onset. This rather restrictive tendency was clearly reinforced in the last ILAE report on classification and terminology (Berg et al., 2010). As a result the terms "benign" and "catastrophic" are no longer recommended. A similar comment was made for the prototype of benign focal idiopathic epilepsies, rolandic epilepsy or BECTS, but a change in the name of the syndrome was not officially suggested.

Obviously the concept of *"benignity"* evolved during the last decade. Epilepsy care is nowadays viewed not only as "control of seizures". Related conditions such as cognition, behaviour, anxiety, depression and/or the underlying etiological substratum need to be considered.

However, the notion of benign was not completely abandoned. The syndrome of "benign familial infantile seizures" is now called "benign familial infantile epilepsy" and is, for a second time, referred as a separate entity next to the sporadic infantile seizures, renamed "benign infantile epilepsy". In clinical practice, but also in publications, the term "benign" is still used when naming syndromes lately better individualized such as: the benign familial neonatal infantile seizures (BFNIS) – with seizure onset after the classical neonatal period and before the age of onset of benign familial infantile seizures; the benign infantile seizures with mild gastroenteritis; the benign infantile focal epilepsy with midline spikes and waves during sleep.

Myoclonic epilepsy of infancy (MEI), which in 2006 "lost" the label of "benign", was not renamed in the recently published update. The proposal to rename the syndrome "idiopathic myoclonic epilepsy of infancy" (IMEI) in order to underscore the good epileptological outcome as compared to other forms of myoclonic epilepsies with uncertain evolution (Dravet and Vigevano, 2007) was not followed as the etiological categories "idiopathic", "symptomatic" and "cryptogenic" were debated and substituted by "genetic", "structural-metabolic" and "unknown". Several sub-forms of MEI especially reflex myoclonic epilepsy of infancy (RMEI – first described by Ricci et al., 1995) have not been recognized as separate entities.

In this chapter we will focus exclusively on three syndromic entities: myoclonic epilepsy of infancy; benign infantile epilepsy; benign familial infantile epilepsy.

With respect to the evolution (2001–2010) of the ILAE recommendations we will discuss for each syndrome the "different qualities that make up the concept of benign":
- good prognosis can be predicted from onset;
- high likelihood of spontaneously remitting at a predictable age;
- easily treated;
- remission without sequelae.

■ Myoclonic epilepsy of infancy (MEI)

A syndrome with good prognosis, which can be predicted from onset or very early?

Such a statement implies that MEI can be correctly diagnosed at seizure onset or soon after, at least by an experienced epileptologist.

To the best of our knowledge, none of the published studies was designed to assess the reliability of the diagnostic process in this syndrome. MEI can be suspected when pure myoclonic seizures start in healthy children between 4 months and 3 years. Myoclonic seizures are expected to be the only seizure type present, exception made for eventual febrile seizures (Dravet and Bureau, 1981; 2005).

From a clinical point of view, MEI can be distinguished from other myoclonic syndromes starting early in life by the topographic distribution of myoclonias, involving particularly upper limbs, neck and chief (Hirano et al., 2009; Darra et al., 2006). Intensity can vary from subtle seizures consisting of *sursum vergens* of the eye globes to classical presentation with sudden flexion of the head and isolated or repeated (usually 1-3) myoclonic events of the upper limbs, responsible for bilateral symmetric abduction and elevation of arms. Rarely some degree of asynchronous, asymmetric myoclonus or, exceptionally, unilateral spontaneous or reflex myoclonias can be observed (Darra et al., 2006; Korff et al., 2009). Falls, reported in up to 18%, are due to massif flexion of inferior limbs (Auvin et al., 2006). Seizures occur in wakefulness; they are facilitated by somnolence and they can be recorded in sleep. Some authors consider that the reflex component is a good clinical marker of the syndrome and should be actively searched (Badinand-Hubert et al., personal communication; Auvin et al., 2006; 2013). Seizures can be organized in clusters but myoclonic status never occurs.

From an EEG point of view, myoclonic seizures occur always time looked to brief (1-3sec) generalized spike and polyspike wave discharges. Of interest, asymptomatic discharges are sparse. The fundamental interictal EEG activity is and remains always normal; rare generalized or focal interictal paroxysms and photosensitivity can occur.

Longer myoclonic seizures with sequences of 3-7 seconds are admitted. In these cases, it might be difficult to evaluate consciousness. Some authors accept a slight alteration of awareness or even some degree of slight absences (Zafeiriou et al., 2003; Caraballo et al., 2011 and 2013). We agree with Guerrini (2012) that in such cases an etiological work up is mandatory, before confirming diagnosis.

In summary: in the absence of a biomarker, the diagnosis remains at present based on electro-clinical features only. We believe that early diagnosis is straightforward in classical presentations, with an even higher degree of certainty when a reflex component is present. Prediction of a favourable epileptological evolution can be made at onset by an experienced epileptologist.

High likelihood of spontaneous seizure remission, at a predictable age?

Currently available data does not allow an "evidence-based" answer to the above question. Publications are rare and usually refer to a small number of patients. We are not aware of any randomized (treated *versus* non treated) studies. In clinical practice most of the children are treated, at least for a short period of time.

One of the seven infants reported in the historical description by Dravet (1981) had ongoing myoclonic seizures (MS) up to age of 8.5 years. Seizures stopped when treatment with clonazepam was started. This drug was not tolerated and was replaced successfully by sodium valproate. Based on this observation, child epileptologists usually introduced treatment for 2-3 years.

Data on follow-up of non-treated MEI patients are rare (Guerrini, 2012). We can add two more observations from our centre. One boy, out of a series of 18, with a mean follow-up of 8 years, started having myoclonic seizures at the age of 12 months; he was diagnosed only at the age of 11 years and subsequently developed JME, responsive to VPA; he presented with a normal cognitive development (Badinand-Hubert et al., 1997; Auvin et al., 2006).

The other child (personal communication from Dr Keo Kosal) experienced brief and subtle myoclonic seizures starting at 6 months. Treatment with sodium valproate was initiated when diagnosed at age 5 years and 9 months. There was excellent seizure control and normal psychomotor development.

These observations might represent one end of a spectrum, with subtle and transient forms at the other end, clearly under reported in the literature. In the series of Auvin (2006), 4 infants were not treated; 2 of them were of the non-reflex form and seizures disappeared spontaneously within 2 months (Badinand-Hubert et al., 1997). In one of the 6 cases described by Zuberi and O'Regan (2006), parents did not wish treatment. Myoclonic seizures started at age of 4 months. Development was normal at age of 13 months. Long-term follow up was not available. In 3 of the 6 cases with reflex MEI reported by Ricci (1995), seizures disappeared spontaneously after an active seizure period of 4-7 months. The mean duration of myoclonic seizures in the 7 untreated patients from the Italian multicenter study on RMEI was 19.4 months *versus* 4.5 months in treated patients, with an age of onset between 3 and 24 months (Verrotti et al., 2013). In the Argentinean follow-up study of 38 MEI patients (Caraballo et al., 2013), 4 RMEI cases were subsequently not treated and the seizures disappeared spontaneously within 8-13 months after seizure onset.

In summary, the likelihood of spontaneous seizure remission in classical MEI seems limited to subtle forms, whereas spontaneous remitting occurs more frequently in the RMEI subtype, within 4-20 months after disease onset.

A syndrome easy to treat?

The high pharmaco-sensitivity of myoclonic epilepsy of infancy was underscored since the very first descriptions of the syndrome. In 2002, Charlotte Dravet and Michèle Bureau found that 55 out of 65 patients (85%) became seizure-free with sodium valproate monotherapy. Ten years later, Guerrini (2012) confirmed in his review that VPA monotherapy was effective in 82.9%. Some of the patients, particularly those also being photosensitive, might need higher VPA plasma levels (Lin et al., 1998; Capovilla et al., 2007).

When reviewing the 4 largest studies accounting for 125 patients (Auvin et al., 2006; Darra et al., 2006; Caraballo et al., 2013; Verrotti et al., 2013) we found that 15 patients (12%) did not require treatment, 13 of those having a reflex form of MEI. In the treated group (110 patients), sodium valproate was the first drug of choice, with 79% of the children considered as responders. In 4 patients (3.6%) seizure freedom was obtained using another AE drug (CBZ, CNZ, ESM) and one patient, initially treated by LTG was seizure-free after VPA substitution which raises the efficacy of an adequate monotherapy to 82.7%. Only 19 patients (17.3%) required a drug association, in most of the cases a combination of a benzodiazepine and ethosuximide. In a very small number a combination of topiramate, levetiracetam or lamotrigine was preferred.

Information is very limited on early relapses, when AE treatment was accidentally interrupted or stopped by parental or medical decision. Dravet (2007) reported, that "the drug treatment must be monitored because an irregular intake can lead to relapse and falsely mimic drug-resistant epilepsy". Caraballo (2013) reported recurrence of MS immediately after treatment discontinuation in 3 cases. Seizure control was good after reinitiating the treatment. Early relapse of essentially myoclonic attacks must be differentiated from occurrence of MS or of another seizure type later in life. The duration of the episodes helps to distinguish between MS in the context of hyperthermia from febrile seizures, which can occur (Dravet *et al.*, 2002; Auvin *et al.*, 2006).

In summary, the 4 largest studies published between 2006 and 2013 (n = 125) confirm that MEI is a pharmaco-responsive syndrome. All patients became seizure-free, more than 80% with an adequate monotherapy. A 12% did not require treatment. The rarity of the syndrome explains the absence of prospective controlled studies and the insufficient data about the effect of newer antiepileptic agents. Treatment guidelines are lacking and expert clinicians empirically treat for a period of 2-3 years.

A syndrome remitting without sequelae?

Among the criteria underlying the concept of "benignity", remission without sequelae is essential. The term "sequelae" was not defined by Engel (2001). Easy to understand in common language, the term is commonly used when referring to seizure disappearance and no or only minimal impact on quality of life. But it is a term not precise enough when one wants to distinguish between immediate and long-term consequences of seizure activity, and/or treatment effects, coincidental pathologies or comorbidities, due to shared genetic factors or environmental influences. Interestingly the term "sequelae" is no longer used in the last update of the ILAE Task Force, which put forward the need to develop more flexible, multidimensional approaches of epilepsies, integrating neuropsychological burden and quality of life (Berg *et al.*, 2010).

Seizure disappearance

The outcome of patients with MEI has been regularly summarized by Dravet (1992; 2002; 2005). Myoclonic seizures usually disappeared in less than one year.

Guerrini (2012) found 10 cases, "mostly not well documented and lost from follow up", with persisting MS despite several treatments. He also reported that in all of the 116 cases with known age at follow up, except one (Prats Vinas *et al.* 2002), myoclonic seizures disappeared. Twenty-three patients were aged 15 years or more with the oldest patient aged 28 years. Since Guerrini's review, more data became available (3 of the 6 patients characterized as BMEI not preceded by generalized tonic-clonic seizures reported by Ito [2012] and 21 of the 38 patients of Caraballo [2013]), raising the total number of published cases with a follow up of at least 15 years to 47. For all disappearance of myoclonic seizures was reported.

Seizures or epilepsies following remission of MEI

Other seizure types may occur after a seizure-free interval of several years. Guerrini (2012) in his review found a risk of subsequent epilepsy in 16% of the 162 patients aged 5 years or more with known follow up. In 17 patients the main seizure type was that of generalized tonic-clonic or clonic with either isolated occurrence, or responding well to treatment. Caraballo (2013) reported on 2 other similar cases. In some rare cases, seizures were induced by intermittent photic stimulation.

Interestingly, in 10 other patients, epilepsy with predominant myoclonic features occurred after a seizure free interval of several years. Four cases were reported as JME (Auvin *et al.*, 2006; Caraballo *et al.*, 2013) and one case with massive photo-induced myoclonias (Darra *et al.*, 2006) or with spontaneous myoclonias preceded by GTCL seizures (Ito *et al.*, 2012). There is one observation of epilepsy with predominantly myoclonic-astatic seizures (MAE) following MEI (Auvin et al., 2012). A familial occurrence of both MAE and MEI has already been reported by Arzimanoglou (1996) in 2 brothers and by Doose in the offspring of a father with MAE (1992). In 3 cases, predominant eyelid myoclonia with absences appeared (Prats Vinas et al., 2002; Capovilla et al., 2007; Moutaouakil et al., 2010). There is one description of classical EAE following MEI (Mangano et al., 2011) and Prats Vinas (2002) reported a case with absence status occurring at age of 10 years. One case with RMEI was followed by a single GTCS and then by complex partial seizures responding to treatment (Auvin et al., 2006).

From an etiological or nosological point of view, the total number of cases remains, however, too small not allowing any definite conclusions. A genetic predisposition can be clearly suspected, in some cases suggesting a continuum within the spectrum of generalized (idiopathic) epilepsies.

Cognitive outcome

Since the very first description of the syndrome, Dravet considered that retarded diagnosis and delayed treatment might lead to impaired psychomotor development. One decade later, only 4 of the 11 cases (36%) had a normal cognitive development at an age between 5 and 15 years; in these cases, MS lasted less than 24 months. Three children had learning difficulties and seizure duration in this group lasted 1 to 3 years. Three had intellectual deficiency and personality disorders. In this group, treatment was initiated later with MS persisting up to 5 to 6 years. One of the patients suffered from trisomy 21 (Dravet, 1990). Subsequent reports confirmed neuropsychological burden (Todt and Muller, 1992; Giovanardi Rossi et al., 1997; Lin et al., 1998).

In her 2002 revision, Dravet reported more details on 69 cases with known psychological evolution: 57 (83%) had a cognitive status considered as normal; 38 were older than 5 years. A mild intellectual disability was found in 10 patients (14%), whereas mental retardation and psychotic evolution was found in 2 cases (3%). Besides importance of early treatment, the possibility of associated factors and familial environment was discussed. Guerrini (2012) actualized the follow-up and discussed psychological outcome only for the 23 patients aged 15 years or older (Guerrini, 1994; Giovanardi Rossi et al., 1997; Lin et al., 1998; Dravet and Bureau, 2005; Prats Vinas et al., 2002; Capovilla et al., 2007; Darra et al., 2006; Auvin et al., 2006). He found 9 cases (39%) with mental retardation, 6 with slight to moderate and 3 with severe deficiency.

A neuropsychological assessment was performed in the patients reported by Giovanardi Rossi (1997), Mangano (2005), Darra (2005), Ito (2012- only the 6 patients with "pure" MEI were considered), Verrotti (2013), in 20 of the 34 patients reported by Auvin (2006) and in the series reported by Caraballo (2013) and Ong (2011). There are significant methodological differences concerning age of testing, type of evaluation scales used for establishing developmental age or formal IQ, instrumental, attention or behavioural disorders. All testing methods confounded, these studies represent a sample of 143 "tested" out of 157 patients. Intellectual deficiency was reported in 13 patients (9%), borderline IQs were not considered. One patient (0.7%) reported by Auvin (2006) had a severe intellectual disability. We did not calculate a cut of age. This amount of cognitive disability is clearly higher than expected in general population.

A good neuropsychological outcome was found in 54.5% to 90% of the above-mentioned series. Only Mangano et al. (2005) found neuropsychological and intellectual disorders in 6 of their 7 cases (86%). All patients underwent a first neuropsychological assessment

(T1) at a mean age of 1.8 years, a second assessment (T2) at a mean age of 4.2 years (after a mean period of 3 years from the onset of seizures) and at the end of follow up (T3), at a mean age of 8 years. At admission, global developmental capacities were within normal ranges in all except one child. At the end of the study, 5 infants had low intellectual performance. Two met criteria of language impairment, 4 showed deficits on 2 subtests assessing expressive and receptive syntax, 2 had very low visual motor abilities and 5 fulfilled the DSM-IV criteria for ADHD. Learning disorders were noticed in 4 patients. School achievement was poor in all but one.

Considering the neuropsychological results of these 143 tested MEI patients, we evaluated that 16.8% had mild neuropsychological problems. Learning difficulties, dyslexia or minor language delay, difficulties in fine motor skills, central auditory processing, stuttering or behavioural difficulties were noticed in 20 patients (14%) and attention deficit disorder, with or without hyperkinesia, was present in 11 patients (mostly overlapping, but referred as an isolated feature in 4 cases).

An age related factor is controversially discussed to explain the frequency of neuropsychological disorders found in MEI when compared with the incidence in the general paediatric population.

Mangano et al. believed that one of the main reasons for unfavourable outcome in their study was the earlier age of seizure onset (mean 15 months; median 12 months; range 7 m-35 m) than those reported by Giovanardi Rossi et al. (1997) and Lin et al. (1998) with a mean age of onset of 1 year and 10 months (range: 3 m-4 y 8 m) and 2 years and 7 months (range 1 y 3 m-3 y 9 m) respectively; these authors mentioned less favourable outcome in 45% and 10% of the patients. Auvin (2006) reported a median age of onset of 12 months and Verrotti et al. (2013) a mean age of onset of 11 months, comparable with Manganos' group. Both authors found excellent outcome in 85%-90% of their series.

Mean age of onset was 19 months (range 3 m-4 y 10 m) in the study of Darra (2006), and only 7 months in patients with predominant reflex myoclonia. She found an excellent outcome in 77% of the infants. Ito (2012) reported a mean age of onset of 2 years and 6 months (range: 1 y 10 m-3 y 6 m) in their BMEI group with no preceding GTCS (BMEI-) and found normal or borderline IQ in 83.3%. Caraballo (2013) reported a mean onset age of 16 months (range 3 m-40 m) and no cognitive problems in 84%.

The interval between onset of MS and onset of treatment is rarely evaluated. It was short in Manganos' study study (2 m 15 d, range: 18 d to 5 m) compared to the studies of Rossi (1997) and Darra (2005) with a mean of 10 months in both. The mean duration of the active phase (interval between treatment onset and seizure control) was 7 m 15 d (range: 10 d to 28 m) in the Mangano study, similar to the active seizure period described by Verrotti (7.8 months). Darra (2006) reported a higher mean duration of 16 months (range: 3 m-4 y); however, 15 out of 18 patients initially treated by VPA were seizure free within 1-6 months (mean: 2 months).

In the BMEI- group reported by Ito (2012), seizure duration was 12 months (range: 3 m-22 m). Seizure control was reported by Caraballo (2013) after a mean treatment duration of 14 months (range: 2 m-34 m); Giovanardi Rossi (1997) mentioned a seizure duration of 1 m-6 months in the group of the 6 patients controlled by VPA monotherapy.

All the above data need to be interpreted very carefully because information about exact age at testing, relation to age of seizure onset, active seizure period, amount of treatment and distance to normalized EEG are only partially available. Also, the standards of "subtle neuropsychological difficulties" vary greatly and, each series taken separately, the number of patients included is rather small. As a result, to our opinion, currently available data do not permit drawing definite conclusions on the respective impact on cognitive functions of epilepsy related factors and or genetic/environmental causes.

Myoclonic Epilepsy of Infancy: conclusive remarks

MEI is a syndrome with a very short active seizure period and with rapid disappearance of related EEG abnormalities. Photosensitivity can occur in some patients. There is a limited risk of developing another type of epilepsy in non-reflex MEI. Typical cases can be easily diagnosed at onset, at least by experienced epileptologists. It would be interesting however to evaluate accuracy of diagnosis in a multicentric longitudinal prospective study.

It is remarkable that 30% of epilepsies following MEI developed seizures with a predominant myoclonic component. This raises the question about not yet identified shared common genetic and/or epigenetic factors. All reported RMEI cases except one (Auvin et al., 2006) did not develop subsequent seizures.

As for cognitive outcome, the majority of follow up studies suggest it is good. However, learning difficulties, behavioural problems and ADHD are consistently reported and are more frequently described in the non-reflex form. This neuropsychological burden is a general problematic in childhood epilepsies and is increasingly a field of research in non-lesional probably genetically determined epilepsies like BECTS, a syndrome for which the term benign is still integrated in its official denomination.

In the absence of prospective longitudinal studies it is still unclear to what extent epilepsy related factors, environmental and associated genetic factors impact the neuropsychological outcome in MEI. The available studies point out that light to moderate intellectual deficiency represents the most frequent related medical condition. Severe mental retardation seems not to be over represented. The number of documented cases followed into adulthood is still unsatisfactory and is probably explained by the rarity of the syndrome.

■ Benign familial epilepsy of infancy (BFEI) & benign epilepsy of infancy (BEI)

Good prognosis, which can be predicted from onset, or very early?

As for MEI early prediction of prognosis implies that there are no or very few diagnostic uncertainties at first clinical presentation or shortly after. Seizures start between 4 months and 2 years with a mean age of onset at 6 months. Some authors consider that in familial forms age of onset clusters in a narrower window between the 4th and 7th months (Vigevano, 2005).

Globally, there are no fundamental phenomenological differences between familial and sporadic forms (Caraballo et al., 2003, 2007; Gautier et al., 1999; Espeche, 2010; Bourel-Ponchel et al., 2011). Clinically there is typically a motion arrest, followed by slow eye and or head version, which can change side within a seizure cluster; there is some degree of hypertonia, apnea, cyanosis, unilateral limb jerking, which can evolve to a bilateral synchronous or asynchronous clonic seizure; the whole lasting 1 to 5 minutes (Vigevano, 2005). In some infants, oro-facial or limb automatisms can occur (Watanabe, 1990).

Early diagnosis can be considered as easy in familial cases, when focal seizures start between the ages of 3 to 10 months with a pick around 6 months, in an infant with normal development, who has no neonatal history, no underlying disorders, no neurological abnormalities, a normal interictal EEG and healthy relatives with similar, transient seizures in infancy. A careful follow up is necessary and diagnosis can be confirmed when seizures remit quickly (within several days or months) in the context of a normal neurological and cognitive development. Genetic testing is more and more accessible and mutations in the *PRRT2* gene are the outstanding cause of these seizures (Heron *et al.*, 2012; Schubert *et al.*, 2012; Zara *et al.*, 2013).

In the absence of familial history, the diagnosis of sporadic cases can be suspected when the above-mentioned electro-clinical criteria are present. The peculiar seizure organization in clusters is helpful clinical information. At onset, there might be isolated seizures, evolving rapidly, within days or several weeks, to clusters but 25% to 47% of infants may experience isolated seizures only (Watanabe and Okumura 2000; Caraballo *et al.*, 2007; Kaleyias *et al.*, 2006; Hrastovec *et al.*, 2012). In the majority of the cases, cluster duration is short (1-4 days) but longer evolutions, lasting between 5 and 15 days have been reported (Capovilla *et al.*, 1998; Gautier *et al.*, 1999; Bourel-Ponchel *et al.*, 2011). Clusters can be isolated or repeated (2-5/d) with 2 to 38 seizures per cluster. Seizure duration is of 1 up to 5 minutes, often longer at the beginning of the cluster; in very rare cases seizure duration was reported to be up to 15-30 minutes (Gautier *et al.*, 1999; Bourel-Ponchel *et al.*, 2011). A post-ictal deficit is not described and the clusters do not evolve to status epilepticus. The description of seizures with alternating gaze and head deviations is an additional valuable clinical symptom. An ictal recording should be attempted, confirming even in apparently secondarily generalized seizures a focal origin, more often over the posterior cortex (Vigevano *et al.*, 1992). Focal discharges arising alternatively from both hemispheres are also a helpful clinical sign together with a normal interictal EEG. Seizures occur in all states of vigilance but are more frequently noticed in wakefulness or drowsiness (Watanabe *et al.*, 1987, 2000; Capovilla *et al.*, 1998; Caraballo *et al.*, 2003; Kaleyias *et al.*, 2006; Hrastovec *et al.*, 2012). However, in all these sporadic cases a structural or metabolic cause must be eliminated.

Two studies, prospectively evaluated the accuracy of the diagnostic process. Okumura (2000) followed 63 patients with epilepsy starting in the first year of life. Inclusion criteria in the group of possible BPEI were: complex partial and/or secondarily generalized seizures; normal psychomotor development and neurologic examination at onset; normal interictal EEGs; normal CT and/or MRI; and no seizures during the first 4 weeks of life. At first presentation, 32 patients were included in the possible BPEI group. At 2 years of age, 7 patients were lost to follow up and 4 patients were excluded because of seizure recurrence or delayed development. These 25 patients were followed up to 5 years when 2 more patients were excluded for the same reasons. Okumura considered that at age of 5 years, 19 patients had definite BPEI. Consequently, it can be considered that in 76% of the cases, diagnosis of definite BPEI could have been established at first presentation (19 of 25) and in 90% of those, who met the inclusion criteria at age of 2 years. He completed the follow up study using a structured telephone-questionnaire at a median age of 11.3 years (all patients were aged 8 years or older). Information from 39 out of 48 patients was available with the diagnosis of possible BPEI at age of 2 years. There were 35 patients with "definite BPEI" at 5 years of age and finally a total of 33 patients with definite BPEI. There were 4 exclusions at age of 5 years and 2 exclusions at age of 8 years. The reasons were: seizure recurrence in 2; Asperger syndrome in one; mild intellectual deficiency in 2; seizures and cognitive problems in one; etiological workup revealed tuberous sclerosis in one and an arterio-venous malformation in another). These data showed that inclusion criteria permitted to establish at age of 5 years a definite diagnosis in most patients; 84.6% of patients diagnosed as possible BPEI at age of 2 years and follow beyond 8 years were correctly assessed (Okumura *et al.*, 2000; 2001; 2006).

Espeche (2010) performed a prospective follow up study in 41 patients with seizure onset between 2 and 12 months, satisfying the diagnostic criteria of BIE. Thirty-five had benign infantile seizures after a median follow up of 69 months. Twenty-six patients had no family history of similar seizures. Patients were evaluated at 2 months, between 1 to 2 years, and at 5 years after diagnosis. At one year of follow up, 2 patients from the "sporadic" group were excluded (one had cortical dysplasia, not detected at inclusion and the other was diagnosed as probably symptomatic); between one and 5 years of follow-up, 2 patients did not complete the study (each in BFEI and BEI group) and 2 from the sporadic group were excluded because of seizure recurrence and intellectual disability. The results are in agreement with the Okumuras' studies (2000; 2001) suggesting that recognition of these two syndromes is possible at the beginning (35 of 41) and easier in familial forms.

In summary, good prognosis is predictable at onset in BFEI. In sporadic cases, early diagnosis is feasible but careful etiological work up is mandatory. Helpful clinical signs are seizure occurrence in clusters and EEG documented seizure onset from both hemispheres, absence of status epilepticus or post-ictal deficits, normal development before seizure onset, normal neurological and neuroradiological investigations and no other etiological factors identified. Diagnosis is possible at 2 years of follow-up with a high diagnostic accuracy. A definite diagnosis should probably not be established before a 5 years follow-up.

High likelihood of spontaneous seizure remission at a predictable age?

The self-limited course of BFEI was demonstrated since the very earliest description of the syndrome. Vigevano (1992) noticed that most of the relatives of the 3 girls and 2 boys affected by BFEI were never treated. Seizure presentation was variable and ranged from an isolated afebrile event at age of 8 months to repeated seizures, starting at 4 or 6 months and lasting 1 to 6 months.

Since this seminal publication, data assessing the temporal course of spontaneously remitting seizures are very limited because treatment is usually started at the first seizure cluster. Isolated seizures or clusters can re-occur with or without treatment, from several per day to one or several seizures within 1 to 12 months (Watanabe et al., 2000; Vigevano et al., 1992; Echenne et al., 1994; Capovilla et al., 1998; Caraballo et al., 2003; Gautier et al., 1999; Bourel-Ponchel et al., 2011). Interictal EEG remains usually normal. In some cases, precipitating factors like fever or mild gastroenteritis (not to confound with FS or benign infantile seizures associated with mild gastroenteritis) were noticed (Capovilla et al., 1998; Okumura et al., 2006a; Saadeldin et al., 2010; Scheffer et al., 2012; Bourel-Ponchel et al., 2011).

Lee *et al.* (1993) considered, in a retrospective study, that 6 out of 23 non-treated children did not experience a more severe presentation. They had recurrent seizures for an average period of 76 days whereas treated patients had recurrent seizures for an average period of 94 days. Outcome was excellent in both.

In the French collaborative study (Gauthier et al., 1999) on benign infantile seizures, 2 familial cases did not receive treatment. One remained seizure-free with a follow-up of 6 years; the second had repeated clusters between one and 3.5 years, but parents did not wish medication. At age of 4 years he developed absence and generalized tonic-clonic seizures. He was treated with sodium valproate for a month; since then he was seizure-free with a follow-up of 7 years.

Watanabe *et al.* (2000) reported remission in some infants with BPEI who were not placed on chronic AE treatment and mentioned a case report with secondarily generalized seizures described by Hattori (1996) with favourable outcome in the absence of medication. Saadeldin *et al.* (2010) noted that in 2 cases without treatment, the seizures stopped spontaneously within 1-5 months (median: 3 months) compared with a median seizure offset of 4.7 months in the treated group. Okumura *et al.* (2006b) compared retrospectively the "seizure cluster" dynamic of 6 non-treated patients with 20 patients on medication. Ages at the first seizure and at the first cluster were similar. There were significantly less seizures per cluster (2 to 4) in the non-treated group compared to patients receiving AEDs (2 to 38 seizures) and cluster duration was significantly lower (6 to 40 hours in the non-treated *vs* 10 to 96 hours in the treated one). All had excellent outcome.

Age of definite seizure offset ranges from several hours to 2 years. In most of the cases, seizures disappeared within a range of 1 to 4 months (Watanabe, 1999; Okumura, 2000; Lee, 1993; Gautier *et al.*, 1999; Nelson *et al.*, 2002; Kaleyias *et al.*, 2006; Zara *et al.*, 2013). Some patients experienced their last seizure at ages 2 to 3 years (Callenbach *et al.*, 2002; Caraballo *et al.*, 2003; Heron *et al.*, 2012; Wang *et al.*, 2013).

Two syndromes easy to treat?

With regard to the self-limited course of this epilepsy, treatment is theoretically not necessary. However, *Table I* rather demonstrates that in clinical practice, it is still difficult to refuse to give medication. One of the main reasons for initiating treatment is probably the high seizure rate per cluster; moreover caregivers and parents may not tolerate longer seizure duration, prolonged up to 10-15 minutes in some cases, usually at the beginning of the serial seizures (Vigevano, 2005). Exceptionally seizures can last up to 30 minutes (Gautier *et al.*, 1999; Bourel-Ponchel *et al.*, 2011). In addition, a variable degree of rather impressive associated vegetative symptoms, with apnea followed by desaturation and cyanosis, can be observed. Usually infants receive a first dose of AE treatment in the emergency unit before a precise personal and familial history can be established. Seizure clusters may not always respond to benzodiazepines (Okumura *et al.*, 2006b; Echenne *et al.*, 1994; Gautier *et al.*, 1999). Okumura *et al.* (2006b) found that phenobarbital was relatively more effective than benzodiazepines; they considered that more than 10 mg/kg/dose may be necessary to stop the seizures and suggested that a more appropriate treatment for clusters, such as midazolam, should be tried.

Carbamazepine is reported to control seizures even at a daily low dose of 5 mg/kg (Matsufuji *et al.*, 2005). Monotherapy with a variety of AEDs (phenobarbital; sodium valproate; carbamazepine; zonisamide; phenytoin or sulthiam) is reported. Obviously this just reflects local practices and not an evidence-based approach. Response to treatment is also reported as good, but in the absence of control studies this could just reflect the fact that treatment may simply not be needed.

Some infants may need an increase in dose or a change of AED (Echenne *et al.*, 1994; Watanabe and Okumura, 2000; Caraballo *et al.*, 2003; Gautier *et al.*, 1999; Espeche, 2010; Hrastovec *et al.*, 2012). The use of a combination of two drugs was reported necessary in two (14%) out of 15 treated patients by Kaleyias *et al.* (2006) and in 1 patient (3%) reported by Espeche (2010). Only Saadeldin *et al.* (2010) reported seizure continuation in all (12/14) treated patients (range 1-9.5 months, median: 4.7 months).

Table I. Percentage of children not treated per study

	Number of patients included	Patients NOT treated
Vigevano et al., 1992	5	
Lee et al., 1998	23	6 (26%)
Echenne et al., 1994	6	
Capovilla et al., 1998	12	
Okumura et al., 2000	19	2 (10.5%)
Gautier et al., 1999	34	2 (5.8%)
Callenbach et al., 2002	43	14 (33%)
Nelson et al., 2002	22	3 (13.6%)
Caraballo et al., 2001	24	9 (37.5%)
Weber et al., 2004	67	
Kaleyias et al., 2006	16	1 (6.25%)
Espeche 2010	35	3 BFEI not after the first cluster, all after seizure recurrence
Bourel-Ponchel et al., 2011	40	4 (10%)
Saadeldin et al., 2010	14	2 (14.2%)
Hrastovec et al., 2012	17	3 (17.5%)
Wang et al., 2013	16	8 (50%)
Heron et al., 2012	77	
Labate et al., 2013	17	
Zara et al., 2013	99	29 (29.3%)

In summary, BFEI and BEI are spontaneously remitting epilepsies with a seizure onset before the age of 2 years (pick about 6 months). The active seizure period is usually very short (1-4 months) and in the majority of the children, seizures disappear before the age of one; in some children seizure offset occurs between the age of 2-3 years. There are no treatment guidelines. When treated, monotherapy is sufficient in the great majority of the patients and overtreatment should be avoided. Treatment experiences and the self-limitied natural seizure evolution suggest that the treatment period could be limited to 6 months in most of the cases.

Two syndromes remitting without sequelae?

As discussed above, the term sequelae is not a well-defined term and should probably be replaced by more specific descriptions of signs and symptoms. In other words, is there any evidence that this very early onset epileptic seizure activity and the related EEG abnormalities lead to ongoing or permanent seizure susceptibility or cognitive impairment? Is there a higher risk of associated relevant medical disorders impacting quality of life?

Seizure disappearance

All follow up studies agree that cerebral hyperexcitability is limited to a very narrow time window. Okumura (2006a) excluded seizure relapses after the age of 2 years in his definition of "definite" BPEI; follow-up studies show that seizures can last occur up to the age of 3 years. The mean duration of follow-up ranged from 15 months to 11 years in the studies performed before 2012, with the exception of the Callenbach et al. (2002) and the Weber et al. (2004) studies providing data up to 25 years. Following the discovery of the major role played by the *PRRT2* mutations, large cohorts (~ 250 patients) have been reviewed in 2012 and 2013 (*Table II*). They provide definite confirmation that BFEI/BEI are self-limited epilepsies. In the largest cohort, accounting for a hundred patients, last assessment was done at a mean age of 26 years (Zara et al., 2013).

Table II. Duration of follow-up per study/or age at last presentation

	Number of patients included	Mean follow-up (year, months)	Range (year, months)
Vigevano et al., 1992	5		24 m-32 m
Lee et al., 1998	23	8.9 y	1.9 y-18.1 m
Echenne et al., 1994	6	6.8 y	3 y-12 y
Capovilla et al., 1998	12	4.2 y	2 y-8.6 y
Watanabe & Okumura 2000	24		3 y-10 y
Okumura et al., 2006	33	11.3 (median)	8 y-20.5 y
Gautier et al., 1999	34		4 y-15 y
Callenbach et al., 2002	43	25.7 y	0.8 y-69 y
Nelson et al., 2002	22	4.4 y	
Caraballo et al., 2007	105	16 y	
Weber et al., 2004	67	25.9 y	0.3-79 y
Kaleyias et al., 2006	16	31 m	13 m-64 m
Espeche 2010	35	69 m (median)	60 m-77 m
Bourel-Ponchel et al., 2011	40	75 m (BFEI); 36 (BEI)	6 m-144 m
Hrastovec et al., 2012	17		
Wang et al., 2013	16	42.4 y	14 y-80 y
Heron et al., 2012	77		
Marini et al., 2012	9	19 y	2.5 y-44 y (family 1)
Steinlein et al., 2012	18		10-17 y in 4 of 5 families
Schubert et al., 2012	49 families and 3 sporadic cases		3 m-82 y
Labate et al., 2013	17	11 y	4 y-28 y
Zara et al., 2013	99	26 y	1 y-9 2 y

Seizures or epilepsies following BFEI/BEI

Febrile seizures or non-specified seizure disorders were occasionally reported in relatives (Vigevano et al., 1992; Caraballo et al., 2003; Kaleyias et al., 2006; Striano et al., 2006a; Saadeldin et al., 2010). Co-occurrence of febrile seizures has been rarely described (Lee et al., 1998; Weber et al., 2004; Bourel-Ponchel et al., 2011). In 2005, Vigevano et al. considered that the incidence of FS and other forms of idiopathic epilepsies does not differ from that of the general population. Currently it is not clear yet whether *PRRT2* mutations contribute to FS or whether the few patients reported to have both BFIS and FS co-segregate (Liu et al., 2012; Labate et al., 2013). In contrast, seizures and epilepsy seems to occur more frequently in the variant of infantile convulsions and choreoathetosis named "ICCA syndrome" (Szepetowski et al., 1997) and in paroxysmal kinesigenic dyskinesia families (Swoboda et al., 2000; Rochette et al., 2008).

Caraballo (2007) reported 3 cases of BEI that developed partial benign epilepsy with centro-temporal spikes. In the French survey on BFEI/BEI, 1 child experienced, at the age of 4 years, absence seizures and generalized tonic-clonic seizures; treated with sodium valproate for only a month he remained seizure free with a follow-up of 7 years. Absence seizures have also been reported in 2 Italian cases, one co-segregating with benign infantile seizures in a family (Marini et al., 2012). The other was a sporadic case, presenting infantile convulsions starting with a seizure cluster at the age of 5 months, followed by 2 isolated seizures at 9 and 20 months and typical, pharmaco-sensitive absence seizures at the age of 5 years (Specchio et al., 2013). One of the patients reported in the Italian multicenter genetic study (Zara et al., 2013) had complex focal seizures at age of 5 years and another patient reported by Labate (2013) developed focal motor seizures at the age of 7 and died at the age of 14 (SUDEP). These cases might be explained by individual genetic or epigenetic factors. The number of subsequent epilepsy in "pure" BFEI/BEI cases seems not higher than in the general population when we consider that currently approximately 750 cases have been reported (establishing the exact number is difficult because of "overlapping" inclusions in the various studies).

Cognitive outcome

Prospective studies including iterative neuropsychological testing are lacking. This is probably due to the fact that clinical evaluation was considered normal. Testing was performed in infants when intellectual disability was suspected and diagnosis of BFEI/BEI revised.

Echenne et al. (1994) reported neuropsychological testing results in 3 patients. One was evaluated using a Brunet-Lezine test (normal) and 2 had a full-scale IQ (120 and 125 respectively) on the Wechsler Intellegence Scale for children-Revised (WISC-R). Specchio et al. (2013) reported normal clinical and neuropsychological findings in 5 families with BFEI or ICCA syndrome and in seven sporadic cases. He mentioned hyperactivity in one case. In his long-term follow-up of 39 "possible" BPEI patients, Okumura (2006) used a structured telephone questionnaire. School performance was excellent in 8, average in 24 and 3 patients "underperformed". There were no major behavioural problems. Hrastovec (2012) tried to confirm favourable evolution based on the results of the SDQ questionnaire. Eight of the 17 concerned families returned the SQD scale. Five of the children had an optimal performance and 3 presented mild signs, essentially in their relation to peers.

Related medical conditions

Dystonic attacks or hemiplegic migraine can appear during childhood or adolescence. In the PRRT2 "era", it is probably obsolete to discuss "pure" BFEI families as overlapping of ICCA families and BFEI may just be a question of size of the family tree.

In large cohorts, as for example in the Italian multicenter study including 29 families diagnosed as BFIS (99 patients), 21 families segregated with *PRRT2* mutations and 5 patients from 3 families developed PKD, with an onset between the ages of 3 and 12 years. One patient had migraine in adulthood, associated to a *SCN2A* mutation. There were no cases with *ATP1A2* mutations with hemiplegic migraine. Espeche *et al.* (2010) reported, in one of the BFEI families studied, hemiplegic migraine in some relatives. Marini *et al.* (2012) confirmed co-occurrence of BFEI with migraine and febrile seizures in 2 families and with hemiplegic migraine in one family related to *PRRT2* mutations. An association of *PRRT2* mutation with migraine was also reported by Steinlein *et al.* (2012) in 1 family.

In summary, cognitive outcome is excellent in both BEI and BFEI. We found no evidence for a higher risk to develop another seizure disorder in BFEI/BEI despite the fact that ICCA syndrome and BFEI are allelic disorders and that in PKD and in ICCA families, the risk of subsequent seizures or epilepsy seems higher. There is no evidence for an associated higher risk of intellectual disability than in the general population. Familial counselling has to be cautious, especially in small families, concerning the risk of subsequent movement disorders.

Benign Epilepsies of Infancy: conclusive remarks

BFEI/BEI are an outstanding example of genetically determined focal epilepsies of very early onset, with short period of seizure expression, who may not need AED treatment or are treated during a very limited period. Seizure and cognitive outcomes are excellent, documented by follow up studies into adulthood.

The actual denomination is not correct, as it does not reflect the focal origin of the seizures.

▪ In conclusion are all the above syndromes always benign?

To answer the above question (see also *Table III* for a comparison of benignity criteria), we first need to agree on what we are referring to: are we dealing with the issue of short- and long-term prognosis of the syndromes or with the most appropriate name to be used in a classification scheme?

From the "prognosis" standpoint we have no doubt that existing data, for the three entities, allows the epilepsy community to consider them as "benign". This can be certified to the families early in the course of the disorder. Exceptions do exist but this is probably always the case in medical practice. One of the reasons for this being that the concept of "benignity" may have several interpretations (Capovilla and Monreale Workshop group, 2008).

For *myoclonic epilepsy of infancy* and *benign infantile epilepsy, familial or sporadic*, existing exceptions are clearly a marginal issue. It is part of our everyday clinical practice to provide some degree of prognosis to our patients and their families and we will keep doing it within the limits of our "reasonable doubts" and independently of all official declarations and definitions. For these syndromes we will keep informing the families that these are benign syndromes.

Table III. Comparison of benignity criteria

	Myoclonic epilepsy of infancy	Benign familial (or sporadic) epilepsy of infancy
Good prognosis predictable at onset	Yes when typical presentation and reflex component	BFEI: yes when typical presentation BEI: with high accuracy at 2 years, definite at 5 years
Remission at a predictable age	~ 4-20 m after onset	~ 1-4 m after onset (hours-3 yrs)
Spontaneous remitting of seizures	In very mild forms more frequent in RMEI	In very mild forms
Easy to treat	Yes	Yes
Self-limited course	Yes	Yes
Related significant medical disorders: – higher subsequent risk of seizures or epilepsy than in the general population – cognitive outcome – most relevant	Yes Yes Good in > 70% ID	Yes No Good PKD, FHM, migraine
Good outcome ascertained by follow up studies into adulthood	Insufficient data	Yes

The answer can be different when debating on the most appropriate denomination of the syndromes. "*Benign*" is a rather magic word in our daily practice. We agree with the statement that identifying a disease as "benign" implies a 100% certainty at onset. From a patient's point of view such a denomination will unavoidably generate a number of questions: will my child be able to attend the usual school path? Will he/she be able to stop AED treatment? Etc. To some of the above questions the answer can easily be "*yes*". However, the most difficult to answer question will then be: Do you think that my child will one day be definitely cured from his epilepsy? This is a much more difficult question to answer, particularly at onset. Parents will be seeking for a "yes" or "no" answer, not for a list of probabilities. As discussed above accuracy of a syndromic diagnosis, immediately following the very first electro-clinical manifestations is not always evident. Similarly, although a favourable evolution in terms of seizure control can easily be certified to the parents, long-term evolution involves several other aspects, not necessarily identifiable at onset. From that point of view one could justify why the term "benign" shall not be part of the denomination of any epilepsy syndrome.

However, we should probably avoid constantly changing the names of the epilepsy syndromes, unless strong, evidence-based and statistically significant, data suggests that a denomination is fundamentally wrong, and can lead to meaningful misinterpretations, from the patients' point of view. Because when doing so, we probably sustain existing confusion, at least for physicians not specialized in epilepsy.

No doubt that terminology and semantic issues are of importance in medical practice and research. However, when discussing current knowledge on prognosis, they should not take the pace over the results of clinical and fundamental research.

References

- Arzimanoglou A, Guerrini R, Aicardi J. *Aicardi's Epilepsy in Children*, 3rd ed. Philadelphia: Lippincott, Williams & Wilkins, 2004.
- Arzimanoglou A, Prudent M, Salefranque F. Épilepsie myoclono-astatique et épilepsie myoclonique bénigne du nourrisson dans une même famille: quelques réflexions sur la classification des épilepsies. *Épilepsies* 1996; 8: 307-15.
- Auvin S, de Bellescize J, Dravet C. Myoclonic epilepsy in infancy: one or two diseases? *Epileptic Disord* 2013; 15: 241-2.
- Auvin S, Lamblin MD, Cuvellier JC, Vallée L. A patient with myoclonic epilepsy in infancy followed by myoclonic astatic epilepsy. *Seizure* 2012; 21: 300-3.
- Auvin S, Pandit F, De Bellecize J, *et al.* And the Epilepsy Study Group of the French Pediatric Neurology Society. Benign myoclonic epilepsy in infants: electroclinical features and long-term follow-up of 34 patients. *Epilepsia* 2006; 47: 387-93.
- Badinand-Hubert N, Isnard H, de Bellescize J, Keo Kosal P, Revol M. Benign myoclonic epilepsy of infancy: 18 cases, a long-term follow-up. Poster Session. *Epilepsia* 1997; 38: S8.
- Berg AT, Berkovic SF, Brodie MJ, *et al*. Revised terminology and concepts for organization of seizures and epilepsies: report of the ILAE Commission on Classification and Terminology, 2005–2009. *Epilepsia* 2010; 51: 676-85.
- Bourel-Ponchel E, Le Moing AG, Delignières A, De Broca A, Wallois F, Berquin P. Familial and non-familial benign infantile seizures: A homogeneous entity? *Rev Neurol* (Paris) 2011; 167: 592-9.
- Callenbach P, De Coo RFM, Vein AA, *et al*. Benign familial infantile convulsions: a study of seven Dutch families. *Eur J Paediatr Neurol* 2002; 6: 269-83.
- Capovilla G, Beccaria F, Gambardella A, Montagnini A, Avantaggiato P, Seri S. Photosensitive benign myoclonic epilepsy in infancy. *Epilepsia* 2007; 48: 96-100.
- Capovilla G, Berg AT, Cross JH, *et al*. Conceptual dichotomies in classifying epilepsies: partial *versus* generalized and idiopathic *versus* symptomatic (April 18–20, 2008, Monreale, Italy). *Epilepsia* 2009; 50: 1645-9.
- Capovilla G, Giordano L, Tiberti S, Valseriati D, Menegati E. Benign partial epilepsy in infancy with complex partial seizures (Watanabe's syndrome): 12 non-Japanese new cases. *Brain Dev* 1998; 20: 105-11.
- Caraballo R, Fejerman N. Benign familial and non-familial infantile seizures. In: Fejerman N, Caraballo R (eds). *Benign Focal Epilepsies in Infancy, Childhood and Adolescence*. Paris: John Libbey Eurotext, 2007; pp. 31-50.
- Caraballo R, Pavek S, Lemainque A, *et al*. Linkage of benign familial infantile convulsions to chromosome 16p12-q12 suggests allelism to the infantile convulsions and choreoathetosis syndrome. *Am J Hum Genet* 2001; 68: 788-94.
- Caraballo RH, Darra F, Fontana E, Garcia R, Monese E, Dalla Bernardina B. Absence seizures in the first three years of life: an electro-clinical study of 46 cases. *Epilepsia* 2011; 52: 393-400.
- Caraballo RH, Flesler S, Pasteris MC, Lopez Avaria MF, Fortini S, Vilte C. Myoclonic epilepsy in infancy: An electroclinical study and long-term follow-up of 38 patients. *Epilepsia* 2013; 54: 1605-12.
- Caraballo, R., Cersosimo, R., Espeche, A., Fejerman, N. Benign familial and non-familial seizures: a study of 64 cases. *Epileptic Disord* 2003; 5: 45-9.
- Commission on Classification and Terminology of the International League Against Epilepsy: proposal for revised classification of epilepsies and epileptic syndromes. *Epilepsia* 1989; 30: 389-99.
- Darra F, Fiorini E, Zoccante L, *et al*. Benign myoclonic epilepsy in infancy (BMEI): a longitudinal electro-clinical study of 22 cases. *Epilepsia* 2006; 47: 31-5.

- Doose H. Benign myoclonic epilepsy. In: Doose H (ed) *EEG in Childhood Epilepsy*. Paris: John Libbey Eurotext, 2003, pp. 133-138.
- Dravet C, Bureau M. Benign myoclonic epilepsy in infancy. In: Roger J, Bureau M, Dravet C, Genton P, Tassinari CA, Wolf P (eds). *Epileptic Syndromes in Infancy, Childhood and Adolescence*, 3rd ed. London: John Libbey, 2002, pp. 69-79.
- Dravet C, Bureau M. Benign myoclonic epilepsy in infancy. In: Roger J, Bureau M, Dravet C, Genton P, Tassinari CA, Wolf P (eds). *Epileptic Syndromes in Infancy, Childhood and Adolescence*, 4th ed. London: John Libbey, 2005, pp. 77-88.
- Dravet C, Bureau M, Roger J. Benign myoclonic epilepsy in infants. In: Roger J, Bureau M, Dravet C, Dreifuss FE, Perret A, Wolf P (eds). *Epileptic Syndromes in Infancy, Childhood and Adolescence*. London: John Libbey, 1992, pp. 67-74.
- Dravet C, Bureau M. The benign myoclonic epilepsy of infancy. *Rev Electroencephalogr Neurophysiol Clin* 1981; 11: 438-44.
- Dravet C, Vigevano F. Idiopathic myoclonic epilepsy in infancy. In: Engel J Jr, Pedley TA (eds). *Epilepsy. A Comprehensive Textbook*, 2nd ed. Philadelphia: Wolters Kluwer/Lippincott Williams & Wilkins, 2007, pp. 2343-2348.
- Dravet C. Les épilepsies myocloniques bénignes du nourrisson. *Épilepsies* 1990; 2: 95-101.
- Echenne B, Humbertclaude V, Rivier F, Malafosse A, Cheminal R. Benign infantile epilepsy with autosomal dominant inheritance. *Brain Dev* 1994; 16: 108-11.
- Engel J. A proposed diagnostic scheme for people with epileptic seizures and with epilepsy: report of the ILAE Task Force on Classification and Terminology. *Epilepsia* 2001; 42:796-803.
- Engel J. Report of the ILAE Classification Core Group. *Epilepsia* 2006; 47: 1558-68.
- Espeche A. Benign infantile seizures: A prospective study. *Epilepsy Res* 2010; 89: 96-103.
- Gauthier A, Pouplard F, Bednarek N, et al. Benign infantile seizures (a French collaborative study). *Arch Pediatr* 1999; 6: 32-9.
- Giovanardi Rossi P, Parmeggiani A, Posar A, Santi A, Santucci M. Benign myoclonic epilepsy: long-term follow-up of 11 new cases. *Brain Dev* 1997; 19: 473-9.
- Guerrini R, Dravet C, Gobbi G, Ricci S, Dulac O. Idiopathic generalized epilepsies with myoclonus in infancy and childhood. In: Malafosse A, Genton P, Hirsch E, Marescaux C, Broglin D, Bernasconi R (eds). *Idiopathic Generalized Epilepsie: Clinical, Experimental, and Genetic Aspects*. London, Paris: John Libbey Eurotext Ltd, 1994, pp. 267-280.
- Guerrini R, Mari F, Dravet C. Idiopathic myoclonic epilepsies in infancy and early childhood. In: Bureau M, Genton P, Dravet C, Delgado-Escueta A, Tassinari CA, Thomas P, Wolf P (eds). *Epileptic Syndromes in Infancy, Childhood and Adolescence*, 5th ed. Paris: John Libbey, Eurotext, 2012, pp. 157-173.
- Hattori H, Higuchi Y, Tsuji M, Furusho K. Spontaneous remission of benign partial epilepsy in infancy. *Tenkan Kenkyu* (Tokyo) 1996; 14: 198-201[Japanese].
- Heron SE, Grinton BE, Kivity S, et al. PRRT2 mutations cause benign familial infantile epilepsy and infantile convulsions with choreoathetosis syndrome. *Am J Hum Genet* 2012; 90: 152-60.
- Hirano Y, Oguni H, Funatsuka M, Imai K, Osawa M. Differentiation of myoclonic seizures in epileptic syndromes: a video-polygraphic study of 26 patients. *Epilepsia* 2009; 50: 1525-35.
- Hrastovec A, Hostnik T, Neubauer D. Benign convulsions in newborns and infants: Occurrence, clinical course and prognosis. *Eur J Paediatr Neurol* 2012; 16: 64-73.
- Ito S, Oguni H, Osawa M. Benign myoclonic epilepsy in infancy with preceding afebrile generalized tonic–clonic seizures in Japan. *Brain Dev* 2012; 34: 829-33.
- Kaleyias J, Khurana DS, Valencia I, Legido A, Kothare SV. Benign partial epilepsy in infancy: myth or reality? *Epilepsia* 2006; 47: 1043-9.
- Korff CM, Jallon P, Lascano A, Michel C, Seeck M, Haenggeli CA. Is benign myoclonic epilepsy in infancy truly idiopathic and generalized? *Epileptic Disord* 2009; 11: 132-5.

- Labate A, Tarantino P, Palamara G, *et al*. Mutations in *PRRT2* result in familial infantile seizures with heterogeneous phenotypes including febrile convulsions and probable SUDEP. *Epilepsy Res* 2013; 104: 280-4.
- Lee WL, Low PS, Rajan U. Benign familial infantile epilepsy. *J Pediatr* 1993; 123: 588-90.
- Lin Y, Itomi K, Takada H, *et al*. Benign myoclonic epilepsy in infants: video-EEG features and longterm follow-up. *Neuropediatrics* 1998; 29: 268-71.
- Liu Q, Qi Z, Wan XH, Li JY, Shi L, Lu Q, *et al*. Mutations in *PRRT2* result in paroxysmal dyskinesias with marked variability in clinical expression. *J Med Genet* 2012; 49: 79-82.
- Mangano S, Fontana A, Cusumano L. Benign myoclonic epilepsy in infancy: neuropsychological and behavioural outcome. *Brain Dev* 2005 ; 27: 218-23.
- Mangano S, Fontana A, Spitaleri C, *et al*. Benign myoclonic epilepsy in infancy followed by childhood absence epilepsy. *Seizure* 2011; 20: 727-30.
- Marini C, Conti V, Mei D, *et al*. PRRT2 mutations in familial infantile seizures, paroxysmal dyskinesia, and hemiplegic migraine. *Neurology* 2012; 79: 2109-14.
- Matsufuji H, Ichiyama T, Isumi H, Furukawa S. Low-dose carbamazepine therapy for benign infantile convulsions. *Brain Dev* 2005; 27: 554-7.
- Moutaouakil F, El Otmani H, Fadel H, El Moutawakkil B, Slassi I. Benign myoclonic epilepsy in infancy evolving to Jeavons syndrome. *Pediatr Neurol* 2010; 43: 213-6.
- Nelson GB, Olson DM, Hahn JS. Short duration of benign partial epilepsy in infancy. *J Child Neurol* 2002; 17: 440-4.
- Okumura A, Hayakawa F, Kato T, Kumo K, Negaro T, Watanabe K. Early recognition of benign partial epilepsy in infancy. *Epilepsia* 2000; 41: 714-7.
- Okumura A, Hayakawa F, Kato T, Kuno K, Negoro T, Watanabe K. Five-year follow-up of patients with partial epilepsies in infancy. *Pediatr Neurol* 2001; 24: 290-6.
- Okumura A, Kato T, Hayakawa F, *et al*. Antiepileptic treatment against clustered seizures in benign partial epilepsy in infancy. *Brain Dev* 2006b; 28: 582-5.
- Okumura A, Watanabe K, Negaro T, *et al*. Long-term follow-up of patients with benign partial epilepsy in infancy. *Epilepsia* 2006a; 47: 181-5.
- Ong HT, Lim K, Tay S, Low PS. Neuropsychological outcome following benign myoclonic epilepsy in infancy. Poster sessions. *Epilepsia* 2011; 52: 23-263.
- Prats-Vinas JM, Garaizar C, Ruiz-Espinoza C. Benign myoclonic epilepsy in infants. *Revista de Neurologia* 2002; 34: 201-4.
- Ricci S, Cusmai R, Fusco L, Vigevano F. Reflex myoclonic epilepsy: a new age-dependent idiopathic epileptic syndrome related to startle reaction. *Épilepsies* 1995; 36: 342-8.
- Rochette J, Roll P, Szepetowski P. Genetics of infantile seizures with paroxysmal dyskinesia: the infantile convulsions and choreoathetosis (ICCA) and ICCA-related syndromes. *J Med Genet* 2008; 45: 773-9.
- Saadeldin IY, Housawi Y, Al Nemri A, Al Hifzi I. Benign familial and non-familial infantile seizures (Fukuyama-Watanabe–Vigevano syndrome): A study of 14 cases from Saudi Arabia. *Brain Dev* 2010; 32: 378-84.
- Scheffer IE, Grinton BE, Heron SE, *et al*. PRRT2 phenotypic spectrum includes sporadic and fever-related infantile seizures. *Neurology* 2012; 79: 2104-8.
- Schubert J, Paravidino R, Becker F, *et al*. PRRT2 mutations are the major cause of benign familial infantile seizures. *Hum Mutat* 2012; 33: 1439-43.
- Specchio N, Terracciano A, Trivisano M, *et al*. PRRT2 is mutated in familial and non-familial benign infantile seizures. *Eur J Paediatr Neurol* 2013; 17: 77-81.
- Steinlein OK, Vilain M, Korenke C. The *PRRT2* mutation c.649dupC is so far most frequent cause of benign familial infantile convulsions. *Seizure* 2012; 21: 740-2.

- Striano P, Lispi ML, Gennaro E, *et al.* Linkage analysis and disease models in benign familial infantile seizures: a study of 16 families. *Epilepsia* 2006a; 47: 1029-34.
- Swoboda KJ, Soong BW, McKenna C, *et al.* Paroxysmal kinesigenic dyskinesia and infantile convulsions. Clinical and linkage studies. *Neurology* 2000; 55: 224-30.
- Szepetowski P, Rochette J, Berquin P, Piussan C, Lathrop GM, Monaco AP. Familial infantile convulsions and paroxysmal choreoathetosis: a new neurological syndrome linked to the pericentromeric region of human chromosome 16. *Am J Hum Genet* 1997; 61:
- Todt H, Muller D. The therapy of benign myoclonic epilepsy in infants. *Epilepsy Res* 1992; 6: 137-9.
- Verrotti A, Matricardi S, Capovilla G, *et al.* Relex myoclonic epilepsy in infancy: a multicenter clinical study. *Epilepsy Res* 2013; 103: 237-44.
- Vigevano F, Fusco L, Di Capua M, Ricci S, Sebastianelli R, Lucchini P. Benign infantile familial convulsions. *Eur J Pediatr* 1992; 151: 608-12.
- Vigevano F. Benign familial infantile seizures. *Brain Dev* 2005; 27: 172-7.
- Wanatabe K, Okumura A. Benign partial epilepsies in infancy. *Brain Dev* 2000; 22: 296-300.
- Wang JL, Mao X, Hu ZM, *et al.* Mutation analysis of *PRRT2* in two Chinese BFIS families and nomenclature of *PRRT2* related paroxysmal diseases. *Neurosci Lett* 2013; 552: 40-5.
- Watanabe K, Miura K, Natsume J, Hayakawa F, Furune S, Okumura A. Epilepsies of neonatal onset: seizure type and evolution. *Dev Med Child Neurol* 1999; 41: 318-22.
- Watanabe K, Yamamoto N, Negoro T, *et al.* Benign complex partial epilepsies in infancy. *Pediatr Neurol* 1987; 3: 208-11.
- Watanabe K, Yamamoto N, Negoro T, Takahashi I, Aso K, Maehara M. Benign infantile epilepsy with complex partial seizures. *J Clin Neurophysiol* 1990; 7: 409-16.
- Weber YG, Berger A, Bebek N, *et al.* Benign familial infantile convulsions: linkage to chromosome 16p12-q12 in 14 families. *Epilepsia* 2004; 45: 601-9.
- Wolf P. History of epilepsy: nosological concepts and classification. *Epileptic Disord* 2014; 16: 261-9.
- Zafeiriou D, Vargiami E, Kontopoulos E. Reflex myoclonic epilepsy in infancy: a benign age-dependent idiopathic startle epilepsy. *Epileptic Disord* 2003; 5: 121-2.
- Zara F, Specchio N, Striano P, *et al.* Genetic testing in benign familial epilepsies of the first year of life: clinical and diagnostic significance. *Epilepsia* 2013; 54: 425-36.
- Zuberi SM, O'Regan ME. Developmental outcome in benign myoclonic epilepsy in infancy and reflex myoclonic epilepsy in infancy: a literature review and six new cases. *Epilepsy Res* 2006; 70 (suppl 1): 110-5.

Fever-susceptibility syndromes
Predicting outcome

Ingrid E. Scheffer[1,2,3], Rosemary Burgess[2], Christopher Reid[1]

[1] *Florey Institute of Neuroscience and Mental Health, Melbourne, Australia*
[2] *Department of Medicine, University of Melbourne, Austin Health, Melbourne, Australia*
[3] *Department of Paediatrics, University of Melbourne, Royal Children's Hospital, Melbourne, Australia*

Febrile seizures (FSs) are the most common seizure disorder. Usually they represent a self-limited disorder without later sequelae. They may, however, herald the onset of epilepsy and an increasing number of epilepsy syndromes associated with FSs is being recognised. These syndromes vary from self-limited and pharmacoresponsive entities to severe epileptic encephalopathies. An understanding of the breadth of disorders associated with FSs facilitates diagnosis which, in turn, informs treatment paradigms, prognostic and genetic counselling.

Here, we will address the self-limited syndromes first of FSs and genetic epilepsy with febrile seizures plus. Then we will review specific epileptic encephalopathies in which FSs play a prominent role.

■ Febrile seizures

FSs occur in 3-5% of Caucasion children with rates of 7% described in Japanese children and 14% in children from Guam (Nelson and Ellenberg, 1976; Verity *et al.*, 1985). FSs are defined as a convulsive seizure associated with a temperature of at least 38 degrees Celsius occurring in an infant or child aged between 6 months and 6 years (Sadleir and Scheffer, 2007; Practice, 1999). The median age of occurrence of FSs is 18 months, with 50% of attacks occurring between one and $2^1/_2$ years (Offringa *et al.*, 1994). There is no evidence to support the oft-quoted view that a FS is more likely to occur during the maximum rate of temperature rise (Berg, 1993).

A diagnosis of a FS can only be made if central nervous system infection and acute electrolyte imbalance have been excluded. A further exclusion criterion is if the child has epilepsy, defined by recurrent afebrile unprovoked seizures (Fisher *et al.*, 2014). In this case their seizure is regarded as a seizure triggered by fever and they do not have FSs per se.

FSs are categorized as simple or complex. Seventy-five percent of FSs are simple with the majority lasting less than two minutes. Although FSs typically comprise generalized tonic clonic seizures, 16% show focal features (Nelson and Ellenberg, 1976; Berg and Shinnar, 1996a; Annegers et al., 1987).

Complex FSs are defined according to three possible criteria. First, duration, where the seizure lasts longer than 15 minutes. This only occurs in 9% FSs (Berg and Shinnar, 1996b). Second, where the seizure has focal features. Third, where multiple seizures occur within 24 hours or within the same illness. Febrile status epilepticus, where the seizure continues for at least thirty minutes, accounts for 5% of cases (Berg and Shinnar, 1996b). Focal features occur in most cases of febrile status epilepticus (Shinnar et al., 2008).

Recurrence of FSs occurs in one-third of cases. Risk factors for recurrence include onset of FSs under 18 months, a lower grade fever (closer to 38 degrees Celsius) with the first FS, a shorter duration (less than an hour) of fever prior to the seizure, and a family history of FSs (Sadleir and Scheffer, 2007). If all these risk factors co-exist, there is a 76% likelihood of recurrence compared with a 4% risk if none is present (Berg et al., 1997).

The aetiology of FSs is multifactorial, and provides an excellent model for examining the interaction of genetic and environmental factors. A family history of FSs is present in 24% of children with FSs and of epilepsy in 4% of children. In terms of molecular data, there are many chromosomal loci reported for FSs but relatively few genes are known. Those that are known encode ion channel genes and include sodium channel subunits and GABA receptor subunits, among others. The underlying gene for FSs has been identified in very few of the rare autosomal dominant families with FS that exist. How an acquired infection interacts to trigger a FS in a child who has a genetic predisposition is not understood.

In recent years, two less common benign entities comprising seizures with fever have been described that occur at a similar age. *Febrile myoclonic seizures* often occur in a baby with a family history of FSs (Narula and Goraya, 2005). They may escape diagnosis as they may be subtle or misinterpreted as rigors.

Another interesting disorder, initially identified in Japanese children, is *convulsions with gastroenteritis* (Uemura et al., 2002). This typically comprises a cluster of convulsions or focal seizures, with or without fever. There is a low risk of recurrence and a family history of seizures is less frequent.

FSs are associated with an excellent outcome. In early studies, it was shown that only 4% of children developed epilepsy by 7 years of age, which meant a doubling of the background frequency of epilepsy (Nelson and Ellenberg, 1976). Where individuals with FSs have been followed until age 25 years, 7% have afebrile seizures (Annegers et al., 1987). This ranges from a low risk of 2.4% in those with a simple FS to 6-8% in those with a complex FS.

Prolonged FSs are often associated with later temporal lobe epilepsy with hippocampal sclerosis (Falconer et al., 1964; Kuks et al., 1993). It is unclear if this is a causal relationship.

Up to 23% of patients with genetic generalized epilepsies (previously called idiopathic generalized epilepsies) have preceding FSs. This is likely to reflect shared genetic determinants (Medina et al., 2012; Thomas et al., 2012).

Genetic epilepsy with febrile seizures *plus* (GEFS+)

Febrile seizures that continue past the age of 6 years or, alternatively, where a child has afebrile convulsions in addition to febrile convulsions, is a syndrome called febrile seizures *plus* (FS+). This was first recognized in a family with the familial epilepsy syndrome of genetic epilepsy with febrile seizures *plus* (GEFS+) (Scheffer and Berkovic, 1997). In this family the most common phenotype was FS+, in addition to some individuals having typical FSs, and others more complex phenotypes. The most common FS+ phenotype is where the febrile seizures do not settle by 6 years and often continue into early adolescence. In some individuals, rare later febrile or afebrile convulsive seizures occur. The less common FS+ phenotype is where afebrile convulsions occur either during the usual age range of FSs or after FSs have abated.

More complex phenotypes are also part of the GEFS+ spectrum, a *familial syndrome characterized by phenotypic heterogeneity*. This includes individuals who have FS/FS+ with other seizure types including focal, absence, myoclonic or atonic seizures, or combinations of these seizure types. In addition, specific epileptic encephalopathies have been identified as part of the GEFS+ spectrum. These include epilepsy with myoclonic-atonic seizures, originally described by Doose (Doose et al., 1970; Scheffer and Berkovic, 1997; Singh et al.; 1999). In addition Dravet syndrome is at the severe end of the GEFS+ spectrum (Singh et al., 2001).

There are now several genes known for GEFS+. These include sodium channel genes encoding the alpha subunits, *SCN1A*, *SCN9A* and possibly *SCN2A*, but the latter requires confirmation (Escayg et al., 2000; Singh et al., 2009; Sugawara et al., 2001). In addition rare families have been described with GABA receptor subunit mutations including *GABRG2* (Wallace et al., 2001; Baulac et al., 2001). The delta subunit of the GABA receptor gene, *GABRD*, is likely to be a susceptibility gene for GEFS+ but this association also requires confirmation (Dibbens et al., 2004).

Epileptic encephalopathies with fever susceptibilty

The prototypical example of an epileptic encephalopathy with fever susceptibility is Dravet syndrome. This disease is not uncommon and classically begins with febrile hemiclonic status epilepticus at around 6 months of age. The hallmark is recurrent episodes of febrile hemiclonic status, which may alternate sides in different attacks. Some children have generalized status epilepticus without hemiclonic attacks. Between 1 and 5 years, children develop other seizure types including focal seizures with impaired awareness, absence and myoclonic seizures and rarely, atonic seizures. Around 90% of children with Dravet syndrome have mutations of the alpha-1 sodium channel subunit gene, *SCN1A*. About 90% of mutations arise *de novo* in the child, and the remainder are often inherited in a dominant fashion in the setting of a family history of GEFS+. While Dravet syndrome is associated with ongoing fever susceptibility into adult life (Catarino et al., 2011), other factors may also trigger seizures, such as vaccination. Vaccination triggers attacks in around one-third of patients with Dravet syndrome (Berkovic et al., 2006; McIntosh et al., 2010).

More recently, it has become clear that there are a number of genetic epileptic encephalopathies that are associated with FSs. The second most common epileptic encephalopathy after Dravet syndrome is *PCDH19* "girls only epilepsy" in which girls present with clusters of brief FSs in a day usually towards the end of the first year of life, and recurring at regular frequencies. While girls may have normal intellect, many develop intellectual disability and a significant proportion have autistic spectrum disorders. The disease is due to mutations in the gene encoding protocadherin 19, *PCDH19*, and it follows an unusual pattern of X-linked inheritance with male sparing. Males are normal transmitting carriers; females are usually affected but may be unaffected carriers. This carries very important implications in terms of genetic counselling. These girls improve with age but many are left with residual learning and behavioural difficulties (Depienne et al., 2009; Dibbens et al., 2011; Higurashi et al., 2013; Higurashi et al., 2012; Hynes et al., 2010; Scheffer et al., 2008).

Very recently *CHD2*, encoding chromodomain-helicase DNA-binding protein 2, has been shown to produce an epileptic encephalopathy. Whilst the initial series of cases did not show any predilection to seizures with fever, a report of three cases specifically noted that all had seizures triggered by fever (Carvill et al., 2013; Suls et al., 2013). It remains unclear what proportion of children with *CHD2* encephalopathy are prone to seizures with fever. It is very likely that many of the many genetic encephalopathies currently emerging will be prone to seizures with fever, as is often the case in infantile and childhood epilepsy.

The outcome of the various epileptic encephalopathies depends on the underlying aetiology. As we learn more about the genes determining these encephalopathies, we will understand more about the prognosis. For example, in Dravet syndrome, approximately half the patients have severe intellectual disability, a quarter moderate and a quarter mild intellectual impairment (Catarino et al., 2011; Jansen et al., 2006). Virtually all patients with Dravet syndrome have ongoing refractory seizures into adult life, although the pattern changes to one of predominantly nocturnal brief convulsions with remission of the episodes of status, apart from those with fever. In terms of the outcome for the other encephalopathies such as *PCDH19* and *CHD2*, and likely many others, the outcome will largely depend on the underlying molecular defect. Thus when a clinician is faced with a child with fever, the most important clinical measure is determining the phenotype of the child. This depends on the age of seizure onset, duration of the FS and nature of additional seizure semiologies. This is then combined with an understanding of their developmental trajectory, MRI and imaging features. If there is a known molecular mutation this will be key in determining the diagnosis and hence the prognosis for the patient.

■ Animal models of febrile seizures

The fundamental biology of seizures triggered by fever in humans remains ill understood. Insights have been afforded by murine models with extensive work on seizures triggered by environmental heating that raises core body temperature (Dube et al., 2009). A number of "syndrome-specific" mouse models of epilepsy based on human mutations have been tested using this method. Specifically, mouse models of Dravet syndrome based on *SCN1A* and *SCN1B* mutations display increased seizure susceptibility (Oakley et al., 2009; Reid et al., 2014). Further, GEFS+ models based on *SCN1B* and *GABRG2* also have heightened seizure susceptibility when exposed to environmental heat (Reid et al., 2013; Wimmer et al., 2010). Such studies have also revealed critical age-dependent effects in terms of seizures evoked by increased temperature, modelling the age-dependent manifestations of FSs (Oakley et al., 2009). The recapitulation of these key clinical hallmarks validates the environmental heating approach as a good method for modelling FS susceptibility.

These animal studies strongly argue that a primary driver of susceptibility in these genetic epilepsies is due to a heat-mediated increase in the excitability of neuronal networks rather than a complex interaction with other immunogenic factors. Syndrome-specific mouse models provide an opportunity to develop a better understanding of the molecular, cellular and neuronal network factors that predispose patients to having FSs. For example, a reduction in GABAergic neuron function in *SCN1A* Dravet syndrome is proposed to cause instability of hippocampal networks (Yu *et al.*, 2006). Also, a heat-sensitive increase in axon initial segment activity is proposed to underlie FS susceptibility in *SCN1B* GEFS+ (Wimmer *et al.*, 2010). More syndrome-specific mouse models will be engineered as we increase our knowledge of the genetic architecture of FS syndromes, further improving our understanding of the fundamental mechanisms of this seizure type. The robustness of the heating method will also allow us to begin to explore environmental factors, such as diet, that could contribute to FS susceptibility. Finally, exposure to environmental heat in early development can initiate epileptogenic cascades that result in later spontaneous seizures. This gives us an opportunity to explore pathological mechanisms underlying temporal lobe epilepsy and other epilepsies associated with a history of FSs (Chen *et al.*, 2001).

References

- Annegers JF, Hauser WA, Shirts SB, Kurland LT. Factors prognostic of unprovoked seizures after febrile convulsions. *N Engl J Med* 1987; 316: 493-8.
- Baulac S, Huberfeld G, Gourfinkel-An I, *et al*. First genetic evidence of GABA(A) receptor dysfunction in epilepsy: a mutation in the gamma2-subunit gene. *Nat Genet* 2001; 28: 46-8.
- Berg AT. Are febrile seizures provoked by a rapid rise in temperature? *Am J Dis Child* 1993; 147: 1101-3.
- Berg AT, Shinnar S. Complex febrile seizures. *Epilepsia* 1996a; 37: 126-33.
- Berg AT, Shinnar S. Unprovoked seizures in children with febrile seizures: short-term outcome. *Neurology* 1996b; 47: 562-8.
- Berg AT, Shinnar S, Darefsky AS, *et al*. Predictors of recurrent febrile seizures. A prospective cohort study. *Arch Pediatr Adolesc Med* 1997; 151: 371-8.
- Berkovic SF, Harkin L, McMahon JM, *et al*. De novo mutations of the sodium channel gene SCN1A in alleged vaccine encephalopathy: a retrospective study. *Lancet Neurol* 2006; 5: 488-92.
- Carvill GL, Heavin SB, Yendle SC, *et al*. Targeted resequencing in epileptic encephalopathies identifies *de novo* mutations in *CHD2* and *SYNGAP1*. *Nat Genet* 2013; 45: 825-30.
- Catarino CB, Liu JY, Liagkouras I, *et al*. Dravet syndrome as epileptic encephalopathy: evidence from long-term course and neuropathology. *Brain* 2011; 134: 2982-3010.
- Chen K, Aradi I, Thon N, Eghbal-Ahmadi M, Baram TZ, Soltesz I. Persistently modified h-channels after complex febrile seizures convert the seizure-induced enhancement of inhibition to hyperexcitability. *Nat Med* 2001; 7: 331-7.
- Depienne C, Bouteiller D, Keren B, *et al*. Sporadic infantile epileptic encephalopathy caused by mutations in PCDH19 resembles Dravet syndrome but mainly affects females. *PLoS Genet* 2009; 5: e1000381.
- Dibbens LM, Feng HJ, Richards MC, *et al*. GABRD encoding a protein for extra- or peri-synaptic GABAA receptors is a susceptibility locus for generalized epilepsies. *Hum Mol Genet* 2004; 13: 1315-9.
- Dibbens LM, Kneen R, Bayly MA, *et al*. Recurrence risk of epilepsy and mental retardation in females due to parental mosaicism of *PCDH19* mutations. *Neurology* 2011; 76: 1514-9.

- Doose H, Gerken H, Leonhardt R, Volzke E, Volz C. Centrencephalic myoclonic-astatic petit mal. *Neuropediatrics* 1970; 2: 59-78.
- Dube CM, Brewster AL, Baram TZ. Febrile seizures: mechanisms and relationship to epilepsy. *Brain Dev* 2009; 31: 366-71.
- Escayg A, MacDonald BT, Meisler MH, *et al*. Mutations of SCN1A, encoding a neuronal sodium channel, in two families with GEFS+2. *Nature Genetics* 2000; 24: 343-345.
- Falconer MA, Serafetinides EA, Corsellis JA. Etiology and pathogenesis of temporal lobe epilepsy. *Arch Neurol* 1964; 10: 233-48.
- Fisher RS, Acevedo C, Arzimanoglou A, *et al*. ILAE official report: a practical clinical definition of epilepsy. *Epilepsia* 2014; 55: 475-82.
- Higurashi N, Nakamura M, Sugai M, *et al*. PCDH19-related female-limited epilepsy: further details regarding early clinical features and therapeutic efficacy. *Epilepsy Res* 2013; 106: 191-9.
- Higurashi N, Shi X, Yasumoto S, *et al*. PCDH19 mutation in Japanese females with epilepsy. *Epilepsy Res* 2012; 99: 28-37.
- Hynes K, Tarpey P, Dibbens LM, *et al*. Epilepsy and mental retardation limited to females with PCDH19 mutations can present *de novo* or in single generation families. *J Med Genet* 2010; 47: 211-6.
- Jansen FE, Sadleir LG, Harkin LA, *et al*. Severe myoclonic epilepsy of infancy (Dravet syndrome): recognition and diagnosis in adults. *Neurology* 2006; 67: 2224-6.
- Kuks JB, Cook MJ, Fish DR, Stevens JM, Shorvon SD. Hippocampal sclerosis in epilepsy and childhood febrile seizures. *Lancet* 1993; 342: 1391-4.
- McIntosh AM, McMahon J, Dibbens LM, *et al*. Effects of vaccination on onset and outcome of Dravet syndrome: a retrospective study. *Lancet Neurol* 2010; 9: 592-8.
- Medina M, Bureau M, Hirsch E, Panayiotopoulos C. Childhood absence epilepsy. In: Bureau M, Genton P, Dravet C, Delgado-Escueta A, Tassinari C, Thomas P, Wolf P (eds). *Epileptic Syndromes in Infancy, Childhood and Adolescence*, 5th ed. Paris: John Libbey Eurotext, 2012, pp. 277-295.
- Narula S, Goraya JS. Febrile myoclonus. *Neurology* 2005; 64: 169-70.
- Nelson KB, Ellenberg JH. Predictors of epilepsy in children who have experienced febrile seizures. *N Engl J Med* 1976; 295: 1029-33.
- Oakley JC, Kalume F, Yu FH, Scheuer T, Catterall WA. Temperature- and age-dependent seizures in a mouse model of severe myoclonic epilepsy in infancy. *Proc Natl Acad Sci USA* 2009; 106: 3994-9.
- Offringa M, Bossuyt PM, Lubsen J, *et al*. Risk factors for seizure recurrence in children with febrile seizures: a pooled analysis of individual patient data from five studies. *J Pediatr* 1994; 124: 574-84.
- Practice. Practice parameter: long-term treatment of the child with simple febrile seizures. American Academy of Pediatrics. Committee on Quality Improvement, Subcommittee on Febrile Seizures. *Pediatrics* 1999; 103: 1307-9.
- Reid CA, Kim T, Phillips AM, *et al*. Multiple molecular mechanisms for a single GABAA mutation in epilepsy. *Neurology* 2013; 80: 1003-8.
- Reid CA, Leaw B, Richards KL, *et al*. Reduced dendritic arborization and hyperexcitability of pyramidal neurons in a Scn1b-based model of Dravet syndrome. *Brain* 2014; 137: 1701-15.
- Sadleir LG, Scheffer IE. Febrile seizures. *BMJ* 2007; 334: 307-11.
- Scheffer IE, Berkovic SF. Generalized epilepsy with febrile seizures plus. A genetic disorder with heterogeneous clinical phenotypes. *Brain* 1997; 120: 479-90.
- Scheffer IE, Turner SJ, Dibbens LM, *et al*. Epilepsy and mental retardation limited to females: an under-recognized disorder. *Brain* 2008; 131: 918-27.

- Shinnar S, Hesdorffer DC, Nordli DR, Jr., et al. Phenomenology of prolonged febrile seizures: results of the FEBSTAT study. *Neurology* 2008; 71: 170-6.
- Singh NA, Pappas C, Dahle EJ, et al. A role of SCN9A in human epilepsies, as a cause of febrile seizures and as a potential modifier of Dravet syndrome. *PLoS Genet* 2009; 5: e1000649.
- Singh R, Andermann E, Whitehouse WPA, et al. Severe myoclonic epilepsy of infancy: Extended spectrum of GEFS+? *Epilepsia* 2001; 42: 837-44.
- Singh R, Scheffer IE, Crossland K, Berkovic SF. Generalized epilepsy with febrile seizures plus: a common, childhood onset, genetic epilepsy syndrome. *Ann Neurol* 1999; 45: 75-81.
- Sugawara T, Tsurubuchi Y, Agarwala KL, et al. A missense mutation of the Na+ channel alpha II subunit gene Na(v)1.2 in a patient with febrile and afebrile seizures causes channel dysfunction. *Proc Natl Acad Sci USA* 2001; 98: 6384-9.
- Suls A, Jaehn JA, Kecskes A, et al. De novo loss-of-function mutations in *CHD2* causes a fever-sensitive myoclonic epileptic encephalopathy sharing features with Dravet syndrome. *Am J Hum Genet* 2013; 93: 967-75.
- Thomas P, Genton P, Gélisse P, Medina M, Serafini A. Juvenile myoclonic epilepsy. In: Bureau M, Genton P, Dravet C, Delgado-Escueta A, Tassinari C, Thomas P, Wolf P (eds). *Epileptic Syndromes in Infancy, Childhood and Adolescence*, 5th ed. Paris: John Libbey Eurotext, 2012, pp. 305-328.
- Uemura N, Okumura A, Negoro T, Watanabe K. Clinical features of benign convulsions with mild gastroenteritis. *Brain Dev* 2002; 24: 745-9.
- Verity CM, Butler NR, Golding J. Febrile convulsions in a national cohort followed up from birth. I–Prevalence and recurrence in the first five years of life. *Br Med J (Clin Res Ed)* 1985; 290: 1307-10.
- Wallace RH, Marini C, Petrou S, et al. Mutant GABA(A) receptor gamma2-subunit in childhood absence epilepsy and febrile seizures. *Nat Genet* 2001; 28: 49-52.
- Wimmer VC, Reid CA, Mitchell S, et al. Axon initial segment dysfunction in a mouse model of genetic epilepsy with febrile seizures plus. *J Clin Invest* 2010; 120: 2661-71.
- Yu FH, Mantegazza M, Westenbroek RE, et al. Reduced sodium current in GABAergic interneurons in a mouse model of severe myoclonic epilepsy in infancy. *Nat Neurosci* 2006; 9: 1142-9.

Infantile spasms semiology and pathophysiology: have we made progress?

Douglas R. Nordli Jr

Epilepsy Center, Ann & Robert H. Lurie Children's Hospital of Chicago, Chicago, USA

William James West described his son's infantile spasms in 1841 (West, 1841). In that famous letter West characterized most of the essential clinical features of spasms including the frequent onset with *sursum vergens* or upward eye deviation, the evolution to flexion spasms – and later extension – movements, the periodicity of the events and most importantly, their association with cognitive regression. West was an astute observer and he left no stone unturned. He took the boy to the finest physicians of the time, wrote to colleagues throughout Europe and when this did not provide a satisfactory answer wrote to the Lancet, imploring the editors to publish his letter (Duncan, 2011).

It is perfectly understandable, therefore, why West's original description has remained the classic clinical description for the past 173 years. It is hard to improve upon the work of a highly motivated and talented professional with excellent observational skills. The only other piece of his eponymic syndrome – the classic interictal EEG correlate termed hypsarhythmia by the Gibbs' – would come many years later, after the advent of clinical electroencephalography (Gibbs, 1954). (We use the original spelling of the term with one "r" as introduced by the Gibbs' in honor of their special contributions.) Gastaut *et al.* (1965) proposed the term West Syndrome in the early 1960's.

West's main tools were his primary senses. Using more advanced techniques unimaginable at the time there have been a broad range of clinical and pathophysiological advances in our understanding of the semiology and cause of infantile spasms. The two are of course related, as clinical observations may inform the basic science and scientific advances in turn provide important direction for clinical work.

Cortical lesions can produce spasms and widespread EEG abnormalities including hypsarhythmia. Removal of isolated cortical lesions can result in complete resolution of symptoms. Clinical experience has shown that many different etiologies located in many different regions of the brain can cause spasms and the common element appears to be a dynamic interaction with deeper structures. Animal models are emerging and offering valuable clues to the pathogeneses. More information is likely to emerge in the near future regarding the shared mechanisms behind these disparate models, but already there are suggestions of common elements including pathology of the interneurons. Infantile spasms and West syndrome can be thought of as a derangement of a network or a system epilepsy. Despite these considerable advances in the cause of the spasms, we poorly understand the precise cause of the accompanying encephalopathy. Here, it is proposed that the background slowing and disruption of the normal brain rhythms may be an important cause of the encephalopathy. In this regard the encephalopathy may also be viewed as a disturbance in brain networks. If borne out by experimental data this may offer different targets for therapy aside from just suppression of the infantile spasms themselves.

This brief review will attempt to develop this point and in the spirit of clinical work informing basic science will propose a new focus for animal models.

■ Detailed semiology of infantile spasms implicates cortical structures in some cases

The widespread availability of video-EEG recording units has allowed a more precise characterization of infantile spasms including details on the varieties of flexion and extension movements, their associated body parts and their frequency. Kellaway et al. (2014) used a time-synchronized video and polygraphic recording system and recorded 5,042 infantile spasms in 24 infants aged 1 to 43 months. They precisely characterized the movements of spasms and found that 33.9% were flexor, 22.5% extensor, and 42.0% mixed flexor-extensor. They noted a period of "akinesia" and apparent diminished responsiveness lasting up to 90 seconds when spasms clustered, a phenomenon that occurred in 78.3%. Spasms were most commonly observed after arousal from sleep. The electroencephalographic seizure pattern was variable, but a marked generalized attenuation of electrical activity was a feature of 71.7% of the attacks (Kellaway, 1979). Concurrent polygraphic recordings can precisely differentiate spasms from other seizures that might appear similar to a firsthand observer. Using surface disc recording electrodes over various muscles one can distinguish spasms from myoclonia, myoclonic-tonic seizures and tonic seizures. Spasms are often accompanied by an electrodecrement with a high voltage slow wave transient at the vertex as well as a rhomboid-shaped complex on EMG. Myoclonia may correlate with electrodecrements as well, but more often have a diffuse spike or polyspike EEG correlates and a quick EMG signature, as the clinical features would suggest. Tonic seizures, often seen with diffuse attenuation with or without low voltage fast activity in infants, have a prolonged rectangular-shaped correlate on EMG. Myoclonic-tonic seizures have an EMG correlate that is a fusion of the last two but often occur with electrodecremental responses.

Gross motor asymmetries or asynchronous movements may be seen in approximately 30% of infants with spasms and if consistent, may be a valuable clinical sign indicating focal structural pathology (Fusco et al., 1993; Gaily et al., 1995). Furthermore, infantile spasms may co-exist with focal seizures in equal number of cases (Donat, 1991). Infantile focal seizures may have a variety of motor manifestations with tonic or clonic features restricted to one part of the body, but even more subtle are focal seizures that present with only a cessation of motor activity and a slight version of the eyes (so-called behavioral arrestversive (BAV) or hypomotor semiology) (Korff et al., 2006). These seizures would have been impossible for West and his contemporaries to accurately detect. BAV seizures often have a rhythmic discharge emanating from the temporal region or posterior quadrant of the brain, making them easy to identify on vEEG. The presence of focal seizures indicates focal, or sometimes multifocal (in the case of varying electrical topographic correlates), cortical grey pathology and hints at an important insight into the pathogenesis of infantile spasms: sometimes focal cortical pathology may trigger infantile spasms. This has been described as an apparent diffusion of the epileptic process to other regions of the brain. Watanabe et al. (2001) carefully studied the clinical and electrographic features of infantile spasms and concluded that there were asymmetric ictal EEG findings in the majority of cases, consistent with involvement of a cortical trigger.

These findings are consistent with some of the animal models of infantile spasms. In one model experimentally induced damage to the cortex can produce a phenotype closely resembling infantile spasms and interictal EEG findings that appear very similar to hypsarhythmia (Lee et al., 2008; Swann et al., 2012). This is caused by infusion of tetrodotoxin (TTX) into one hemisphere. Another animal model of infantile spasms involving the ARX mouse produces movements that closely resemble infantile spasms and it is believed to be caused, at least in part, by involvement of GABA interneurons (Olivetti, 2012).

A large group of diverse cortical pathologies can result in infantile spasms

Frost and others have enumerated at least 200 serious pathological processes affecting the brain that are capable of producing infantile spasms during the vulnerable months of infancy (Pellock et al., 2010; Frost, 2003). Trauma, infections, certain autosomal dominant conditions and hypoxic-ischemic injuries may be evident from the history. Some conditions, like major chromosomal abnormalities or phakomatoses, to name just two, may be evident from the physical examination. High quality brain MR imaging provides valuable clues to the presence of cortical malformations, cryptic intrauterine injuries and sometimes metabolic conditions. Newborn tandem mass spectroscopy has led to the automatic detection of a number of important treatable and next generations sequencing has provided a wealth of data allowing us to diagnose conditions that were completely obscure only years, or sometimes months ago. This technology is transforming our clinical protocols, and has resulted in a large number of important conditions that need to be considered in any patient with infantile spasms of unknown cause.

A central paradox is how can such a diverse group of conditions impacting many different regions of the brain results in a syndrome with such consistent clinical features?

Independent subcortical and brainstem involvement in infantile spasms

Hrachovy, Frost et al. (1989) suggested that the common mechanism involved in diverse cases of infantile spasms might be brainstem pathology. They found abnormal sleep patterns in infantile spasms patients and proposed a loss of the normal reciprocal relationship between the inhibitory noradrenergic neurons of the locus ceruleus, the serotonergic neurons of the dorsal raphe, and the excitatory cholinergic neurons in adjacent pontine regions. The net effect was predicted to decrease output of the cholinergic system. Infantile spasms would result from intermittent interference with descending pathways that control spinal reflex activity, whereas abnormal activity in the ascending tracts from these same pontine regions that project widely to the cerebral cortex would lead to the electrodecremental EEG responses, and possibly cognitive dysfunction as well. The ability of the brainstem and deeper structures to produce clinical spasms is evident from the observation of an infant with hydranencephaly: they may demonstrate infantile spasms clinically identical to those seen in infants with completely intact nervous systems (Neville, 1989). Brainstem pathology has also been implicated in infantile spasms using MRI studies and evoked potentials (Miyazaki et al., 1993). Subcortical and brainstem injury in neonates with hypoxic-ischemic injury appears to be associated with later development of infantile spasms (Gano et al., 2013).

Despite the supportive evidence this model did not precisely explain the above-mentioned focal EEG features or the associated cortical abnormalities. Furthermore, pharmacological attempts to modulate these pathways did not result in a satisfactory response in the majority of patients (Frost, 2005).

A dynamic interaction between the cortex and subcortical structures

Through a series of astute clinical observations investigators came to the conclusion that in a subset of infants suffering spasms a focal epileptogenic cortical grey lesion may cause infantile spasms and that removal of this lesion can result in immediate and lasting freedom from disabling attacks (Chugani et al., 1993). This observation was confirmed in other centers (Hwang, 1996). The concept here is that spasms could be triggered by an interaction between the cortical grey and subcortical structures (Chugani et al., 1990). This nociferous dynamic once established, allows the subcortical regions, brainstem, or both to become generators of infantile spasms (Hrachovy, 2008). Early PET studies revealed a consistent pattern of hypermetabolism in the lenticular nuclei and sometimes in the brainstem (Chugani et al., 1992). Descending volleys from the deep structures produce the motor manifestations of spasms whereas ascending volleys are responsible for the electrodecremental correlate. Although there are many features to electrodecremental responses the high voltage slow wave transient, which is often maximal at the vertex, is one of the most common, and might conceivably arise from deep-seated structures (Fusco, 1993).

Frost et al. (2005) revised their original model and speculated that infantile spasms are caused by a developmental desynchronization of pathways with widespread projection between the brainstem and cortex. In this manner they incorporated their earlier concept of brainstem involvement with the emerging data suggesting cortical pathology. Pathology anywhere in the brain could conceivably disrupt the normal balance between various critical pathways and during a vulnerable period of life produce infantile spasms.

A network or system epilepsy

Lado et al. (2013) observed that the presence of two animal models of infantile spasms involving widespread damage in one, and focal cortical injury in the other corresponded nicely with the observations in infants and matched the model of a dynamic interaction between cortical and subcortical structures. Specifically, a region of epileptogenic cortex interacting with subcortical regions including serotonergic, catecholaminergic and cholinergic pathways could explain the pathogenesis. The ascending pathways could reduce cortical activity, and encephalopathy could be due to this suppression, independent cortical derangements, or both. In a related publication, Capovilla et al. (2013) argue that infantile spasms cannot be adequately explained either as a focal or generalized epilepsy and are better described by the concept of a system epilepsy.

In summary, our understanding of the pathogenesis of infantile spasms has evolved considerably. We have moved from a simple dialectic of considering cortical or brainstem sources to a more nuanced view where disruptions in widely distributed networks at a particular stage of development cause the distinctive EEG and clinical features. The importance of thinking of the brain in terms of networks is also evident when we consider the source of the encephalopathy.

The epileptic encephalopathy

The early literature indicates that perhaps the most important aspect of West Syndrome is not the infantile spasms themselves. Many years after the resolution of the spasms James Edwin West had an enduring and devastating encephalopathy that resulted in his institutionalization. What causes this encephalopathy?

It seems highly unlikely that it is the spasms themselves. As many who have personally seen infantile spasms can testify spasms are relatively brief, cause only a momentary EEG change, are almost never associated with oxygen desaturation, and often there is a quick resumption of the EEG background, with no lasting post-ictal attenuation or slowing. In short, other than their upsetting appearance, they seem to have little immediate clinical or EEG post-ictal effect. In fact, the profound EEG abnormalities of high voltage slow waves and multifocal spikes often diminish during the cluster of spasms. Furthermore, there are rare but important patients with periodic spasms whose seizures are nearly identical in every respect to infantile spasms (save one- they usually do not have hypsarhythmia). Although originally described in children with some form of neurological dysfunction our group and others have seen those who develop well despite having daily clusters of epileptic spasms (Gobbi et al., 1987; Goldstein, 2008).

Secondly, rare but critical serial observations of infants at risk for spasms have taught us that development of an encephalopathy precedes the appearance of the spasms themselves. Philippi et al. (2008) demonstrated this in a series of careful observations of at-risk very young infants who clearly began having difficulty with visual interaction prior to the development of the spasms themselves.

If the seizures are not clearly the cause of the encephalopathy, is it the spikes? Momentary disruptions have been found but interestingly, sometimes appear to correlate more with the slow wave component of the spike-wave complex than the spike itself (Shewmon, 1988). In clinical practice we not infrequently see children with abundant, sometimes continuous spikes without any cognitive impact, neither lasting nor even transient. Still, others speculate that continuous spikes during sleep could alter the slow wave activity of sleep and cause cognitive dysfunction (Tassinari, 2006). Hernan et al. (2014) reported that an artificially created spike focus in the prefrontal cortex of an animal was associated with attention and socialization issues, raising the possibility that spikes could produce long-term consequences. ACTH treatment improved the outcome without significantly impacting the spike frequency, raising some doubt as to whether the spikes themselves were the culprit.

Working with an animal model of atypical absence seizures, Chan et al. (2006) showed that low levels of a GABAB antagonist restored cognitive function but did not influence the frequency of spikes or seizures. This suggests that cognitive function could be independent of these variables, in at least some circumstances.

The cause of epileptic encephalopathy:
EEG slowing, disorganization, and lack of normal rhythms

If not the spasms themselves, or the spikes, what else could cause the associated encephalopathy in West Syndrome? Are there any other clues offered by the EEG? Children with encephalopathy and epilepsy often have profoundly slowebackground activity on EEG (Lado et al., 2013). In those with severe epileptic encephalopathies in addition to being slowed the EEGs often contain electrodecrements and epochs of discontinuity (Nordli, 2014). In short, they are profoundly disorganized and lack the normal sustained rhythms seen in age-matched children. There is also a clinical spectrum of epileptic encephalopathies including Early Infantile Epileptic Encephalopathy, West Syndrome, Late Infantile Epileptic Encephalopathy and Lennox-Gastaut Syndrome where the clinical and EEG expression is likely modulated by developmental processes (Yamatogi, 1981; Nordli, 2012). In all of these cases the awake and sleep EEGs have marked disruptions of the normal architecture, organization and continuity. (Interestingly, Japaridze et al. used dynamic imaging of coherent sources or DICS and argued that the generator of the delta range activity seen in hypsarhythmia stemmed from a circuit involving the brainstem, putamen, posterior parietal cortex and occipital cortex. These findings are consistent with the discussion regarding pathogenesis of infantile spasms themselves.)

From one perspective background slowing and lack of the normal organization may be viewed as an etiologically non-specific markers of cerebral dysfunction but looked at another way, could they actually be the cause or strong contributors to the encephalopathy?

Scientific support for this concept comes from the work on place cells in the rodent hippocampus. In order for spatial information to be encoded there must be an orderly and well-maintained theta rhythm. The rodent cannot process spatial information unless it occurs in a specific relationship to the underlying sine wave. If this inherent rhythm is disrupted memory is also markedly impaired (Yamaguchi et al., 2007). If this concept can be extended to other brain activity it would imply that disruption of the underlying brain rhythms could lead to more widespread cognitive disruption. Faster rhythms in the 20-40 Hz range have been noted in various cortical areas associated with increased alertnesss to stimuli in animals and humans and proposed to contribute to cognitive recognition (Brandeis, et al., 2009).

One may speculate that the ongoing work on resting state and neurocognitive networks may shed some light on the epileptic encephalopathy. In 2001 Gusnard et al. (2001) described a default mode of brain function. Using PET, they determined that certain regions of the brain de-activate during tasks compared to baseline suggesting that brain activity was suspended in these regions and that the brain at rest had an intrinsic organization of activity. The normal background EEG clearly demonstrates that the brain at rest is actually very active and Laufs et al. (2008) were able to show that these default mode networks correlated with the power in different frequency bands of the EEG. Network analysis of EEG is a growing rapidly field in neuroscience that has attracted investigators from a wide spectrum of disciplines including magnetoelectroencephalography, electroencephalography and functional MRI (Cabral et al., 2014). All of these techniques have generated convincing data that the brain has widespread coherent networks, even at rest and several theoretical models have evolved to explain the observations. The precise function of these networks is an evolving story, but there is an emerging understanding that these resting states can influence the perception of stimuli. One could hypothesize that disruption of these networks could underlie the apparent lack of visual perception seen in infants with hypsarhythmia. This conjecture could be further extended to state that disruption of the resting state networks of the brain by chaotic brain activity could be responsible for the global cognitive dysfunction seen in children with epileptic encephalopathies.

Conclusion

There has been substantial new information regarding the EEG features, causative factors and pathogenesis of West Syndrome in the 173 years following the original description. Discussions have moved from original attempts to localize the pathology to a specific brain region towards a broader, more nuanced concept of a network or system epilepsy where dysfunction is the result of the disruption of widely distributed circuits in a developmentally susceptible brain. West is now considered a prototypic epileptic encephalopathy, where the epilepsy itself contributes to the encephalopathy, thereby making effective treatment an urgent matter. The specific cause of the encephalopathy is not precisely known, but just as the concept of pathogenesis has evolved to networks, so too should our scope of investigation broaden to include the impact of EEG network disruption upon cognition.

The recent appearance of relevant animal models have raised the hope that there will be further pathophysiological insights and novel treatments (Scantlebury *et al.*, 2010). At the same time, animal models should be used to study the impact of the condition on cognition so that this important aspect of West Syndrome can be better understood and treated.

References

- Brandeis D, Michel CM, Amzica F. From neuronal activity to scalp potential fields. In: Michel CM, Koenig T, Brandeis D, Gianotti LRR, Wackermann J, eds. *Electrical Neuroimaging*. Cambridge: Cambridge University Press, 2009, pp. 1-24.
- Cabral J, Kringelbach ML, Deco G. Exploring the network dynamics underlying brain activity during rest. *Progress in Neurobiology* 2014; 114: 102-31.
- Capovilla G, Moshe SL, Wolf P, Avanzini G. Epileptic encephalopathy as models of system epilepsy. *Epilepsia* 2013; 54 (suppl 8): 34-7.
- Chan KF, Burnham WM, Jia Z, Cortez MA, Snead OC, 3rd. GABAB receptor antagonism abolishes the learning impairments in rats with chronic atypical absence seizures. *European Journal of Pharmacology* 2006; 541: 64-72.
- Chugani HT, Shewmon DA, Sankar R, Chen BC, Phelps ME. Infantile spasms: II. Lenticular nuclei and brain stem activation on positron emission tomography. *Ann Neurol* 1992; 31: 212-9.
- Chugani HT, Shewmon DA, Shields WD, *et al.* Surgery for intractable infantile spasms: neuroimaging perspectives. *Epilepsia* 1993; 34: 764-71.
- Chugani HT, Shields WD, Shewmon DA, Olson DM, Phelps ME, Peacock WJ. Infantile spasms: I. PET identifies focal cortical dysgenesis in cryptogenic cases for surgical treatment. *Ann Neurol* 1990; 27: 406-13.
- Donat JF, Wright FS. Simultaneous infantile spasms and partial seizures. *Journal of Child Neurology* 1991; 6: 246-50.
- Dulac O, Chiron C, Robain O, Plouin P, Jambaque II, Pinard JM. Infantile spasms: a pathophysiological hypothesis. *Seminars in Pediatric Neurology* 1994; 1: 83-9.

- Duncan R. Infantile spasms: the original description of Dr West. 1841. *Epileptic Disord* 2001; 3(1): 47-8.
- Frost JD, Jr., Hrachovy RA. *Infantile Spasms: Diagnosis, Management, and Prognosis*. Boston: Kluwer Academic Publishers, 2003.
- Frost JD, Jr., Hrachovy RA. Pathogenesis of infantile spasms: a model based on developmental desynchronization. *J Clin Neurophysiol* 2005; 22: 25-36.
- Fusco L, Vigevano F. Ictal clinical electroencephalographic findings of spasms in West syndrome. *Epilepsia* 1993; 34: 671-8.
- Gaily EK, Shewmon DA, Chugani HT, Curran JG. Asymmetric and asynchronous infantile spasms. *Epilepsia* 1995; 36: 873-82.
- Gano D, Sargent MA, Miller SP, et al. MRI findings in infants with infantile spasms after neonatal hypoxic-ischemic encephalopathy. *Pediatric Neurology* 2013; 49: 401-5.
- Gastaut H, Roger J, Soulayrol R, Salamon G, Regis H, Lob H. [Infantile myoclonic encephalopathy with hypsarrhythmia (West's syndrome) and Bourneville's tuberous sclerosis]. *J Neurolog Sci* 1965; 2: 140-60.
- Gibbs EL, Fleming MM, Gibbs FA. Diagnosis and prognosis of hypsarhythmia and infantile spasms. *Pediatrics* 1954; 13: 66-73.
- Gobbi G, Bruno L, Pini A, Giovanardi Rossi P, Tassinari CA. Periodic spasms: an unclassified type of epileptic seizure in childhood. *Developmental Medicine and Child Neurology* 1987; 29: 766-75.
- Goldstein J, Slomski J. Epileptic spasms: a variety of etiologies and associated syndromes. *Journal of Child Neurology* 2008; 23: 407-14.
- Gusnard DA, Raichle ME, Raichle ME. Searching for a baseline: functional imaging and the resting human brain. *Nat Rev Neurosci* 2001; 2: 685-94.
- Hernan AE, Alexander A, Lenck-Santini PP, Scott RC, Holmes GL. Attention deficit associated with early life interictal spikes in a rat model is improved with ACTH. *PloS One* 2014; 9: e89812.
- Hrachovy RA, Frost JD, Jr. Infantile spasms: a disorder of the developing nervous system. In: Kellaway P, Noebels JL, eds. *Problems and concepts in developmental neurophysiology*. Baltimore: Johns Hopkins University Press, 1989, pp. 131-47.
- Hrachovy RA, Frost JD, Jr. Severe Encephalopathic Epilepsy in Infants: Infantile Spasms (West Syndrome). In: Pellock JM, Bourgeois BFD, Dodson WE, eds. *Pediatric Epilepsy: Diagnosis and Therapy*, 3rd ed. New York: Demos Medical Publishing, LLC, 2008, pp. 249-68.
- Hwang PA, Otsubo H, Koo BK, et al. Infantile spasms: cerebral blood flow abnormalities correlate with EEG, neuroimaging, and pathologic findings. *Pediatric Neurology* 1996; 14: 220-5.
- Japaridze N, Muthuraman M, Moeller F, et al. Neuronal networks in West Syndrome as revealed by source analysis and renormalized partial directed coherence. *Brain Topogr* 2013 Jan; 26(1): 157-70; doi: 10.1007/s10548-012-0245-y. Epub 2012 Aug 4. PubMed PMID: 23011408.
- Kellaway P, Hrachovy RA, Frost JD, Jr., Zion T. Precise characterization and quantification of infantile spasms. *An Neuro* 1979; 6: 214-8.
- Korff CM, Nordli DR, Jr. The clinical-electrographic expression of infantile seizures. *Epilepsy research* 2006; 70 (suppl 1): S116-31.
- Lado FA, Rubboli G, Capovilla P, Avanzini G, Moshe SL. Pathophysiology of epileptic encephalopathies. *Epilepsia* 2013; 54 (suppl 8): 6-13.
- Laufs H. Endogenous brain oscillations and related networks detected by surface EEG-combined fMRI. *Human Brain Mapping* 2008; 29: 762-9.
- Lee CL, Frost JD, Jr., Swann JW, Hrachovy RA. A new animal model of infantile spasms with unprovoked persistent seizures. *Epilepsia* 2008; 49: 298-307.
- Lee YJ, Berg AT, Nordli DR, Jr. Clinical spectrum of epileptic spasms in children. *Brain Dev* 2014.

- Miyazaki M, Hashimoto T, Tayama M, Kuroda Y. Brainstem involvement in infantile spasms: a study employing brainstem evoked potentials and magnetic resonance imaging. *Neuropediatrics* 1993; 24: 126-30.
- Neville BG. The origin of infantile spasms: evidence from a case of hydranencephaly. *Dev Med Child Neurol* 1972; 14: 644-7.
- Nordli DR. Pediatric Epilepsy Syndromes. In: Ebersole JS, Husain AM, Nordli DR, eds. *Current Practice of Clinical Electroencephalography*, 4th ed. Philadelphia: Wolters Kluwer Health, 2014, pp. 283-314.
- Nordli DR, Jr. Epileptic encephalopathies in infants and children. *J Clin Neurophysiol* 2012; 29: 420-4.
- Olivetti PR, Noebels JL. Interneuron, interrupted: molecular pathogenesis of ARX mutations and X-linked infantile spasms. Current opinion in neurobiology 2012; 22: 859-65.
- Pellock JM, Hrachovy R, Shinnar S, *et al*. Infantile spasms: a U.S. consensus report. *Epilepsia* 2010; 51: 2175-89.
- Philippi H, Wohlrab G, Bettendorf U, *et al*. Electroencephalographic evolution of hypsarrhythmia: toward an early treatment option. *Epilepsia* 2008; 49: 1859-64.
- Scantlebury MH, Galanopoulou AS, Chudomelova L, Raffo E, Betancourth D, Moshe SL. A model of symptomatic infantile spasms syndrome. *Neurobiol Dis* 2010; 37: 604-12.
- Shewmon DA, Erwin RJ. The effect of focal interictal spikes on perception and reaction time. II. Neuroanatomic specificity. *Electroencephalography and Clinical Neurophysiology* 1988; 69: 338-52.
- Swann JW, Moshe SL. On the Basic Mechanisms of Infantile Spasms. In: Noebels JL, Avoli M, Rogawski MA, Olsen RW, Delgado-Escueta AV, eds. *Jasper's Basic Mechanisms of the Epilepsies*, 4th ed. Bethesda: National Center for Biotechnology Information, 2012.
- Tassinari CA, Rubboli G. Cognition and paroxysmal EEG activities: from a single spike to electrical status epilepticus during sleep. *Epilepsia* 2006; 47 (suppl 2): 40-3.
- West WJ. On a peculiar form of infantile convulsions. *Lancet* 1841; 1: 724-5.
- Yamaguchi Y, Sato N, Wagatsuma H, Wu Z, Molter C, Aota Y. A unified view of theta-phase coding in the entorhinal-hippocampal system. *Current Opinion in Neurobiology* 2007; 17: 197-204.
- Yamatogi Y, Ohtahara S. Age-dependent epileptic encephalopathy: a longitudinal study. *Folia Psychiatr Neurol Jpn* 1981; 35: 321-32.

Trials for the treatment of infant seizures: theory, practice, ethics and potential future trends

Andrew Lux[1], Finbar J. K. O'Callaghan[2]

[1] Department of Paediatric Neurology, Bristol Royal Hospital for Children, Bristol, United Kingdom
[2] Section of Clinical Neurosciences, Institute of Child Health, University College London, London, United Kingdom

---

With the exception of the benign infantile epilepsy syndromes, seizures in infancy are generally a marker of a serious underlying metabolic, structural or genetic pathology. Many such cases have the features of an epileptic encephalopathy: that is, a seizure disorder that is associated with behavioural and developmental regression coincident with the onset of seizures and in some way attributable to the epilepsy. Clinicians are strongly motivated to find effective treatments that will improve seizure control and also improve neurodevelopmental outcomes, and in order to improve the evidence for treatment interventions, we need clinical studies with robust designs and that are capable of effective implementation.

There are many challenges associated with studying infantile seizures, and in particular where the aim is to study treatment interventions by means of randomized-controlled trials. In terms of study design, it is necessary to decide upon reliable case definitions, the most important and valuable outcome measures, and whether the focus of the trial design is upon effectiveness or efficacy. Investigators need to validly and coherently present, interpret, and explain data obtained from the trial, and the first step in this process is to ensure that statistical inference is sound. Among practical issues, it is necessary to perform a statistical power calculation to ensure that clinically important differences in outcome are likely to be detected. There might be theoretical or practical issues relating to research ethics and research governance, particularly where there are studies being performed across institutional or national boundaries. And there might be specific issues relating to risk or potential harm, some of which might become apparent during the course of a clinical study and require changes in protocol.

This chapter examines key aspects of these theoretical, practical, and ethical challenges in the context of infantile seizures, and in particular for infantile spasms (West syndrome), which is the form of epilepsy in infancy that has been subjected to most interventional studies. The chapter concludes by discussing potential directions for future studies of infantile seizures.

Theoretical issues relating to clinical trial design

Case definitions

As well as the challenges related to the many features that may constitute the semiology or phenomenology of a seizure, it can be difficult to categorize cases into seizure types, and by combining the seizure types with electrographic (EEG) features, to categorize into epilepsy syndromes. Practical help can come from home video, perhaps captured on mobile phone, the greater availability of video-EEG telemetry, and combined monitoring of EEG with surface EMG (electromyography), which can help to identify and distinguish seizure types – for example, distinguishing myoclonus from epileptic spasms – on the basis of duration of muscle activity. Using these other forms of capturing information about semiology provides some assurance that studies are valid and reliable.

The EEG provides a surfeit of information from which key data require abstraction, and readers will require assurance that there has been reliable and reproducible interpretation. Ideally, assessors blinded to treatment exposure will perform EEG categorisation, and many studies will have more than one EEG reviewer and some statement of inter-rater reliability. The most relevant EEG features may be ictal or interictal. In the case of infantile spasms, the most characteristic EEG pattern is hypsarrhythmia and is generally found between, rather than during, the clinical attacks of clustered spasms.

For infantile spasms, there has been an international initiative by the West Delphi group to define cases of infantile spasms (Lux and Osborne, 2004). The group, which consisted of 31 members from 15 countries, felt during its first round that it would be easy to reach agreement on the core features of hypsarrhythmia and to provide a succinct definition, but by the end of the study they realised that this was more challenging than had initially been thought.

Outcomes and outcome measures

The West Delphi group (Lux and Osborne, 2004) also sought clear definitions for key outcomes and outcome measures. The most radical departure from previous practice was the consensus definition of *cessation of spasms*, which unless otherwise qualified, should be defined as the absence of any witnessed spasm for at least 28 consecutive days, with that cessation starting within 14 days of the treatment intervention.

One of the key advantages of a community of practice defining standardized outcomes and outcome measures for clinical studies is that subsequent aggregation of data and meta-analysis is not subject to the added heterogeneity of different outcome measures, and that any clinician reading a collection of studies can be clearer about what a positive outcome really means.

Efficacy and effectiveness paradigms for clinical studies

A challenging area of consensus and classification within epilepsy relates to aetiological classification. Where specific underlying etiologies are not identified, there has been a practice of categorizing cases into symptomatic, idiopathic, and cryptogenic groups. More recent proposals for classification have taken a different approach, but the underlying principle of aggregating disparate specific etiologies into aetiological categories remains (Osborne et al., 2010). Where aetiological categories cover a broader range of etiologies, the underlying mechanisms of epilepsy are likely to be more heterogeneous, and there is the possibility that effective treatment interventions will be subject to dilutional bias where some other specific etiologies are not effectively treated because of the different mechanism(s) underlying the epilepsy.

Therefore, when one is designing a study of infantile seizures, where it is likely that there are different underlying etiologies, there may be disagreement around this issue of "lumping or splitting". For the sake of clarity, one way to frame this challenge is to consider the distinction between studies of efficacy and studies of effectiveness (Piantadosi, 1997). Although this is not an absolute distinction, it is useful way of clarifying the underlying issues.

In general terms, an efficacy study sets out to test a biological question by identifying a cohort that is as homogenous as possible. Data are collected in detail, eligibility criteria are strict, and there is a strong focus on the internal validity of the data. In contrast, an effectiveness study addresses the pragmatic question of whether a treatment intervention improves outcomes in a broader cohort of patients that have more heterogeneous underlying etiologies. The focus is more on external validity of the data, which are collected on a larger group that has more relaxed eligibility criteria, and the data are generally collected in less detail.

In the case of infantile spasms, for example, a study focusing on efficacy might restrict eligibility to cases where the underlying cause is tuberous sclerosis. This would allow a more effective investigation of whether a treatment intervention works on a specific mechanism of epilepsy due to tuberous sclerosis than would a study that included infantile spasms with other underlying etiologies. However, where the treatment decision precedes the identification of a specific underlying aetiology, as is often the case with infantile spasms, the pragmatic question becomes, "How many of my patients will respond to this treatment irrespective of the underlying cause that we might identify later?"

The effective use of information from clinical studies

In planning clinical trials, it is necessary to consider a balance between gathering detailed information and gathering sufficient information for the needs of answering the most pertinent questions. If the scope of data gathering is too broad and the detail too fine, it is likely that investigators will be overwhelmed and there will be a loss of practical efficiency. If insufficient data are gathered, then it might be that the effort and cost of the study is not rewarded with the capability to perform analyses that address the initial questions alongside questions that arise after the study is completed. Should there be an unexpected finding or some apparent bias or confounding for which a post hoc analysis might wish to control, then the value of a broader scope of data may become apparent too late in the day.

In statistical terms, continuous data contain more information when analysed by means of a statistical test designed for continuous data than when the data are collapsed into categories and analysed by a test designed for categorical data. For example, if the duration of seizures (in days) prior to a treatment intervention is used as a predictor variable that is analysed for an independent effect upon later neurodevelopmental scores, analysis of that duration in number of completed days would provide more information, and therefore greater discriminatory power within a statistical test, than if these same data were collapsed into categories of duration, such as up to 7 days, between 8 and 14 completed days, and

15 days or longer. However, in practical terms there is added cost associated with collecting the data with more precision (in days) than in three simple categories, and in practice there is often a great deal of uncertainty about the exact number of days for which a symptom, such as seizures, has occurred. In this instance, the challenge of study design is to identify a pragmatic and informed balance between collecting data with great precision and collecting data in a fashion that is sufficient to answer questions that are known and that are likely to arise following the initial data analysis.

An illustration of this issue lies in several studies of lead-time to treatment intervention for infantile spasms. Retrospective studies by Eisermann and colleagues, studying cases with Down syndrome, and by Kivity and colleagues, studying idiopathic cases of infantile spasms, reported the effects upon neurodevelopment of treatment delays of more than 2 months and more than 1 month, respectively (Eisermann et al., 2003; Kivity et al., 2004). In the case of the United Kingdom Infantile Spasms Study, it was possible to categorise the collected data by duration of epileptic spasms prior to treatment intervention into five periods of duration: fewer than 8 days; between 8 and 14 days; between 15 days and 1 month; between 1 and 2 months; and longer than 2 months (O'Callaghan et al., 2011). This approach allowed a visual analysis of trends in the overall group, in the group with identified symptomatic etiologies, and in the group with no identified underlying cause, and the analysis showed a clear trend in Vineland Adaptive Behavior Scales (VABS) in this last group. Analysis was by means of a linear regression model with the outcome variable being the VABS score and the predictor variables including the lead-time as a categorical predictor variable. By including etiological categories and the treatment intervention, it was possible to demonstrate that lead-time to treatment independently predicts neurodevelopmental outcome.

Effect estimates, confidence intervals, and P-values

A large study with high statistical power is able to detect a smaller difference than a smaller study with the same study design. Therefore, a statistically significant difference may indicate a relatively small effect or a relatively large effect, and is therefore of limited value in itself to a clinician attempting to interpret the findings of a clinical study. The reporting and interpretation of a study is more valuable if it provides effect estimates and confidence intervals than if it provides solely P-values (Altman, 1991).

Taking the example of the UKISS study of lead-time to treatment, the statement that lead-time had a statistically significant P-value within the linear regression model is less informative than the interpretation given in terms of its effect estimate: in other words, that for each increase in duration of spasms by one of the categories of duration used in the study, there was an average decrease in developmental quotient of 3.9 points (O'Callaghan et al., 2011). Presenting the interpretation in this fashion allows the clinician to evaluate the magnitude of the effect and to decide whether it is clinically important.

■ Practical issues relating to clinical trial design

Trial size and duration

The incidence of the infantile epilepsies is relatively low. Therefore, there are a number of practical difficulties in conducting trials to evaluate treatment. The numbers needed to adequately power clinical trials means either that trials have to take place over a number of years or that they involve multiple countries. For these reasons, most studies in this area have been underpowered or have been unable to answer the most fundamental questions about neurodevelopment. The International Collaborative Infantile Spasm Study (ICISS EudraCT Number: 2006-000788-27) has recently finished recruiting after collecting sufficient numbers to have more than 80% power to answer its two primary outcome questions regarding seizure cessation and development. It took 7 years and has involved 5 countries to recruit the 377 cases needed to answer the research questions. If future progress is to be made in this area there will need to be multinational research and funding agencies prepared to fund long-term projects.

Blinding and masking

The gold standard for clinical trials is that both the patients (and their families) and the doctors should be blinded to the treatment being allocated. However, with infantile epilepsies this is often difficult. In the area of infantile spasms, hormonal treatments (ACTH or prednisolone) are one of the most commonly studied treatment modalities. ACTH needs to be given via injection, and it is generally considered unethical to give placebo injections to infants in the other treatment arm. Moreover, because the side effects of hormonal therapy are often evident to observers even where they are blinded to the treatment intervention, attempts at blinding are often rendered futile. It is feasible, however, that those assessing treatment effects remain blinded wherever possible to treatment allocation. Unfortunately, in 18 RCTs analysed in the Cochrane Review of Infantile Spasms, only 6 RCTs had assessors who were blinded to treatment allocation (Hancock et al., 2013).

■ Ethical and safety issues relating to clinical trial design

Equipoise

Ethically, it has been considered a *sine qua non* of clinical trials in all areas of practice that researchers are in a state of equipoise about which treatment is best. In essence, the concept of equipoise indicates that the clinician has a balanced belief about whether the treatment, either in itself or relative to another treatment, is as likely to do harm as good, or to do no better or worse than its comparator (Fried, 1974).

In the field of infantile seizures, there is relatively little evidence about which treatments are most effective, and yet it is often the case that individual equipoise does not exist. In the specific area of infantile spasms, for example, there are influential advocates who would argue that vigabatrin, ACTH, and even nitrazepam, is the most appropriate first-line treatment. If the community of clinicians managing these epilepsy conditions is to make progress, it is necessary for those clinicians to acknowledge that, even where not every individual clinician is in a state of equipoise, it remains ethical, and we would argue necessary, to be prepared to participate in clinical trials where the clinical community as a whole is in equipoise in order to identify which is the most effective treatment (Freedman, 1987).

In the context of infantile epilepsy, the scientific community should be in an almost permanent state of equipoise for many treatment comparisons because the evidence base for treatment is so thin. However, there are threats to the equipoise of the clinical community. Firstly, dominant opinion makers can disrupt equipoise by forcefully championing a particular treatment even when strong or relevant evidence for effectiveness does not exist. Secondly, equipoise is vulnerable if clinicians fail to critically evaluate the evidence that is presented to them. For example, vigabatrin is considered by many as the most appropriate treatment for infantile spasms in tuberous sclerosis complex (TSC) predominantly on the basis of one scientific paper (Chiron et al., 1997). This paper reported a small, unblinded trial that compared vigabatrin against hydrocortisone as first-line therapy for infantile spasms in TSC. Although this paper showed a clear advantage for vigabatrin, the comparison treatment, hydrocortisone, is one that is not used broadly for this indication and that does not have substantial published evidence of effectiveness.

It seems that community equipoise has now been lost in this area to the extent that it would currently be difficult to investigate any other treatment modalities for infantile spasms in TSC. For example, it is for this reason that the UKISS and ICISS RCTs excluded TSC patients; a decision related to study design that one can argue has perpetuated the notion that the advantage of vigabatrin in TSC has been proven.

The use of placebo controls

It is often impossible to randomize treatments against placebo. Many of the infantile epilepsies that we wish to study are thought to be epileptic encephalopathies and it seems unethical to delay an active treatment – by allocating one treatment arm to interventional monotherapy and the other treatment arm to a placebo – that may ameliorate the devastating effects of the encephalopathy. This would certainly be true in an area such as infantile spasms, where there is at least some evidence for effective treatment. But it might seem less relevant in the case of other epileptic encephalopathies, such as early myoclonic encephalopathy (EME) and early infantile epileptic encephalopathy (Ohtahara syndrome; EIEE), where there is currently no substantial published evidence of an effective treatment, either in terms of seizure reduction or in terms of improved neurodevelopmental outcome. Placebo controls can certainly be used in adjunctive (add-on) trials of therapy. The study by Chiron and colleagues of Dravet syndrome elegantly showed how the addition of stiripentol – to a combination treatment of sodium valproate with clobazam – improved seizure control in comparison to an arm that added a placebo to the combined existing treatment (Chiron et al., 2000). In this scenario, neither treatment arm in the trial is being denied an "active" treatment.

The benefit-risk balance and potential causes of harm in clinical studies

One consequence of the reluctance in studies of epilepsy to use a placebo control is that differences in neurodevelopmental outcome can be interpreted in several ways: as a chance occurrence; as evidence that one treatment is associated with an improvement in neurodevelopment; or that the other treatment is associated with a poorer outcome.

For example, in the UKISS study it was found that neurodevelopmental outcomes at 14 months of age in the group with no identified underlying aetiology, for whom the effect of treatment intervention upon neurodevelopment was expected to be most evident, was with borderline statistical significance relatively better in study participants enrolled to receive hormonal treatments rather than vigabatrin (Lux et al., 2005). In this case, one needs to consider the scenario of a chance occurrence, of a protective effect of hormonal treatment, or of a potential harm upon neurodevelopment related to vigabatrin. If there were studies relating to the natural history of neurodevelopmental outcomes with this specific epilepsy syndrome, or a collection of outcome measures from similar studies with different treatment interventions, then by comparison with those existing data, some inference might be made about the likely benefits or harms with the current study. This also provides a further argument for the value of standardisation of outcome measures between studies.

Potential risks and trial stopping rules

Because clinical trials are associated with the risk of interventions worsening rather than improving outcomes, and also because a trial might unexpectedly identify a larger difference in treatment effects between two interventions than anticipated, many trials will plan interim analyses, and all trials of treatment intervention will have some form of safety monitoring and reporting for serious adverse events (SAEs). A problem with most trials in the area of infantile seizures is that there are small numbers of study participants. A consequence of this is that serious adverse events of moderate or low probability are unlikely to be encountered during the clinical trial, and it may be difficult to attribute causality to the treatment intervention. Another problem is that, because any interim analysis requires some form of "spending function" of the P-value in order to adjust for the effect of repeated analyses, both the interim analysis and the final analysis will suffer a further diminution in statistical power (DeMets, 1994).

Future directions for clinical studies

To date most studies in the area have focused on comparing single anticonvulsant therapies as treatments for the infantile epilepsies. Recently, novel approaches and treatment modalities have been suggested and investigated.

Combination therapy

Finding an effective monotherapy is an understandable goal in the treatment of those with epilepsy, but in the more difficult epilepsies it is likely that the best treatment effect will be obtained by modifying more than one mechanism by means of combination therapy. This idea forms the basis for many oncology trials and may be applicable in the field of infantile epilepsy.

In Dravet syndrome, for example, there is RCT evidence that the combination of sodium valproate, clobazam and stiripentol is more effective at reducing seizure frequency than valproate and clobazam alone (Chiron et al., 2000). In the UKISS study, it was clear that some patients who had failed first-line treatment (either vigabatrin or hormonal therapy) responded rapidly when switched to the alternative trial therapy (Lux et al., 2005). This observation suggests that there are subpopulations of patients, unidentifiable on the basis of our current knowledge at the start of the trial, which will respond better to one or other drug. This observation led to the hypothesis that combination therapy with both vigabatrin and hormonal therapy would be more effective at abolishing seizures than monotherapy alone, and that this earlier control of spasms would result in better neurodevelopmental outcome. And this hypothesis has in turn informed the study design of the International Collaborative Infantile Spasms Study (ICISS), which has recently finished recruiting and might soon provide an answer to this question.

Presymptomatic treatment

As epileptic encephalopathies with onset in infancy are thought to have the potential to damage development from a time preceding the onset of the epilepsy, there has been considerable interest in whether prophylactic treatment in high-risk patients might improve prognosis. The best example of this is in TSC, where there is a high risk of developing infantile spasms that can often be identified before the onset of epilepsy. Jozwiak et al. reported a study comparing a group of TSC patients who were treated with vigabatrin as soon as epileptic discharges were seen on EEG, but before the onset of clinical seizures, against a group who were treated conventionally and only after the onset of clinical seizures (Jozwiak et al., 2011). They observed that the prophylactic group had a significantly better neurodevelopmental outcome, a lower incidence of subsequent drug-resistant epilepsy and less need for later polytherapy, and a higher incidence of subsequent seizure freedom. The study has methodological issues that require the results to be treated with caution, but the questions it poses and starts to address certainly merit further study, and indeed are now the focus of a multicentre European trial.

Potential value of modifying the mTOR (mammalian target of rapamycin) pathway

The mammalian target of rapamycin (mTOR) signaling pathway regulates cell growth, proliferation, and differentiation. Dysregulation of this pathway has been implicated in several genetic conditions, such as neurofibromatosis type 1 (NF1) and tuberous sclerosis complex (TSC), which have clinical phenotypes that can include epilepsy (Tee et al., 2002; Johannessen et al., 2005). Dysregulation of mTOR has also been implicated in focal cortical dysplasias and hemimegalencephaly, which are associated with intractable focal epilepsy (Ljungberg et al., 2006; Lee et al., 2012). Therefore, there is much interest in exploring whether mTOR inhibition will interfere with epileptogenesis and improve cognitive outcome for those suffering early onset epilepsies.

Evidence from studies of mice with disrupted mTOR signaling does suggest that mTOR inhibition can prevent epilepsy and ameliorate the underlying pathology. In the multiple hit animal model of infantile spasms, treatment with the mTOR inhibitor rapamycin suppresses spasms and improves cognitive outcome (Raffo et al., 2011). Similarly in a mouse-model of focal cortical dysplasia, treatment with the mTOR inhibitor rapamycin suppressed the development of neuronal hypertrophy and seizures (Ljungberg et al., 2009). In post-status epilepticus models of temporal lobe epilepsy, mTOR inhibition may suppress mossy fibre sprouting and reduce future seizures, although the timing of administration of mTOR inhibition may be crucial and there is the possibility that there can be a paradoxical effect of increased mTOR activation if mTOR inhibition occurs too close to the timing of brain injury (Buckmaster et al., 2009; Buckmaster and Lew, 2011). If mTOR over-activation is epileptogenic, then the implication is that, for mTOR inhibition is to be a sustainably effective intervention, then it is necessary for it to be administered long-term.

Inhibition of mTOR may, however, be a double-edged sword: preventing epileptogenesis but having detrimental effects on brain development and recovery from brain injury (Zeng et al., 2010). The PI3K-Akt-mTOR pathway is critical in brain development with mTOR activation promoting neuronal differentiation, dendrite elongation, and branching and synapse development (Murakami et al., 2004). Animal models with significantly reduced mTOR activity are either lethal or result in significantly reduced brain size (Guertin et al., 2006; Thomanetz et al., 2013). Therefore long-term inhibition could theoretically have a negative effect on development. mTOR activation has been implicated in improved recovery from brain injury by promoting angiogenesis, neuronal regeneration and synaptic plasticity (Chen et al., 2012). Moreover, mTOR inhibitors have predictable and unpleasant side effects outside the CNS, with risks that include immunosuppression, hyperlipidaemia and mucosal ulceration.

Interventions involving neuroprotection

If we accept the concept of infantile encephalopathy, then it is logical to explore not only whether there are effective anti-epileptogenic agents and anticonvulsants, but also whether there are any agents that can protect the brain against injury. Carmant et al. explored whether there was a neuroprotective effect in infantile spasms from supplementation of standard anticonvulsant treatment with the calcium-channel blocking drug flunarizine (Bitton et al., 2012). They reported no difference in cognitive outcome between the groups receiving flunarizine or placebo with the exception of children with no identified aetiology for their spasms. At 24 months of age and assessed by means of Vineland Adaptive Behavior Scales (VABS) and Bayley Scales, the ten flunarizine-treated children with no identified etiology had a better outcome than the eight controls (VABS 84.1 ± 11.3 vs 72.3 ± 9.8; $P = 0.03$; and Bayley Scale 87.6 ± 14.7 vs 69.9 ± 25.3; $P = 0.07$).

There is a growing body of clinical and experimental evidence that neuroinflammation is involved in the pathophysiology of a number of epilepsies. Patients who have undergone epilepsy surgery for drug-resistant epilepsies show increased expression of proinflammatory molecules in resected tissue (Das et al., 2012). In infantile spasms investigators have noted increased levels of interleukin-2, interferon-alpha and tumour necrosis factor-alpha when compared with matched controls (Liu et al., 2001). The apparent relative effectiveness of anti-inflammatory and immunomodulatory therapies such as steroids and immunoglobulins in treating epileptic encephalopathies such as Infantile Spasms, Landau-Kleffner syndrome, Lennox-Gastaut syndrome and Rasmussen's Encephalitis is also suggestive that inflammation plays a key role in epilepsy. Inflammatory mediators such as tumour necrosis factor and interleukins may therefore be promising targets for future antiepileptic treatments in the infantile epileptic encephalopathies.

■ Conclusions

The infantile epilepsies are often associated with a poor outcome and there is an understandable need to discover the most effective treatments. Assessing treatments in this area using clinical trial methodology has both ethical and practical problems. However, the problems can be overcome provided investigators can agree about case definitions and standardized outcomes measures and collaborate on an international scale. And for progress to be made there has to be an acceptance that it is appropriate to study treatment options when the clinical community is in equipoise even if individual equipoise does not exist. The interest already being shown in new combination treatment regimens, mTOR inhibitors, and in neuroprotective and immunomodulatory therapies means that more effective treatment modalities may be imminent.

References

- Altman DG. Principles of statistical analysis. In: *Practical Statistics for Medical Research*. New York: Chapman and Hall, 1991, pp. 152-78.
- Bitton JY, Sauerwein HC, et al. A randomized controlled trial of flunarizine as add-on therapy and effect on cognitive outcome in children with infantile spasms. *Epilepsia* 2012; 53: 1570-6.
- Buckmaster PS, Ingram EA, et al. Inhibition of the mammalian target of rapamycin signaling pathway suppresses dentate granule cell axon sprouting in a rodent model of temporal lobe epilepsy. *J Neurosci* 2009; 29: 8259-69.
- Buckmaster PS, Lew FH. Rapamycin suppresses mossy fiber sprouting but not seizure frequency in a mouse model of temporal lobe epilepsy. *J Neurosci* 2011; 31: 2337-47.
- Chen H, Qu Y, et al. Role of mammalian target of rapamycin in hypoxic or ischemic brain injury: potential neuroprotection and limitations. *Rev Neurosci* 2012; 23: 279-87.
- Chiron C, Dumas C, et al. Randomized trial comparing vigabatrin and hydrocortisone in infantile spasms due to tuberous sclerosis. *Epilepsy Res* 1997; 26: 389-95.
- Chiron C, Marchand MC, et al. Stiripentol in severe myoclonic epilepsy in infancy: a randomised placebo-controlled syndrome-dedicated trial. STICLO study group. *Lancet* 2000; 356: 1638-42.
- Das A, Wallace GCT, et al. Hippocampal tissue of patients with refractory temporal lobe epilepsy is associated with astrocyte activation, inflammation, and altered expression of channels and receptors. *Neuroscience* 2012; 220: 237-46.
- DeMets DL, Lan KK. Interim analaysis: the alpha spending function approach. *Stat Med* 1994; 13: 1341-52.
- Eisermann MM, DeLaRaillere A, et al. Infantile spasms in Down syndrome – effects of delayed anticonvulsive treatment. *Epilepsy Res* 2003; 55: 21-7.
- Freedman B. Equipoise and the ethics of clinical research. *N Engl J Med* 1987; 317: 141-5.
- Fried C. *Medical Experimentation: Personal Integrity and Social Policy*. Amsterdam, The Netherlands: North Holland Press, 1974.
- Guertin DA, Stevens DM, et al. Ablation in mice of the mTORC components raptor, rictor, or mLST8 reveals that mTORC2 is required for signaling to Akt-FOXO and PKCalpha, but not S6K1. *Dev Cell* 2006; 11: 859-71.
- Hancock EC, Osborne JP, et al. Treatment of infantile spasms. *Cochrane Database Syst Rev* 2013; 6: CD001770.
- Johannessen CM, Reczek EE, et al. The NF1 tumor suppressor critically regulates TSC2 and mTOR. *Proc Natl Acad Sci USA* 2005; 102: 8573-8.
- Jozwiak S, Kotulska K, et al. Antiepileptic treatment before the onset of seizures reduces epilepsy severity and risk of mental retardation in infants with tuberous sclerosis complex. *Eur J Paediatr Neurol* 2011; 15: 424-31.
- Kivity S, Lerman P, et al. Long-term cognitive outcomes of a cohort of children with cryptogenic infantile spasms treated with high-dose adrenocorticotropic hormone. *Epilepsia* 2004; 45: 255-62.
- Lee JH, Huynh M, et al. De novo somatic mutations in components of the PI3K-AKT3-mTOR pathway cause hemimegalencephaly. *Nat Genet* 2012; 44: 941-5.
- Liu ZS, Wang QW, et al. Serum cytokine levels are altered in patients with West syndrome. *Brain Dev* 2001; 23: 548-51.
- Ljungberg MC, Bhattacharjee MB, et al. Activation of mammalian target of rapamycin in cytomegalic neurons of human cortical dysplasia. *Ann Neurol* 2006; 60: 420-9.
- Ljungberg MC, Sunnen CN, et al. Rapamycin suppresses seizures and neuronal hypertrophy in a mouse model of cortical dysplasia. *Dis Model Mech* 2009; 2: 389-98.

- Lux AL, Edwards SW, *et al*. The United Kingdom Infantile Spasms Study (UKISS) comparing hormone treatment with vigabatrin on developmental and epilepsy outcomes to age 14 months: a multicentre randomised trial. *Lancet Neurol* 2005; 4: 712-7.
- Lux AL, Osborne JP. A proposal for case definitions and outcome measures in studies of infantile spasms and West syndrome: consensus statement of the West Delphi group. *Epilepsia* 2004; 45: 1416-28.
- Murakami M, Ichisaka T, *et al*. mTOR is essential for growth and proliferation in early mouse embryos and embryonic stem cells. *Mol Cell Biol* 2004; 24: 6710-8.
- O'Callaghan FJ, Lux AL, *et al*. The effect of lead time to treatment and of age of onset on developmental outcome at 4 years in infantile spasms: evidence from the United Kingdom Infantile Spasms Study. *Epilepsia* 2011; 52: 1359-64.
- Osborne JP, Lux AL, *et al*. The underlying etiology of infantile spasms (West syndrome): information from the United Kingdom Infantile Spasms Study (UKISS) on contemporary causes and their classification. *Epilepsia* 2010; 51: 2168-74.
- Piantadosi S. The Study Cohort. *Clinical Trials: A Methodologic Perspective*. New York: Wiley, 1997, pp. 186-202.
- Raffo E, Coppola A, *et al*. A pulse rapamycin therapy for infantile spasms and associated cognitive decline. *Neurobiol Dis* 2011; 43: 322-9.
- Tee AR, Fingar DC, *et al*. Tuberous sclerosis complex-1 and -2 gene products function together to inhibit mammalian target of rapamycin (mTOR)-mediated downstream signaling. *Proc Natl Acad Sci USA* 2002; 99: 13571-6.
- Thomanetz V, Angliker N, *et al*. Ablation of the mTORC2 component rictor in brain or Purkinje cells affects size and neuron morphology. *J Cell Biol* 2013; 201: 293-308.
- Zeng LH, McDaniel S, *et al*. Regulation of cell death and epileptogenesis by the mammalian target of rapamycin (mTOR): a double-edged sword? *Cell Cycle* 2010; 9: 2281-5.

The role of ketogenic diet

Giangennaro Coppola

Child and Adolescent Neuropsychiatry,
Faculty of Medicine and Surgery, University of Salerno, Italy

---

Ketogenic diet is a high fat, adequate protein and low carbohydrate diet, which has proved effective for over a century in patients with refractory epilepsy (Wilder, 1921).

Even then, this author linked the benefits of the diet to the production of ketone bodies, similarly to what happens in prolonged fasting. Over the decades, the effectiveness of the diet has been confirmed in numerous case studies and one recent systematic review showed complete cessation of seizures in 16% of children, greater than 90% reduction in 32%, and more than 50% in 56% with the use of the ketogenic diet (Kossoff *et al.*, 2009).

The diet globally has shown effective in various types of seizures, perhaps with a certain prevalence in those of generalized type (Maydell *et al.*, 2001) and in subjects of younger age (Coppola *et al.*, 2001), although positive results are possible in adolescents and adults too (Mady *et al.*, 2003). Over the years, in order to make the diet more effective in the sense of ketogenic, it was supplemented with MCT oil (MCT diet by Huttenlocher, 1971), then modified with a reduction of the MCT oil from 60% to 30% to make it more palatable (modified MCT diet). More recently, other diets, with lower percentages of fat, have been developed such as the MAD and the LGIT, in order to make less severe and more acceptable this type of diet, especially by older children and young adults (see further details at page 8 of this chapter).

In recent years there is a tendency to introduce as early as possible the diet in combination with drug therapy, especially in younger children with epileptic encephalopathies of the first years of life.

The ketogenic diet is not only an alternative treatment for refractory epilepsies, but is indicated as primary option for metabolic disorders such as abnormal carbohydrate metabolic pathway.

KD is, conversely, contraindicated in other conditions and metabolic disorders (*Table I*).

Table I. Potential indications and contraindications for dietary therapy

Probable benefit (at least two publications)
Glucose transporter protein-1 (GLUT-1) deficiency
Pyruvate dehydrogenase deficiency (PDHD)
Myoclonic-astatic epilepsy (Doose syndrome)
Tuberous sclerosis complex
Rett syndrome
Severe myoclonic epilepsy of infancy (Dravet syndrome)
Infantile spasms
Selected mitochondrial disorders
Children receiving only formula (infants or enterally fed patients)
Suggestion of benefit (one case report or series)
Landau–Kleffner syndrome
Lafora body disease
Combined use with vagus nerve stimulation
Combined use with zonisamide
Children with recently worsened seizures in the past month
Contraindications (*relative)
Pyruvate carboxylase deficiency
Porphyria
Beta-oxidation defects
Primary carnitine deficiency
Inadequate ability to maintain nutrition or comply with the KD restrictions
Combined use with phenobarbital*
Children with a clear focal lesion potentially resectable*
Severe gastroesophageal reflux*

From Kossoff *et al.* (2013).

■ Ketogenic diet in epileptic encephalopathies

KD is mainly indicated for the treatment of epileptic encephalopathies, starting in the first years of life, for some of which it may represent a "first choice treatment". All these epileptic syndromes and conditions may be, of course, distinguished as more or less responsive to the dietary therapy. Among the first, there are the epileptic infantile spasms, the epilepsy with myoclonic-astatic seizures (Doose syndrome), the spasms and focal seizures due to tuberous sclerosis, Dravet syndrome, Lennox-Gastaut syndrome and some encephalopathies caused by mitochondrial disorder. Among the latter, Landau-Kleffner syndrome, migrating malignant partial seizures in infancy, and Ohtahara syndrome/EME must be included.

In the present paragraph the main data on the efficacy of the KD for the treatment of epileptic encephalopathies will be reported, by listing them according to age of onset.

As to *Ohtahara syndrome*, reports of single cases or patients have to be searched in larger series. Recently, Ishii *et al.* (2011) reported a male infant with OS who failed serial trials of high-dose pyridoxal phosphate, antiepileptic drugs, sodium valproate, phenobarbital, clonazepam, and clobazam in various doses and combinations, ACTH, TRH, and gamma globulin. Then, the KD diet was tried and found effective in controlling seizures. In other sporadic cases from large series (Coppola *et al.*, 2009), results have been poorly satisfying as to seizure outcome.

Recently, in two of 3 patients with *early myoclonic encephalopathy (EME)* secondary to non ketotic hyperglycinemia, a > 50% seizure reduction was reported wih KD therapy, while a third patient showed a mild improvement only. No significant adverse effects were seen (Cusmai *et al.*, 2012).

Epilepsy with malignant migrating focal seizures in infancy (MMPSI) has been poorly sensitive to KD adjunctive treatment in the few cases reported so far (Francois *et al.*, 2003; Marsh *et al.*, 2005; Okuda *et al.*, 2000; Lee *et al.*, 2012), although some cases more responsive to the diet have been described recently (Thammongkol *et al.*, 2012).

For *infantile spasms*, data in the literature are not only larger, but also more encouraging as regards the use of KD.

In a prospective single-center experience in 104 consecutive infants with infantile spasms treated with ketogenic diet, Hong *et al.* (2010) reported their experience with KD given between 1996 and 2009. Previous treatment for these patients included a mean of 3.6 anticonvulsants, 71% including corticosteroids or vigabatrin. At 6 months follow-up, 64% of children showed a more than 50% spasm decrease; such improvement increased by 77% after 1-2 years. Thirty-eight (37%) became spasm-free for at least a 6-month period within a median 2.4 months from starting the KD. Furthermore, 62% showed a psychomotor improvement, while 29% were able to reduce concurrent anticonvulsant drugs.

Overlapping data have been reported by Eun *et al.* (2006) in 43 children with intractable infantile spasms. More recently, Lee *et al.* (2013) reported that ketogenic diet overall increased by 10% the rate of spasm-free group within their series of 69 children with drug-resistant infantile spasms. Ketogenic may also be considered as first-choice treatment for new-onset infantile spasms. In a retrospective study comparing the results of all infants on the KD *versus* high-dose ACTH for new-onset IS, Kossoff *et al.* (2008) reported as spasm-free within 1 month about 62% (8/13) of infants treated with the KD compared to 90% (18/20) treated initially with ACTH.

When effective, median time to spasm freedom was similar between ACTH and the KD (4.0 *versus* 6.5 days). Those treated with ACTH were more likely to have a normal EEG at 1 month (53% *versus* 9%); however, KD led to EEG normalization within 2-5 months in all 8 who became spasm-free in the KD-treated group.

Such a delay in EEG normalization with not well defined persisting EEG abnormalities may arise some concerns and criticisms on the opportunity of KD as first-line treatment especially in idiopathic form of infantile spasms in subjects with normal psychomotor development before spasm-onset.

The modified Atkins diet, which is a simpler and easier-to-administer version of the ketogenic diet, has also been reported to be effective in children with infantile spasms refractory to hormonal therapy and/or vigabatrin. The EEG showed resolution of hypsarhythmia at 3 months and the diet was well tolerated in these young children.

There is equally encouraging data regarding the use of KD in *Dravet syndrome*. Fejerman et al. (2005) first reported a significant response (50-100% control of seizures) in 9 of 17 patients with DS after a 2-years follow-up; in 2 patients only a decline in efficacy of the diet was described over time and in 4 a persisting seizure improvement even after KD was discontinued. Caraballo et al. (2005) offered the ketogenic diet to 20 out of 52 patients meeting the criteria for DS. KD was given in conjunction with 1-3 AEDs. Thirteen (65%) of the 20 patients remained on the diet 1 year after initiation. A > 75% seizure reduction was reported in 10 (77%) children with 2 (15%) becoming seizure-free. Currently, Caraballo and collegues offer the KD after failing 3 adequate AEDs including stiripentol, in children with DS (Caraballo, 2011).

In another multicentric study, Kang et al. (2005) found similar results in 14 patients with DS. More recently, Nabbout et al. (2011) reported a ≥ 75% decrease in seizure frequency in 10 patients out of 15 who had failed trial of multiple anticonvulsant drugs including stiripentol. Nonetheless, efficacy tended to decrease over time and 5 patients only remained on KD for over 12 months. KD was also found to be beneficial on behaviour disturbances including hyperactivity, inattention, impulsiveness, and aggression. Laux et al. (2013) confirmed KD to be effective in about 65% of their 20 patients, thus providing further evidence on the use of ketogenic diet in this syndrome.

Another condition for which KD has shown particular efficacy as reported in several series of patients is *epilepsy with myoclonic atonic seizures (Doose syndrome)*. Oguni et al. (2002) reported KD as the most effective in stopping seizures followed by ACTH and ethosuccimide, in a large series of 218 patients with this syndrome. In their cohort, 26 patients were treated with KD and 15/26 (58%)achieved excellent outcome, while 9 (35%) had a 50% seizure reduction. According to this data, Caraballo and Fejerman (2006) reported after a 18-month follow-up a ≥ 50% seizure reduction in 6 out of 11 patients, aged 4 to 9 years (mean age 5 years) of whom 2 became seizure-free. Overlapping results were obtained by Kilaru and Berqvist (2007) in 5 out of 10 patients who were seizure-free on KD, but only 3 had follow-up longer than 6 months. In the remaining 5 children, 3 had no change in seizure frequency, 1 developed pancreatitis leading to discontinuation of the diet and 1 had a significant reduction in seizures.

Interestingly, Mullen et al. (2011) showed that 5% of children with EMAS have glucose transporter-1 deficiency with mutations in *SLC2A1*. The presence of *GLUT1* deficiency suggests that KD should be considered early in the treatment with potential beneficial effects on seizure control and neurodevelopmental outcome.

All the studies assessing the effectiveness of the KD in MAE confirm that this is probably one of the most sensitive syndromes to KD treatment; that is why it should be considered as early as possible, also allowing for reduction and tapering of antiepileptic medication.

As to *Lennox-Gastaut syndrome*, the first reports on potential improvement in some patients were by Freeman and Vining (1999) followed by Wheless et al. (2001) and Moreno Villares et al. (2001). Recently, Lemmon et al. (2012) performed a retrospective review of 71 children with LGS fed with KD at the Johns Hopkins Institute from 1994 to 2010. The median age at initiation of diet was 3 years 6 months (range 18 m–18 y).

Sixty-five children (92%) had daily seizures, including atonic, tonic, atypical absence, and myoclonic seizures. The median number of anticonvulsants tried before ketogenic diet initiation was 6 (range 1–13). Twenty-five children (35%) had a lesional etiology for their LGS, including both focal structural abnormalities and generalized brain malformations. Using an intent-to-treat analysis, after 6 months, 36 (51%) achieved more than 50% seizure reduction, 16 (23%) experienced more than 90% seizure reduction, and 1 (1%) achieved seizure freedom. Thirty-two children (45%) were able to reduce concurrent anticonvulsant use while being treated with the ketogenic diet. Results were similar after 12 months. Age, sex, side effects, valproate use, and history of infantile spasms were not predictive of more than 90% seizure reduction. In the literature, 88 of 189 (47%) children with LGS treated with KD, as reported in eighteen studies in the last 20 years, had more than 50% seizure reduction after 3 to 36 months of ketogenic diet treatment. Lemmon et al. (2012) underpin that there was no significant difference in the rate of more than 50% seizure reduction between their data and those shown in the literature (51% *vs* 47%, p = 0.32). In contrast, their patients experienced a lower rate of seizure freedom (1% *vs* 16%, p < 0.001). The ketogenic diet seems thereby a good option in these patients.

Ketogenic diet may be successful in the management of refractory seizures due to *tuberous sclerosis*. In one of the first works 12 patients with TSC were studied, aged between 8 months and 18 years (Kossoff et al., 2005). In 9/12 (75%) children there was a history of infantile spasms but they all had daily focal seizures at the time of diet initiation. The majority (8/12, or 67%) had been treated with vigabatrin prior to the start of the diet and spasms had resolved in 3. At 6 months on the diet, 11/12 (92%) had a > 50% reduction in seizure frequency and 8/12 (67%) had a > 90% response. Five children achieved seizure-freedom for 5 months. The children remained on the diet for a mean period of 2 years (2 months-5 years). Eight of 12 (67%) were able to reduce their AEDs while on the diet.

Similar results were reported in 3 boys with refractory focal discognitive seizures by Coppola et al. (2006). The patients had previously tried 5-7 AEDs. The first patient after 14 months on the KD was completely seizure-free. The second patient remained seizure-free on the KD for 31 months without adverse side effects and all AEDs were weaned. The third patient after being on the diet for 15 months had > 50% decrease in seizures, with seizures becoming briefer and less intense. That child underwent surgical removal of left frontal lobe tubers. All patients were more alert on the KD.

Interestingly, Martinez et al. (2007) reported seizure recurrence in 3 children with TSC soon after discontinuing ketogenic diet and thereby suggest to go on with the diet even after 2 years of seizure- freedom. As our personal experience suggests, children with TSC and refractory focal seizures can be safely shifted from KD to an alternative diet as LGIT. In conclusion, the KD should be considered as a therapeutic option for children with TSC and intractable epilepsy.

Ketogenic diet was then tried in several other epileptic conditions and epileptic encephalopathies starting in the first years of life such as Landau-Kleffner syndrome and CSWSS, Angelman syndrome (Stein et al., 2010), epilepsia partialis continua associated with Alpers encephalopathy (Joshi et al., 2009), multifocal epileptic encephalopathy with spasms and tonic seizures (Coppola et al., 2006), and refractory status epilepticus (Nabbout et al., 2010; Sorte et al., 2013; Strzelczyk et al., 2013).

A few patients with Landau-Kleffner and CSWSS have been treated with KD. In 1999 Berqvist et al. reported on 3 patients with LKS refractory to traditional treatments who were successfully treated with the KD; all 3 patients had lasting improvement of their language, behaviour and seizures for 26, 24 and 12 months, respectively. More recently, Nikanorova et al. (2009) assessed the clinical and EEG efficacy after 24 months on the KD in 5 children aged between 8 and 13 years with refractory CSWSS.

Only 1 case responded with complete CSWSS disappearance, while in another one the effect was partial and intermittent. In 3 patients no response had been observed. Furthermore, the ketogenic diet did not appear to influence the neuropsychological outcome.

Metabolic disorders with epilepsy and ketogenic diet

GLUT1 deficiency syndrome is another condition responsible of refractory infantile seizures, developmental delay, acquired microcephaly, hypotonia, spasticity, and a complex movement disorder consisting of ataxia and dystonia. Over the years, beyond this "classical phenotype" subdivided into early-onset and late-onset subtypes, other phenotypes including mental retardation and movement disorder without epilepsy or adult cases with minimal symptoms have been described.

Recognizing glucose transporter-1 deficiency syndrome as early as possible is important, because prompt initiation of KD in childhood is crucial for an effective etiological therapy (De Giorgis and Veggiotti, 2013). Milder phenotypes of GLUT1 deficiency have been described in children with early-onset absence epilepsy and/or movement disorders and mild learning difficulties (Anand et al., 2011). Recently, a modified Atkins diet has been successfully tried in some patients (Ito et al., 2008; Haberlandt et al., 2013).

Mechanism of action

There are more than 100 years that the mechanisms of action of the KD remain unclear. Over time, several hypotheses have arisen with varying degrees of success, such as changes in brain pH, changes in electrolyte and water balance, direct inhibitory actions of fatty acids (iePUFAs), neurotransmitters alterations, changes in energy metabolism.

The role of ketone bodies, whose production level in the blood has been linked to the effectiveness and fine-tuning of KD, remains somewhat controversial both clinically and experimentally.

The effectiveness of alternative diets such as MAD and LGIT which result in a low or no production of serum ketone bodies may be further confounding. Conflicting data also emerge for the role of blood glucose level while on KD. The experimental data in animals and *in vitro* argue for an inhibitory role on seizure activity and/or neuronal excitability played by calorie restriction, increase in CSF levels of amino acids and neurotransmitters (GABA-A and glutamate), activation of potassium ATP channels, adenosine, inhibition of glycolysis, a direct effect on excitability by PUFAs and ketone bodies (especially acetoacetate). Currently, much interest is focused on glucose metabolic pathways relevant to KD mechanisms.

Several compounds that act along this pathway have shown ability to inhibit seizure activity such as 2DG, FDP and anaplerotic compounds such as thriheptanoin which can "refill" the seizure induced deficiency of tricarboxilic acid cycle (TRA) intermediates.

Results from studies on KD, 2DG, FDP and anaplerosis suggest that a modification of glycolsis may represent a novel mechanism and strategy of seizure treatment. So far, it seems clear that these metabolic substrates are players on a more complex arena (Rho and Strafstrom, 2012).

Other alternative diets

Although the KD is the most well-established dietary therapy for epilepsy, it is too restrictive and associated with a number of adverse side effects. For such reason, alternative more liberal diets with a lower percentage of fats such as the Medium Chain Trygliceri-des-Ketonic Diet (MCT-KD), the modified Atkins diet (MAD) and the low-glycemic index diet (LGIT) have been developed (*Tables II and III*).

Table II. Comparison of MAD and LGIT

MAD Low carbohydrate – adequate (high) protein – high fat diet	LGIT Low carbohydrate – adequate protein – high fat diet
Carbohydrate restriction 10 (–15–20) g/d All carbohydrates allowed Ratio fat: protein and carbohydrate count, otherwise, free but high fat encouraged Moderate to high ketosis Stable BS (how compared with KD?)	Carbohydrate restriction 40–60 g/d Only low-glycaemic carbohydrates (GI < 50) Ratio fat: protein and carbohydrates: ≤ 1:1 Dietician guidance with calorie, protein (20-30%) and fat goal (60%) Low ketosis Stable blood sugar (compared with KD?)

g: gram; KD: classical ketogenic diet; LGIT: low glycaemic index diet; MAD: modified Atkins diet.
(From Miranda et al., 2012.)

As to MCT KD, it was the first alternative diet to be used since the 1970s (Huttenlocher et al., 1970), designed to allow for more carbohydrates and protein by utilizing more of the extremely ketogenic oil containing medium chain tryglicerides (60% of the diet).

Because of its poor palatability and frequent gastrointestinal side effects, it was successively modified by Schwartz et al. (1989) and MCT fat was then reduced to 30% and LCT fat provided further 30% of energy.

Recently, Neal et al. (2008) suggested a flexible scale of MCT fat between 30% and 60%, according to the needs of patient, tolerance and ketosis. The remaining calories are provided by protein (10%) and carbohydrate (15-19%).

The modified Atkins diet (MAD) was first introduced by Kossoff et al. (2003) by deriving it from the Atkins diet, largely known in the US for the management of obesity. Unlike the Atkins diet, the modified Atkins encourages a higher fat intake and lower carbohydrate content (10 g per day for children, 20 g per day for adults, indefinitely). The true goal of MAD is not weight loss, but a beneficial effect on epileptic seizures. Protein is then allowed freely and fat is encouraged. Although the carbohydrate is long-term restricted, this represents a more liberal regimen than the classical KD.

MAD is also started as an outpatient without a fast, but does not restrict calories, fluid, or protein. The MAD ratio of fat/protein and carbohydrates is estimated on average to be 1:1, while KD ratio in the classical KD is 3-4:1. Ketosis is induced by MAD regimen but is generally lower than KD.

Table III. Comparison of the 5 diets: normal, LGIT, MAD, MCT and KD

	Normal	LGIT	MAD	MCT	KD
Fat	30% (-35%)	60%	60-70%	MCT: 30-60% LCT: 11-45%	90%
Protein	20% (10-15%)	20-30%	20-30%	10%	6-8%
Carbohydrates	50%	10%	6%	15-19%	2.4%
Ratio	0.2-0.3:1	1:1	1:1	NA	3-4:1

KD: ketogenic diet; LGIT: low glycemic index treatment; MAD: modified Atkins diet; MCT: medium chain tryglicerides. (From Miranda et al., 2012.)

The low glycemic index diet (LGIT) was first published by Thiele and Pfeiffer (2005) in order to create a more liberal diet, alternative to KD. It is inspired by diets used for the management of obesity and diabetes such as the South Beach and Zona diets, which prefer carbohydrates having a low glycemic index. The glycemic index (GI) is a measure of how much a particular food will elevate the blood glucose compared to an equivalent amount of glucose (Jenkins et al., 1981). The use of low GI carbohydrates (e.g., whole gree, berries, green vegetables) produces a smaller increase in post-prandial blood glucose and a much more stable glucose levels throughout the day.

With respect to KD, the LGIT allows 40 g/day of GI < 50 carbohydrates, total calories are roughly limited by carbohydrate limitation, a rough meal portion control. In addition, ketone bodies are not elevated in LGIT, blood glucose is still in normal range, although relative lower and there is no significant acidosis. So it is substantially unknown how this diet works.

■ Are alternative diets as effective as classical ketogenic diet?

In this regard we must consider the following questions: 1) are the different types of diets comparable for efficacy? 2) Shifting from a diet to another is equally safe and effective? 3) Which type of diet should we start with?

For the first question, there are currently no RCT studies comparing the efficacy of KD with that of MAD or LGIT. Recently, 2 small studies compared KD and MAD in uncontrolled fashion (Porta et al., 2009; Miranda et al., 2011). The first one showed that there was a significant difference in efficacy (> 50% seizure reduction) at 3 months (p = 0.03); however, the difference was no longer significant at 6 months (7/17, 41% versus 2/10, 20%, p = 0.24). In the second trial, Miranda et al. (2011) reported > 50% seizure improvement at 6 month in 60% of their patients compared with 39% on MAD (p = 0.06). However, this difference tended to lower once the younger patients in the KD group were excluded from comparison, so KD and MAD groups were age-comparable.

As to shifting from a diet to another, several studies and clinical evidence suggest that KD can be successfully transitioned to the MAD (Kossoff et al., 2003), or the LGIT (Pfeiffer and Thiele, 2005) without loss of seizure control.

In general, after a first phase of 1-3 months of "stricter" dietary treatment, KD ratio can be reduced with a KD or a MAD, and this is compatible with maintaining efficacy (Seo et al., 2007; Miranda et al., 2012). Conversely, the transition from MAD to KD may improve seizure control in some children (Kossoff *et al.*, 2010). This may be true, for example during some epileptic syndromes particularly sensitive to KD, such as myoclonic-astatic epilepsy (MAE).

Which diet to choose first?

Although the effectiveness of alternative diets as MAD is close to that of classical KD, evidence seems to suggest that an initial (1-3 months) diet with higher intakes of fat and lower carbohydrate is linked to better outcomes (Kossoff *et al.*, 2007).

It is also true that, in the case of inefficacy of an alternative diet, the chances of getting a result shifting to a classical KD are very low (Kossoff *et al.*, 2010).

This figure, however, leaves us with a question, *i.e.* whether it is true that starting with a stricter diet (*i.e.* with the classical KD) may produce better results compared to its secondary shift from a more liberal diet.

In addition, the choice of a diet should be done on an individual basis, bearing in mind the child's age, the type and severity of epileptic syndrome, the family compliance, the need to obtain immediate clinical results according to the patient's context.

A protocol of choice based on criteria as those suggested by Thiele *et al.* (2005) and Miranda *et al.* (2012) is shown schematically in *Figure 1*.

Figure 1 shows the following indications: 1) all children below 2 years should be initiated on the KD, as well as all children with an enteral feeding tube; 2) children with myoclonic astatic epilepsy (MAE) should be offered first the ketogenic diet (Kossoff *et al.*, 2010); 3) GLUT-1 patients should be initiated on the KD, unless older children with poor individual and/or family compliance; 4) children between 2 and 6 years of age should first be given more liberalized diet, unless particular conditions including epilepsy type and severity. It is good to bear in mind the potential benefit of a "strict" start with high fat and lower carbohydrate daily amount in the first 1-3 months (*i.e.* 10 g/day in the MAD); 5) older children, teenagers and adults should primarily be treated with MAD or LGIT. Switching from KD to MAD or LGIT is possible without loosing efficacy.

Adverse side effects

Currently, the elimination of the initial prolonged fasting and a more gradual introduction of the diet in clinical practice, resulted in a much lower incidence of early side effects such as dehydration, and gastrointestinal disturbances such as obstinate constipation, hypoglycemia, abnormal serum electrolytes and metabolic acidosis. Also, some of the most frequent adverse effects, such as hypercholesterolemia, mineral deficits, acidosis, constipation, and weight loss are treatable or, better, preventable. This fact has been made possible through a more extensive use of initial alternative diets, the early supplementation of calcium, carnitine, selenium, zinc, vitamin D and oral polycitra. As to the effects in the longer term, the possible shift from a KD after years towards MAD or LGIT could minimize the risk of kidney stones, bone fractures and decreased linear growth, although definite data are still lacking in this regard.

Recent data from Patel *et al.* (2010) have also determined that in children who were on KD years before (but have discontinued it) there are no obvious long-term effect on growth, cholesterol or cardiac health. More recently, Coppola *et al.* (2014) reported that

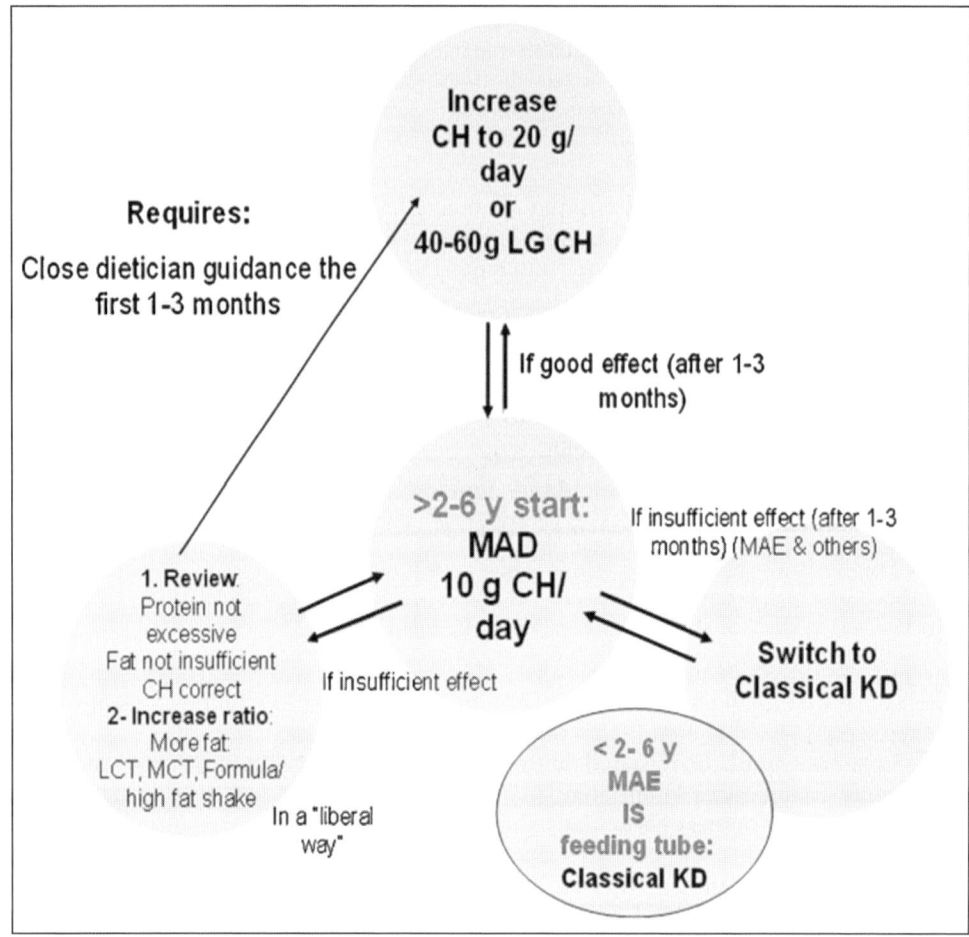

Figure 1. Proposed diagram of a future algorithm about how using the ketogenic diets. (From Miranda et al., 2012, modified.)

subjects treated with ketogenic diet had higher arterial stiffness parameters, including AIx and β-index and higher serum levels of cholesterol or triglycerides compared to those who had never been on the diet (control group) ($p < 0.001$). The authors state arterial stiffness to be increased in children and young adults treated with the ketogenic diet, before the increase of the intima media thickness. This supports that arterial stiffness is an early marker of vascular damage.

■ Are there factors predicting a favourable response to ketogenic diet therapies?

One thing several studies seem to agree upon is that about 40% of patients treated with the KD will show a ≥ 50% seizure reduction after 3-month follow-up and that a "probable benefit" will be more likely reported by patients with early-onset epileptic syndromes as Dravet syndrome, epilepsy with myoclonic-astatic seizures, infantile spasms, and refractory seizures in tuberous sclerosis.

Predicting factors of a favourable response to KD treatment might undoubtedly help decreasing the number of patients uselessly fed with the diet and giving priority to those most likely to respond. This might allow a better understanding of the mechanisms behind dietary treatments, and so optimise clinical application of KD, *e.g.* decreasing the daily dietician load.

Recently, Schoeler *et al.* (2013) carried out a literature review to identify factors that may influence response to KD. Twenty-one factors were identified. They were divided in 5 groups (A to E) depending on the consistency of evidence across studies. In group A, defined as "strong evidence for an effect on response to KD", no factors were identified as having a good or bad effect on response to KD. Group B, defined as "mixed findings", included other biochemical markers, seizure type and epilepsy cause and syndrome. Evidence regarding these factors is almost equally divided in literature, so it is difficult to draw conclusions.

In group C (weak evidence), although findings are conflicting, evidence is strongest for factors such as age at diet initiation (a better response to KD in children younger than 6-8 years), diet type (KD is better than MAD in some series, while in others efficacy of KD, MAD and MCT KD is quite similar), EEG (worse outcome associated with temporal discharges, secondary bilateral synchrony, hypsarrhythmia and multifocal spikes), and ketosis (higher the ketosis, better the clinical response to KD). No correlations at all were found for other factors including age at seizure onset, number of previous antiepileptic drugs, body mass index, diet ratio and seizure frequency.

In group D (strong evidence for no effect on response to KD), were included gender and developmental delay/cognitive impairment. In group E (limited data), conflicting or limited data are relative to the role of blood glucose levels, genetics and structural brain abnormalities at MRI. In conclusion, no strong evidence for any specific factors that affect response has been found so far.

■ Perspectives and concluding remarks

According to what is stated in this chapter, the most significant change over the past ten years is the expansion of diets offered, alternative to KD, more liberal and better accepted by patients, especially older children, teenagers and adults.

Another fact is the almost overlapping effectiveness of diets such as the more palatable MAD compared to KD. Today, the clinician has the opportunity to shift from one diet to another, and the choice of the diet should be always based on an individual basis with its variables.

Several questions still remain open about those that are the main diets, namely KD, MAD and LGIT.

First, there are no RCTs comparing the effectiveness of KD with the other diets. Still, is there an ideal age when to shift from KD to the other diets? On the opposite, does shifting from MAD or LGIT towards the KD hinder the effectiveness of the latter? What are the long-term side effects of MAD and LGIT, whereas even for the KD exhaustive data are still lacking in this regard?

Only further clinical trials, accurate in method and selection of cases, will improve the decision making of the clinician, perhaps contributing to the understanding of the basic mechanisms of dietary treatment of epilepsy.

References

- Anand G, Padeniya A, Hanrahan D, et al. Milder phenotypes of glucose transporter type 1 deficiency syndrome. *Dev Med Child Neurol* 2011; 53: 664-8.
- Bergqvist AG, Chee CM, Lutchka LM, Brooks-Kayal AR. Treatment of acquired epileptic aphasia with the ketogenic diet. *J Child Neurol* 1999; 14: 696-701.
- Caraballo RH, Cersosimo RO, Sakr D, Cresta A, Escobal N, Fejerman N. Ketogenic diet in patients with Dravet syndrome. *Epilepsia* 2005; 46: 1539-44.
- Caraballo RH, Cersósimo RO, Sakr D, Cresta A, Escobal N, Fejerman N. Ketogenic diet in patients with myoclonic-astatic epilepsy. *Epileptic Disord* 2006; 8: 151-5.
- Caraballo RH. Nonpharmacologic treatments of Dravet Syndrome: Focus on the ketogenic diet. *Epilepsia* 2011; 52 (suppl 2): 79-82.
- Coppola G, Klepper J, Ammendola E, et al. The effects of the ketogenic diet in refractory partial seizures with reference to tuberous sclerosis. *Eur J Paediatr Neurol* 2006; 10: 148-51.
- Coppola G, Verrotti A, Ammendola E, et al. Ketogenic diet for the treatment of catastrophic epileptic encephalopathies in childhood. *Eur J Paediatr Neurol* 2009; 14: 229-34.
- Coppola G, Natale F, Torino A, et al. The impact of the ketogenic diet on arterial morphology and endothelial function in children and young adults with epilepsy: a case-control study. *Seizure* 2014; 23: 260-5.
- Cusmai R, Martinelli D, Moavero R, et al. Ketogenic diet in early myoclonic encephalopathy due to non ketotic hyperglycinemia. *Eur J Paediatr Neurol* 2012; 16: 509-13.
- De Giorgis V, Veggiotti P. GLUT1 deficiency syndrome 2013: Current state of the art. *Seizure* 2013; 22: 803-11.
- Eun SH, Kang HC, Kim DW, Kim HD. Ketogenic diet for treatment of infantile spasms. *Brain Dev* 2006; 28: 566-71.
- Fejerman N, Caraballo R, Cersosimo R. Ketogenic diet in patients with Dravet syndrome and myoclonic epilepsies in infancy and early childhood. *Adv Neurol* 2005; 95: 299-305.
- François LL, Manel V, Rousselle C, David M. Ketogenic regime as anti-epileptic treatment: its use in 29 epileptic children. *Arch Pediatr* 2003; 10: 300-6.
- Freeman JM, Vining EP. Seizures decrease rapidly after fasting: preliminary studies of the ketogenic diet. *Arch Pediatr Adolesc Med* 1999; 153: 946-9.
- Haberlandt E, Karall D, Jud V, et al. Glucose transporter type 1 deficiency syndrome effectively treated with modified Atkins diet. *Neuropediatrics* 2014; 45: 117-9.
- Hong AM, Turner Z, Hamdy RF, Kossoff EH. Infantile spasms treated with the ketogenic diet: prospective single-center experience in 104 consecutive infants. *Epilepsia* 2010; 51: 1403-7.
- Huttenlocher PR, Wilbourn AJ, Signore JM. Medium-chain triglycerides as a therapy for intractable childhood epilepsy. *Neurology* 1971; 21: 1097-103.
- Ishii M, Shimono M, Senju A, Kusuhara K, Shiota N. The ketogenic diet as an effective treatment for Ohtahara syndrome. *No To Hattatsu* 2011; 43: 47-50.
- Ito S, Oguni H, Ito Y, Ishigaki K, Ohinata J, Osawa M. Modified Atkins diet therapy for a case with glucose transporter type 1 deficiency syndrome. *Brain Dev* 2008; 30: 226-8.
- Jenkins DJ, Wolever TM, Taylor RH, et al. Glycemic index of foods: a physiological basis for carbohydrate exchange. *Am J Clin Nutr* 1981; 34: 362-6.
- Joshi CN, Greenberg CR, Mhanni AA, Salman MS. Ketogenic diet in Alpers-Huttenlocher syndrome. *Pediatr Neurol* 2009; 40: 314-6.
- Kang HC, Kim YJ, Kim DW, Kim HD. Efficacy and safety of the ketogenic diet for intractable childhood epilepsy: Korean multicentric experience. *Epilepsia* 2005; 46: 272-9.

- Kilaru S, Bergqvist AGC. Current treatment of myoclonic astatic epilepsy: clinical experience at the Children's hospital of Philadelphia. *Epilepsia*. 2007; 48: 1703-7.
- Klepper J, Leiendecker B. Glut1 deficiency syndrome and novel ketogenic diets. *J Child Neurol* 2013; 28: 1045-8.
- Kossoff EH, Thiele EA, Pfeifer HH, McGrogan JR, Freeman JM. Tuberous sclerosis complex and the ketogenic diet. *Epilepsia* 2005; 46: 1684-6.
- Kossoff EH, McGrogan JR, Bluml RM, Pillas DJ, Rubenstein JE, Vining EP. A modified Atkins diet is effective for the treatment of intractable pediatric epilepsy. *Epilepsia* 2006; 47: 421-4.
- Kossoff EH, Turner Z, Bluml RM, Pyzik PL, Vining EP. A randomized, crossover comparison of daily carbohydrate limits using the modified Atkins diet. *Epilepsy Behav* 2007; 10: 432-6.
- Kossoff EH, Hedderick EF, Turner Z, Freeman JM. A case-control evaluation of the ketogenic diet *versus* ACTH for new-onset infantile spasms. *Epilepsia* 2008; 49: 1504-9.
- Kossoff EH, Zupec-Kania BA, Amark PE, *et al*. Optimal clinical management of children receiving the ketogenic diet: recommendations of the International Ketogenic Diet Study Group. *Epilepsia* 2009; 50: 304-17.
- Kossoff EH, Bosarge JL, Miranda MJ, Wiemer-Kruel A, Kang HC, Kim HD. Will seizure control improve by switching from the modified Atkins diet to the traditional ketogenic diet? *Epilepsia* 2010; 51: 2496-9.
- Kossoff EH, Wang HS. Dietary Therapies for Epilepsy. *Biomed J* 2013; 36: 2-8.
- Laux L, Blackford R. The Ketogenic Diet in Dravet Syndrome. *J Child Neurol* 2013; 28: 1041-4.
- Lee EH, Yum MS, Jeong MH, Lee KY, Ko TS. A case of malignant migrating partial seizures in infancy as a continuum of infantile epileptic encephalopathy. *Brain Dev* 2012; 34: 768-72.
- Lee J, Lee JH, Yu HJ, *et al*. Prognostic factors of infantile spasms: role of treatment options including a ketogenic diet. *Brain Dev* 2013; 35: 821-6.
- Lemmon ME, Terao NN, Ng Y, Reisig W, Rubenstein JE, Kossoff EH. Efficacy of the ketogenic diet in Lennox-Gastaut syndrome: a retrospective review of one institution's experience and summary of the literature. *Dev Med Child Neurol* 2012; 54: 464-8.
- Mady MA, Kossoff EH, McGregor AL, Wheless JW, Pyzik PL, Freeman JM. The ketogenic diet: adolescents can do it too. *Epilepsia* 2003; 44(6): 847-51.
- Marsh EB, Freeman JM, Kossoff EH, *et al*. The outcome of children with intractable seizures: a 3- to 6-year follow-up of 67 children who remained on the ketogenic diet less than one year. *Epilepsia* 2006; 47: 425-30.
- Martinez CC, Pyzik PL, Kossoff EH. Discontinuing the ketogenic diet in seizure-free children: recurrence and risk factors. *Epilepsia* 2007; 48: 187-90.
- Miranda MJ, Mortensen M, Povlsen JH, Nielsen H, Beniczky S. Danish study of a modified Atkins diet for medically intractable epilepsy in children: can we achieve the same results as with the classical ketogenic diet? *Seizure* 2011; 20: 151-5.
- Miranda MJ, Turner Z, Magrath G. Alternative diets to the classical ketogenic diet–can we be more liberal? *Epilepsy Res* 2012; 100: 278-85.
- Moreno Villares JM, Oliveros-Leal L, Simón-Heras R, Mateos-Beato F. The return to the ketogenic diet. What role does it play in the treatment of refractory seizures of infancy? *Rev Neurol* 2001; 32: 1115-9.
- Mullen SA, Marini C, Suls A, *et al*. Glucose transporter 1 deficiency as a treatable cause of myoclonic astatic epilepsy. *Arch Neurol* 2011; 68: 1152-5.
- Nabbout R, Mazzuca M, Hubert P, *et al*. Efficacy of ketogenic diet in severe refractory status epilepticus initiating fever induced refractory epileptic encephalopathy in school age children (FIRES). *Epilepsia* 2010; 51: 2033-7.
- Nabbout R, Copioli C, Chipaux M, *et al*. Ketogenic diet also benefits Dravet syndrome patients receiving stiripentol: a prospective pilot study. *Epilepsia* 2011; 52: e54-7.

- Neal EG, Chaffe H, Schwartz RH, et al. The ketogenic diet for the treatment of childhood epilepsy: a randomised controlled trial. *Lancet Neurol* 2008; 7: 500-6.
- Nikanorova M, Miranda MJ, Atkins M, Sahlholdt L. Ketogenic diet in the treatment of refractory continuous spikes and waves during slow sleep. *Epilepsia* 2009; 50: 1127-31.
- Oguni H, Tanaka T, Hayashi K, et al. Treatment and long-term prognosis of myoclonic-astatic epilepsy of early childhood. *Neuropediatrics* 2002; 33: 122-32.
- Okuda K, Yasuhara A, Kamei A, Araki A, Kitamura N, Kobayashi Y. Successful control with bromide of two patients with malignant migrating partial seizures in infancy. *Brain Dev* 2000; 22: 56-9.
- Patel A, Pyzik PL, Turner Z, Rubenstein JE, Kossoff EH. Long-term outcomes of children treated with the ketogenic diet in the past. *Epilepsia* 2010; 51: 1277-82.
- Pfeifer HH, Thiele EA. Low-glycemic-index treatment: a liberalized ketogenic diet for treatment of intractable epilepsy. *Neurology* 2005; 65: 1810-2.
- Porta N, Vallée L, Boutry E, Auvin S. The ketogenic diet and its variants: state of the art. *Rev Neurol* 2009; 165: 430-9.
- Schwartz RH, Eaton J, Bower BD, Aynsley-Green A. Ketogenic diets in the treatment of epilepsy: short-term clinical effects. *Dev Med Child Neurol* 1989; 31: 145-51.
- Schoeler NE, Cross JH, Sander JW, Sisodiya SM. Can we predict a favourable response to Ketogenic Diet Therapies for drug-resistant epilepsy? *Epilepsy Res* 2013; 106: 1-16.
- Seo JH, Lee YM, Lee JS, Kang HC, Kim HD. Efficacy and tolerability of the ketogenic diet according to lipid:nonlipid ratios–comparison of 3:1 with 4:1 diet. *Epilepsia* 2007; 48: 801-5.
- Stein D, Chetty M, Rho JM. A "happy" toddler presenting with sudden, life-threatening seizures. *Semin Pediatr Neurol* 2010; 17: 35-8.
- Strzelczyk A, Reif PS, Bauer S, et al. Intravenous initiation and maintenance of ketogenic diet: proof of concept in super-refractory status epilepticus. *Seizure* 2013; 22: 581-3.
- Thammongkol S, Vears DF, Bicknell-Royle J, et al. Efficacy of the ketogenic diet: which epilepsies respond? *Epilepsia*. 2012; 53: e55–e59.
- Thiele EA. Assessing the efficacy of antiepileptic treatments: the ketogenic diet. *Epilepsia* 2003; 44 (suppl 7): 26-9.
- Wheless JW, Baumgartner J, Ghanbari C. Vagus nerve stimulation and the ketogenic diet. *Neurol Clin* 2001; 19: 371-407.
- Wilder RM. The effects of ketonemia on the course of epilepsy. *Mayo Clin Proc* 1921; 2: 307-8.

Optimizing treatment for neonatal and infantile seizures
Do guidelines have a role in management?

Jo M. Wilmshurst[1], J. Helen Cross[2]

[1] Department of Paediatric Neurology, Red Cross War Memorial Children's Hospital, School of Child and Adolescent Health, University of Cape Town, South Africa
[2] Neurosciences Unit, UCL Institute of Child Health, London, United Kingdom

---

Many changes occur in the developing brain, inferring a susceptibility to external influences as well as a greater degree of plasticity than at any other time in life. However, despite considerable advances in diagnostic evaluation, great uncertainty remains with regard to optimized treatment regimes. With advances in genetics, in some children we are able to consider targeted treatments, but in the majority existing antiepileptic drugs remain our only option. Guidelines are potentially very powerful tools used to enable informed decisions and to improve patient outcomes. They are used to lobby local government for better facilities and capacity to deliver health care. As a result the content and logistics of such guidelines bear great responsibility to be useful, accurate and viable across all sectors and regions of health care.

Schemes are in place to ensure that guidelines are evidence based with presented data graded using numerous different systems from the GRADE, to the American Academy of Neurology (Atkins *et al.*, 2004a; Edlund *et al.*, 2004). However, the major lack of class 1 studies in the infantile and neonatal age ranges means that either no recommendation can be made or working groups must accept and revert to the less accepted method of consensus based on "expert-opinion". There is no point in developing guidelines if there are either not read, cannot be implemented or are not relevant to a region. Despite being of high quality the National Institute for Clinical Excellence (NICE) guidelines for epilepsy have received significant scrutiny and as a result adaptions to the roll-out of this tool have been reviewed (Dunkley and Cross, 2006).

The preceding chapters have provided the state of the art screens and interventions, the most current and future concepts, and understandings in the fields of neonatal and infantile seizures. Much of this data is research based, experimental or hypothetical and has some way to go before becoming part of current recommended standard practice. The lack of large randomized controlled studies in these areas generally means that such data will not be included in a standard practicing guideline at this time.

■ Optimal treatment for neonatal seizures

Neonatal seizures continue to provide the greatest challenge to management in day to day practice (also refer to chapters by Hellström-Westas (page 39); Ikonomidou (page 71); Boylan and Low (page 81); Campistol and Plecko (page 105) of the present volume). Most are acute symptomatic in their aetiology, and consequently although acute treatment is required, it is not likely to be continued in the majority beyond the neonatal period. Hypothermia has not only proven neuroprotective, but also has reduced the seizure burden in acute hypoxic ischaemic encephalopathy (Low et al., 2012; Orbach et al., 2013; Glass et al., 2014). However, despite advances in understanding of the neonatal brain, we remain limited in our choice of AEDs. Further questions also remain, not least when are we required to treat (at risk vs overt seizures) should we treat the EEG vs clinical seizures, and does treatment actually make a difference to longer term outcome? There is still a requirement for a concerted effort at consistency to treatment utilising the least toxic agents, with standardized collection of relevant clinical therapeutic information.

In 2011 a working group, with collaborators from the ILAE, the International Bureau of Epilepsy (IBE), the World Health Organisation (WHO) and the Institute for Research on Mental Retardation and Brain Aging (IRCCS), completed a document on the "Guidelines on Neonatal Seizures" (<http://apps.who.int/iris/bitstream/10665/77756/1/9789241548304_eng.pdf>).

The guidelines were intended for use by all health care professionals who may be part of the management of neonates with seizures. The aim of the document was to ensure that there was relevance for those based in primary through to tertiary settings.

Eleven key questions were identified, two of which related to epidemiology and aetiologies of neonatal seizures and the remainder considered priority issues in the management of neonatal seizures. The Grading of Recommendations Assessment, Development, and Evaluation (GRADE) approach was used to analysis the quality of the evidence supporting a recommendation (Atkins et al., 2004a).

From the management recommendations produced, there was strong evidence to support that seizures in neonates should be treated if they lasted longer than 3 minutes or were recurrent. There was strong evidence to support that electrical seizures should also be treated, it was acknowledged that this would be a major resource limitation since few centres would have access to EEG monitoring technology. However, putting the statement in this context remains extremely important to enable centres to refer to it when motivating for expanded and improved capacity to deliver care. These findings have been further supported by subsequent well designed studies and are described in more detail in chapter "Clinical and electrographical neonatal seizures – To treat or not treat" (Kontio et al., 2013; van Rooij et al., 2010). There was strong evidence to support that all clinical seizures should be confirmed by an electroencephalogram but that other investigations should be performed only to attempt to confirm the underlying aetiology in the neonate with seizures. As access to a EEG becomes more widely available detection of, and early intervention for, neonatal seizures should improve.

The document reported that all neonates should have hypoglycaemia excluded before antiepileptic drugs are instituted, this was supported by strong evidence. Since some centres may lack the capacity to screen for hypoglycaemia, in this setting empirical treatment was recommended, this was based more on expert opinion (common sense) as the level of evidence was weak. Where there were clinical signs suggestive of sepsis or meningitis, a lumbar puncture to exclude central nervous system infection was recommended, and where found, treatment with antibiotics commenced. But many centres, especially in resource poor countries, are unable to perform lumbar punctures, and in this case empirical treatment with antibiotics, in neonates suspected to have sepsis, or meningitis, was recommended, based on weak, context-specific evidence. There was strong evidence to support the screening of all neonates with seizures for hypocalcaemia, with correction of levels if confirmed. Initiation of pyridoxine treatment before commencing antiepileptic drugs was recommended, based on weak evidence, in the setting of exclusion of hypoglycaemia, hypocalcaemia, meningitis and other obvious causes for seizures, such as hypoxic ischaemic encephalopathy, in centres with the capacity to administer the treatment.

Phenobarbitone remained the first line agent recommended to treat neonatal seizures, and the document promoted that the agent should be readily available in all settings. This was supported by strong evidence but the quality of the studies (directness and consistency) was very low. However, this statement in the guidelines is extremely important as it can be used for lobbying in resource poor countries to ensure access to therapy is maintained.

Once the first intervention is attempted with optimal loading with phenobarbitone the management becomes more complex and there was little data to direct the next step in treatment. The recommendation had to be made based on weak evidence of a very low quality. The group suggested as second line intervention that either a benzodiazepine, phenytoin or lidocaine be administered. For the latter two they would need cardiac monitoring, but such monitoring equipment is rarely readily available in resource poor settings (Wilmshurst et al., 2011).

Those neonates with a normal neurological examination, and/or electroencephalogram, could have their antiepileptic drugs stopped if they had been seizure-free for greater than 72 hours. The importance of this statement highlighted that at this stage these neonates are not labelled as having epilepsy and as such should not require long-term antiepileptic drug therapy. The potential long-term sequelae of early high dose anti-epileptic drug usage is believed to influence the outcomes of brain maturation, and as a result the less medication administered the better (Bittigau et al., 2002; Forcelli et al., 2012). If further seizures occurred after removal of the AED then therapy could be recommenced. Based on the available literature this was supported as a weak statement based on a very low quality of evidence. This decision would be dependent on a trained health care professional being competent in the findings of a normal neonatal neurological examination of a normal neurological examination. Specific training in the normal neurodevelopmental milestones, and neurological findings, of neonates is lacking in many parts of the world. The latest data relating to the treatment of neonatal seizures with AEDs is addressed in chapter "Treatment of neonatal seizures with antiepileptic drugs".

Where seizures were controlled with a single AED, the therapy could be withdrawn abruptly without a reducing scale, for those on more than one agent the therapy could be stopped sequentially with phenobarbitone as the last agent to be removed. This recommendation was again more expert opinion from the group as the strength of evidence to support this common practice was weak. For neonates compromised by hypoxic ischaemic encephalopathy the practice in many units has been to give prophylactic phenobarbitone prior to any seizure occurrence, the group were able to confirm that this practice could not be supported based on strong strength of evidence and moderate quality of data.

As regards the role of radiological investigations, including ultrasound, computed tomography and magnetic resonance imaging, of the brain, the group concluded that these had no role in the identification of clinical seizures, or to evaluate the efficacy of treatment with antiepileptic drugs. There was strong evidence to support this. However, radiological investigations could be done as part of a comprehensive evaluation of the aetiology of neonatal seizures to assist with the prognostic assessment. This recommendation was based on a weak level of evidence. This area is covered in detail in chapter "Neuro-imaging in neonatal seizures".

This report provides a useful guide where there is a specific question to be addressed, where the clinician is experienced enough to source the data and as such is aware that it exists. However, for the average clinician in clinical practice the management of neonates with seizures is far more practical, and more likely to be based on the need for a clear directive of a step by step guide to optimal care. In most parts of the world, the locations where neonates with seizures will be managed, will be settings which lack key resources whereby many of the screening and interventions recommended are beyond the clinicians centre's capacity. The guideline written by Co *et al.* provides a more "user friendly" approach which follows the step by step approach, and is relevant to resource poor countries (Co *et al.*, 2007). Whilst the recommendations themselves are predominantly based on common practice and expert opinion the algorithms in the report may be considered are useful aids to practicing clinicians (*Figures 1-3*).

■ Optimal treatment for infantile seizures

Seizures in the infantile period have the highest incidence of all age groups with ranges of 90-212 per 100,000 of a population reported (Camfield *et al.*, 1996; Doose and Sitepu, 1983; Dura-Trave, Yoldi-Petri and Gallinas-Victoriano, 2008; Freitag *et al.*, 2001; Granieri *et al.*, 1983; Kurtz, Tookey and Ross, 1998; Olafsson *et al.*, 2005; Verity, Ross and Golding, 1992). Recognition of seizures in this population can be challenging. There are many mimics of seizures and it is important to consider and exclude these (Alam and Lux, 2012; Capovilla, 2011). However, the epilepsies in this age group remain amongst the most challenging to manage, with little evidence base with regard to AEDs, and many remaining difficult to treat with high rates of later comorbidity. This aside advances in our understanding of some aetiologies have given greater insight into a possible targeted treatments, *e.g.* ketogenic diet in GluT 1 transporter deficiency (*SLC2A1* mutations). Over time, genotype phenotype correlations are being clarified, so perhaps greater insight can be gained into specific treatments that may be useful (or contraindicated) in specific phenotypes. Ongoing from this, we need to clarify whether pre-treatment of infants at risk, *e.g.* tuberous sclerosis complex, post-hypoxia ischaemic encephalopathy utilising EEG markers, lead to improve longer term outcome, as well as the relative role of the concept of "epileptic encephalopathy" – how much can we really influence, *i.e.* improve, neurodevelopmental outcome?

Evidence based guidelines which clarify the optimal management of seizures in the infantile period do not exist, most are based on unit preferences and expert panel opinion. A committee was recruited in 2011 by the ILAE to review this, which consisted of child

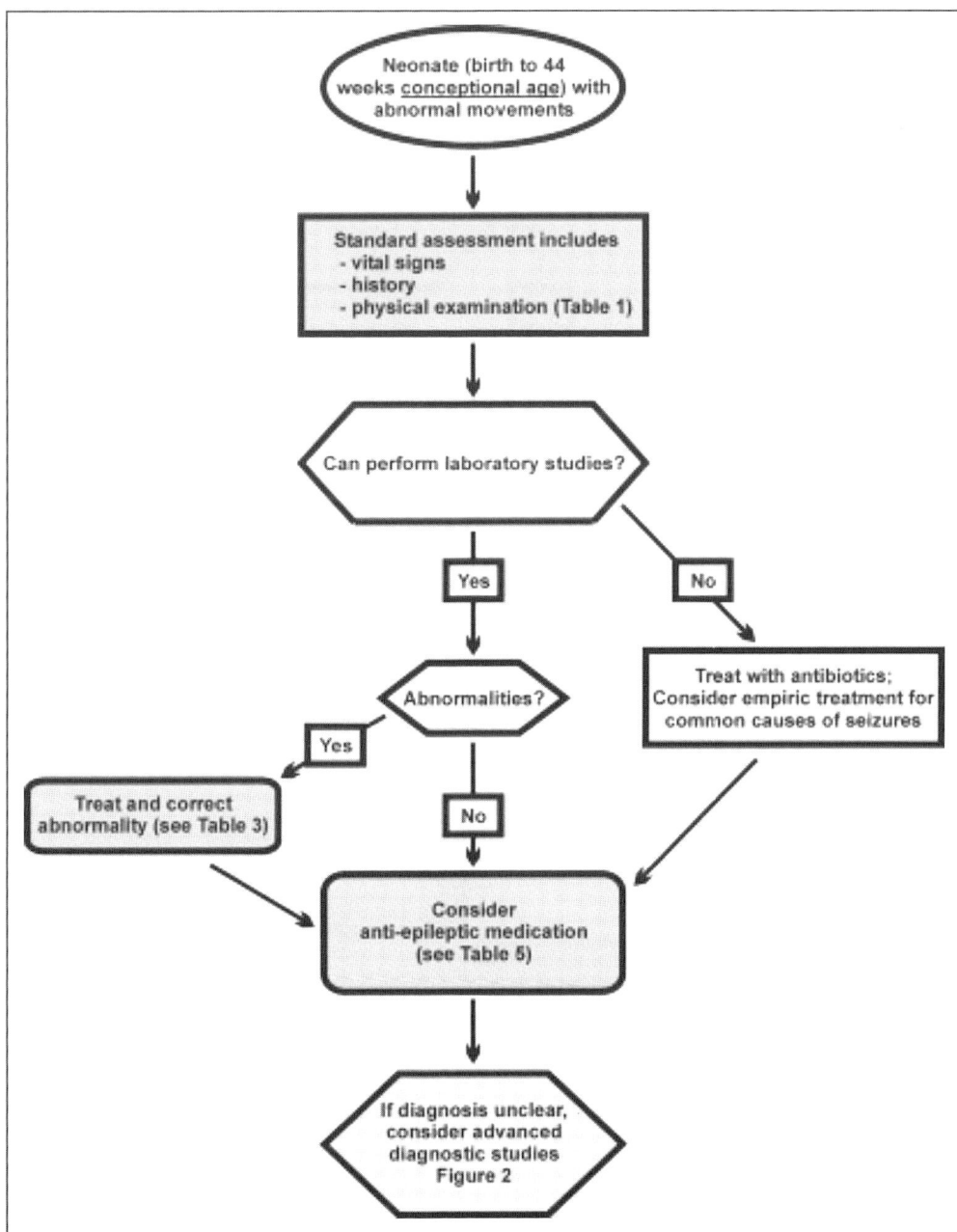

Figure 1. Proposal of an algorithm for diagnosis and treatment of neonatal seizures in developing countries. (According Co et al., 2007.)

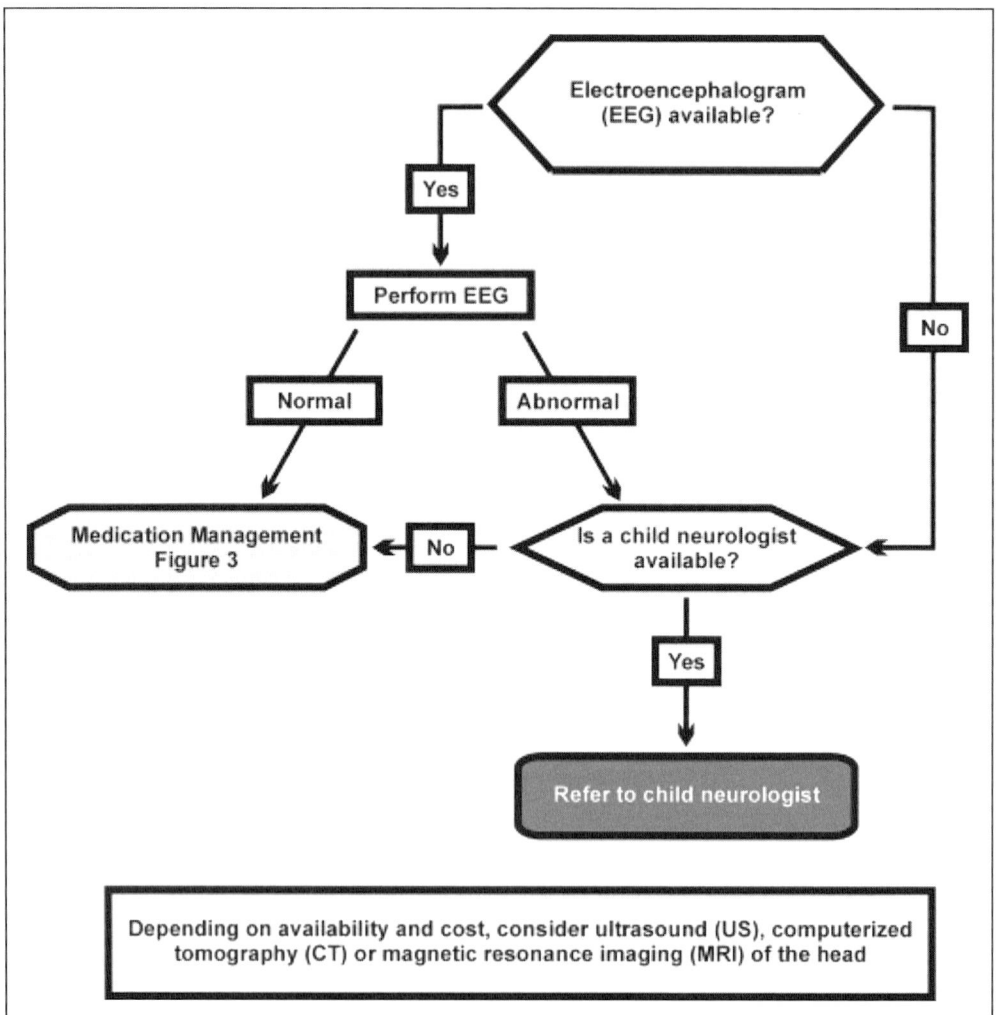

Figure 2. Proposal of an algorithm for diagnosis and treatment of neonatal seizures in developing countries. (According Co et al., 2007.)

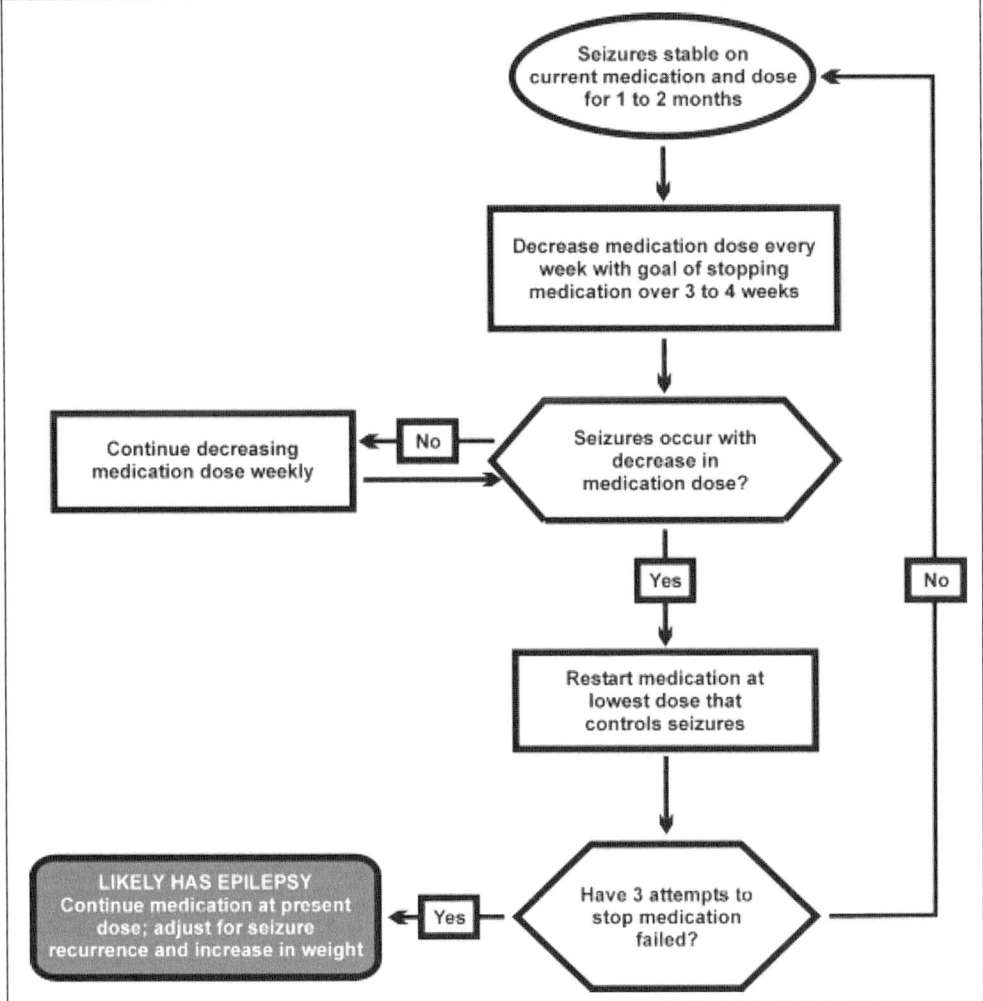

Figure 3. Proposal of an algorithm for diagnosis and treatment of neonatal seizures in developing countries. (According Co et al., 2007.)

neurologists with worldwide expertise. The aim would be to recommend a logical, and a viable, approach to the standard and the optimal management of the infant with seizures, wherever possible according to evidence based data.

Recommendations were graded as to the level of the evidence. Where no evidence was available the committee acknowledged that these recommendations were based on "expert opinion" and "standard practice". As per recommended practice, level of evidence was graded using a combination of the GRADE system and the American Academy of Neurology (AAN) Practice Parameters (Atkins et al., 2004b; Edlund et al., 2004; Gronseth and French, 2008). Comparison studies were assessed via the AAN practice parameters and descriptive studies via the GRADE system.

The committee formulated the recommendations under the headings of standard and optimal care, as would be recommended at primary/secondary and tertiary/quaternary facility level. Standard care was defined as the interventions which would be appropriate for all infants regardless of which centre they attended, and would equate to safe care. Specifically this was to address the challenges in resource poor countries (RPC). The committee were aware that some of these recommendations may be infrequently available in many RPCs. Children should be entitled to appropriate health care to enable them to reach their full potential. Without documenting the "standard" care for such infants, the centres providing care are left without a tool with which to lobby for improved facilities. The committee also developed the concept of optimal care, which was the "state of the art" management for infants with seizures considering progress made to date in defining aetiology, and optimising metabolic and AED care.

Diagnosis

Seizures presenting in between one month and 2 years of age were used as the inclusion age range. Febrile seizures (also refer to the chapter by Scheffer et al. page 205 of the present volume) and infantile spasms (also refer to the chapter by Nordli, page 213, of the present volume) were addressed in separate sections. The former because it is the most common seizure event to occur in the infantile period, the key factors relevant to the management of epilepsy in infants with febrile seizures were addressed. The latter, because it represented the major group in the epidemiology of epilepsy in the infantile period.

First steps in the clinical management would be to recognise an abnormal movement or behavior as an epileptic seizure, to characterise the type of seizure, and to make an electro-clinical diagnosis of a particular epileptic syndrome. It was recognized that patients should be referred from primary/secondary level (a centre able to provide basic clinical assessment – history, examination and interpretation –, baseline investigations – infection and electrolyte screens – and identification of an infant who would benefit from referral to the next level of care) to tertiary/quaternary level (centres with access to doctors with experience in the management of infants with epilepsy, with access to specific investigations relevant to understanding the etiology of the epilepsy and access to relevant extended AEDs and alternative treatments) after failure of one AED. It is hoped this system would then capture children treated with the incorrect agent or who have a complex form of epilepsy and from this that correct management may be offered without delay (Expert opinion, Level of evidence U). There is no data to support when an infant should commence regular AEDs. The likelihood of recurrence for non-provoked seizures is higher in the infantile period than for other age time periods (Hirtz et al., 1984; Shinnar et al., 1996) Certain epilepsy syndromes may have improved outcome if control of seizures is attained earlier, for example epileptic spasms and Dravet syndrome (Brunklaus et al., 2012). In an otherwise well infant, a policy of "wait and see" is reasonable after the first afebrile seizure. In reality this is a rare event, as such close monitoring is essential as the risk of recurrence is high in infants with epilepsy. At this stage, as a standard level of care, urgent referral to a specialist and plan to initiate therapy should be considered.

Simple febrile seizures (SFS) are the most common seizures in the first 2 years of life.

Children with complex/complicated febrile seizures (CFS) are defined as those infants with a focal, or prolonged seizure (of a duration greater than 15 minutes), or recurring within 24 hours (Berg and Shinnar, 1996; Capovilla et al., 2009). The clinician must differentiate from acute symptomatic seizures secondary to CNS infection or seizures triggered by fever in children with epilepsy. However, a seizure with fever can be the onset of an epilepsy syndrome. Examples are Dravet syndrome and epilepsy associated with *PCDH19* mutations.

Children with complex febrile seizures are at higher risk of developing epilepsy. There are trends to support the relationship between history of early prolonged FS or FS status, hippocampal sclerosis and the development of temporal lobe epilepsy. Although anti-epileptic drugs can prevent recurrent febrile seizures, they do not alter the risk of subsequent epilepsy. (Offringa and Newton, 2012). The association between FS and TLE probably results from complex interactions between several genetic and environmental factors (Hesdorffer et al., 2013). There is evidence to support that the intervention of prolonged FS (*i.e.*, longer than 10 minutes of seizing) with benzodiazepines will reduce the subsequent development of TLE. This is illustrated by the reduction of TLE/MTS in adults since this intervention has been used (expert opinion). Acute intervention at the time of SFS does not alter the subsequent development of epilepsy (Class 1 evidence). Antipyretic intervention does not affect the recurrence rate of subsequent FS (Class 1 evidence) (Baumann and Duffner, 2000).

There is no indication for initiation of prophylactic AEDs for SFS (Class 1 evidence). In the acute treatment it is important to treat seizures lasting 10 minutes or longer. Although initial management of these children is often at the primary or secondary level, infants with CFS should be regarded with a low threshold for referral to tertiary setting for further management and exclusion of underlying etiologies (level of evidence U, expert opinion).

An EEG record is recommended in the case of a paroxysmal event occurring in a child at this age (Eisermann et al., 2013; Flink et al., 2002) EEG is not helpful in the management of simple febrile seizures. EEG is a very important tool which can confirm a diagnosis and characterise a syndrome (including interictal and ictal patterns). In a facility with staff trained to perform and interpret EEG studies on infants, and with access to reliable equipment, data from such studies can be of great benefit to the management (also refer to the chapter by Bast, page 163 of the present volume).

In any child with undiagnosed repeated abnormal events, where EEG analysis has failed to delineate the condition, video EEG monitoring is recommended (Yu et al., 2013) This should be regarded as standard care at tertiary and quaternary level. At primary and secondary level carers are strongly encouraged to video events on home based systems such as cell phone devices (level of evidence U; expert opinion).

Neuroimaging is recommended at all levels of care for infants presenting with epilepsy (Gaillard et al., 2009; also refer to chapters by Weeke et al. (page 27) and Gaillard et al. (page 171), in the present volume). At a primary or secondary level of care optimal care would be MRI screening, but could be limited to CT scan imaging (standard care) (Eltze et al., 2013; Hsieh et al., 2010). At tertiary or quaternary level MRI is recommended as the standard investigation (level A) (Gaillard et al., 2009). Although inborn errors of metabolism are found in a relatively small proportion of patients with epilepsy, a significant proportion of patients with inborn errors of metabolism will experience regular epileptic seizures and consequently have a diagnosis of epilepsy. Metabolic disorders should therefore be considered in any infant who presents with a seizure disorder for which there is no structural explanation as the primary cause for the seizures, or who has unexplained electrolyte derangement, and who does not fulfil a known syndrome diagnosis (Bahi-Buisson et al., 2006; Surtees and Wolf, 2007). A number of metabolic conditions if identified early in the course can respond well to specific interventions (Wolf, Bast and Surtees, 2005). The level of evidence for the suggested screens in Tables I and II – weak recommendation, level B – based mainly on case reports and expert centre opinions. For interventions in any infant with suspected reversible metabolic disease, or with an acute clinical presentation empirical treatment should be initiated as soon as possible independently of disease confirmation (also refer to the chapter by Campistol and Plecko, page 105 of the present volume).

There is a role for genetic evaluation as part of optimal care in children where an aetiology for the epilepsy is not evident from preliminary investigation (also refer to chapters by Cilio (page 49), Fusco (page 61) and Lemke (page 95) of the present volume); a review of the benefits and risks of genetic testing in the field of epilepsies is represented by the Report of the ILAE Genetics Commission (Class IV: expert opinion) (Ottoman et al., 2010). Genetic counselling is defined as the process of helping people understand and adapt to the medical, psychological and familial implications of genetic contributions to disease. This process integrates the following: interpretation of family and medical histories to assess the chance of disease occurrence or recurrence; education about inheritance, testing, management, prevention, resources and research, counselling to promote informed choices and adaptation

Table I. Metabolic screens and interventions for infants with seizures

Primary/secondary levels of facilities	Tertiary/quaternary facilities
Standard practice:	Standard practice:
Glucose Basic haematological screening Liver function tests including ammonia, urine analysis pH and arterial blood gas, plasma electrolytes (sodium (Na), potassium (K), chloride (Cl) for anion gap measurement) CSF and plasma lactate CSF glucose (paired with blood glucose).	Amino acid and organic acid chromatography or tandem mass spectrometry Specific enzymatic studies and molecular quantifications Genetic workup Liver, skin, muscular and bone marrow biopsies
	Optimal practice
	Extended definitive markers to make genetic closure which enables disease severity to be predicted.
Standard practice:	Standard care:
Maintain adequate pH Hydro electrolyte balance High metabolic glucose flow Protein restriction	Disease specific treatments initiated
Refer tertiary center	
(where specific studies and interventions are possible).	

Table II. Metabolic screens for infants with hypoglycaemia and seizures

Primary/secondary levels of facilities	Tertiary quaternary facilities
Refer to tertiary for "work-up"	Standard practice
	Blood glucose
	β-hydroxybutrate
	Free fatty acids
	Lactate
	Amino acids
	Acyl-carnitine esters
	Ammonia
	Insulin
	Growth hormone
	Cortisol
	Urine ketones and organic acids

to the risk or condition (National Society of Genetic Counsellors' Definition Task Force et al., 2006). Basic training in genetic counselling is an important primary health care tool and access should be promoted with training in basic genetic understandings implemented.

Some resource equipped centres are able to routinely extend their genetic screening to explore underlying aetiologies for infants with infantile spasms without a known cause and other epileptic encephalopathies such as Ohtahara syndrome. Genetic screening should not be undertaken at a primary or secondary level of care. Standard care should permit genetic counselling by trained personnel to be undertaken at all levels of care (primary to quaternary). Early diagnosis of some mitochondrial conditions may alter long term outcome and as such there may be a case for such screening at quaternary level (level of evidence U, expert opinion).

Treatment

No data exists to assess the optimal initiating time and differing drug pharmacokinetics limit the capacity to set fixed guidelines of optimal dosages beyond the standard recommendations. Seizures in the infantile period often differ to other times of life as events may be more severe, aggressive and medically intractable. As such rapid initiation may be necessary for conditions such as epileptic spasms and Dravet syndrome (Brunklaus et al., 2012; Go et al., 2012). Rapid introduction of incremental AED doses should be considered for infantile epileptic encephalopathies. Treatment should be coordinated as standard practice through a tertiary/quaternary centre but introduction of therapy not delayed. Optimal tertiary care would permit the infant to remain as an in-patient or daily review to monitor the response to therapy acute (expert opinion; level of evidence U).

There is no high level evidence to support any of the current agents used. Most research is now focused on the newer generation AEDs. It is not possible to draw conclusions for AEDs used in RPC, e.g. phenobarbitone, phenytoin, valproate and carbamazepine. Even using evidence based studies there is frustratingly little in the literature to guide the optimal therapy for infants with different seizure types. Of concern agents such as phenobarbitone, the main agent most widely available and prescribed worldwide is rarely assessed in AED studies and even less so for those in the infantile period. Most studies are add-on methodology in patients with intractable focal onset epilepsy.

Owing to the lack of evidence relating to therapeutic interventions for the epilepsies in this age group a survey was sent to members of the ILAE, the International Child Neurology Association, the European Paediatric Neurology Society, the Child Neurology Society, the Asian and Oceanic Child Neurology Association and the Japanese Society of Child Neurology. The survey invited practitioners who regularly cared for children with neurological diseases to answer some simple questions relating to their standard day to day practice in the management of infants with seizures. Whilst this was not considered as a true evidence base, it was felt relevant to establish trends on a geographical level. Seven hundred and thirty three unique responses were captured from 96 different countries. Countries were grouped into geographical regions based on the World Bank (Europe and Central Asia, North America, South America and the Caribbean, Sub-Saharan Africa, North Africa and the Middle East, Asia and Oceania). Of the respondents 93% were either child neurologists or epileptologists.

Although some of the statements may assist guiding therapeutic decisions, the literature is incomplete and the range of studies do not comprehensively allow for strong recommendations to be made as to whether there is a role for the safe use of agents such as phenobarbitone, or whether a strong case should be made to motivate for second generation AEDs. With the advent of generics, the cost and availability of these agents will improve world-wide, but studies related to the efficacy of AEDs currently is directed based on pharmaceutical company needs and do not include agents such as phenobarbital. The summary of the evidence based data (graded *via* the AAN practice parameters) and the common practice results (gauged from the international survey) for AED prescribing for infants with seizures are documented in *Table III*.

Most centres recommend a slow incremental gradual approach to therapy with the lowest dose resulting in the best seizure control and the least side effects. There is no data to support the optimal duration of time required for treatment of an infant with epilepsy. Decisions are situation and epilepsy type specific. From the survey this was divided according to seizure type. For focal seizures occurring in infants most regions would medicate for 2 years before consideration of weaning, a quarter of North American respondents would consider weaning at 3-6 months. The need to be situation specific in the decision to wean medication was noted *i.e.* according to structural changes, persistent EEG changes, developmental status, etc. For generalized seizures the majority of respondents from all regions recommended 2 years medication before weaning. Other most likely options were "situation specific" and considering weaning at 3-6 months (especially Oceania). For infants with myoclonic seizures, most regions suggested 2 years seizure free before weaning AEDs, although there was some variation across regions. With regard to Dravet syndrome, 60% of respondents accepted that therapy was most likely lifelong and about 30% referred to the 2 year therapy trial.

For infants with epileptic spasms, the suggestions from Europe varied greatly from a short course of ACTH to lifelong therapy, this was often situation specific but even adjusting for this there was very little consistency apparent. Respondents from North America were more decisive; half opted for 3 to 6 months of AEDs and a number supported a shorter course (2-10 weeks).

With regard to other interventions for infants with epilepsy there is insufficient evidence to determine if a ketogenic diet is effective and safe in general or when differentiated dependent on seizure types and syndromes (also refer to the chapter by Coppola, page 235 of the present volume). Conversely, KD is the treatment of choice for the glucose

Table III. Summary of Evidence based (graded via the AAN practice parameters) and common practice (gauged from an international survey) AEDs prescribed for infants with seizures

Seizure type	Evidence based data supporting efficacy	Survey (common practice) Overall (Regional deviations)	Survey Second line (Regional deviations)	Survey Third line (Regional deviations)	Comment
Focal seizures	Levetiracetam effective	Overall: CBZ/oxcarbamezepine (N. America: Levetiracetam)	levetiracetam (28%) valproate (20%)		
Generalized seizures	levetiracetam, sodium valproate, lamotrigine, topiramate clobazam possibly effective, weak evidence	Overall: Valproate (North America: (63%) Oceania levetiracetam)	Levetiracetam (N. America Topiramate)		
Myoclonic seizures	NA	Valproate (Oceania/ North America benzodiazepines)	Benzodiazepines Levetiracetam		Vitamin replacement trials Exclusion of mitochondrial pathology
Severe myoclonic epilepsy of infancy	Stiripentol, strong evidence topiramate, zonisamide, sodium valproate, bromide ketogenic diet, weak evidence Exacerbation of seizures lamotrigine, carbamazepine phenytoin strong evidence	Valproate (North America Levetiracetam or valproate)	Europe: Clobazam or clonazepam Other regions clobazam/ clonazepam, levetiracetam, valproate, topiramate	Europe/Oceania Topiramate Other regions Levetiracetam Topiramate	Consider also stiripentol, ketogenic diet bromides/sulthiam. Many use stiripentol between 1st and 3rd line.
Epileptic spasms	Steroids/ACTH Strong evidence Vigabatrin for Tuberous sclerosis complex Strong evidence	ACTH	Vigabatrin		Aetiology driven i.e. different practice in the setting of TSC
Ohtahara syndrome	Poorly controlled topiramate, conventional AEDs, ACTH, prednisolone pyridoxine weak evidence				

transporter 1 deficiency syndrome (Glut1 DS) and pyruvate dehydrogenase deficiency (PDHD) (Freeman et al., 1998), both associated with cerebral energy failure (level 1). KD should be offered to infants with selected epileptic encephalopathies and a sub-set with medically refractory seizures at optimal level care at tertiary/quaternary facilities based on expert opinion and standard practice (level of evidence U).

There is insufficient data to conclude if there is a benefit from intervention with vagal nerve stimulation in infants with seizures. Infants with medically refractory seizures who are not suitable candidates for epilepsy surgery, may be considered for vagal nerve stimulation based on expert opinion and standard practice (Orosz et al., 2014). This would be optimal level care at tertiary/quaternary facilities.

Infants with focal onset seizures, particularly those with a unilateral structural brain abnormality, or those with persistent seizures despite two AEDs should be assessed in a specialist epilepsy unit with access to epilepsy surgery (Cross et al., 2006). The identification of patients as potential candidates for epilepsy surgery should be part of standard practice at primary/secondary level care, whilst the actual evaluation or detailed screening as to whether they could be an epilepsy surgery candidate is the role of tertiary/quaternary settings. Depending on the resources of the region this may be regarded as a standard level of care, whilst in resource limited settings this may be limited to an optimal level of care at quaternary level facilities only. The recommendation is that such interventions are only undertaken in facilities with appropriate capacity and experience to provide a safe level of care.

Epileptic spasms

No major studies have been published since the last Cochrane reviews on this topic (Hancock et al., 2008; Hancock et al., 2013). The American Academy of Neurology/ Practice committee of the Child Neurology Society have recently updated this data (Go et al., 2012). They concluded that when steroids were compared to ACTH, it was not possible to comment on which was the optimal therapy. Low-dose ACTH was found to be equally effective to high-dose ACTH. ACTH is more effective than vigabatrin in the short term, excluding patients with tuberous sclerosis. Early intervention results in better outcome (O'Callaghan et al., 2011).

Based on the most recent Cochrane review (Hancock, Osborne and Edwards, 2013) few well-designed RCTs have considered the treatment of infantile spasms, and the numbers of patients enrolled have been small. In the majority, methodology has been poor, hence it is not clear which treatment is optimal in the treatment of this epilepsy syndrome. Hormonal treatment resolves spasms in more infants than vigabatrin, but this may or may not translate into better long-term outcomes. If prednisolone or vigabatrin is used, high dosage is recommended. Vigabatrin may be the treatment of choice in tuberous sclerosis. Resolution of the EEG features may be important, but this has not been proven. Further research using large studies with robust methodology is required.

As regards the overall outcomes of infants with seizures current studies suggest, that epilepsy, autism, intellectual disability commonly co-exist. In addition, these recent studies suggest that early onset seizures may index a group of infants at high risk for developing autism, usually with associated intellectual deficits. Screening for Autism Spectrum Disorders, as recommended by the American Academy of Pediatrics (American Academy of Pediatrics Council on Children With Disabilities, 2007) in this high-risk population is strongly suggested.

Overall certain concepts at this stage can be agreed in the management of seizures with onset in infancy, not least in our ability to diagnose and monitor such infants, our ability to increasingly diagnose the clause, and to target treatment in some infants. However, there remains a fair bit to unravel, not least how we constructively go about increasing our evidence base for practice. We need to unify our practice for data collection, in order to delineate further phenotype and treatment response as well as utilise newer methodologies to study response in this group of patients.

■ Do guidelines have a role in the management of neonatal and infantile seizures?

The aim of guidelines should be to enable informed decisions and to improve outcomes. However many existing guidelines are based on anecdotal preferences and the views of "expert panels". Even those with apparent evidence based approaches, when screened by tools such as Appraisal of Guidelines for Research and Evaluation (AGREE), are found to be lacking (www.agreetrust.org). However, the lack of well-designed studies in the neonatal and the infantile age groups results in major gaps in management when only implementation based only on level 1 evidence is taken.

Most RCTs are driven by pharmaceutical companies and focus on the newer generation agents. There are few comparative studies with phenobarbitone or phenytoin specifically in neonatal seizures and no useful studies for phenobarbitone *versus* these newer generation AEDs. As such most guidelines are more recommendations based largely on "expert opinion" and common practice. The "informed decisions" we are given are driven by evidence based medicine established from the current pool of RCTs. They do not necessarily reflect the optimal intervention, or the day to day clinical situations, and challenges most clinicians are working with.

In many resource poor countries (RPCs) guidelines are impossible to follow. Management is based on the assumption that the diagnosis of epilepsy is accurately made. In a Kenyan study 89% of children in a community survey, who were found to have epilepsy, had either not been diagnosed with the disease, or were not receiving medication (Mung'ala-Odera et al., 2008). That in itself is challenging due to the lack of clinical skills (training) in RPC and the recommendations for use of scare tools such as EEG. The recommended AEDs are not available, or supply is unreliable, with a treatment gap reported in rural areas of RPCs of 73.3%, and in urban regions of 46.8% (Mbuba et al., 2008; Wilmshurst et al., 2011). Health care workers are not equipped to manage neonates or infants presenting with seizures, they often have no knowledge of how to recognize a seizure or what and when to initiate an AED. This potentially leads to a two tiered system of practice and recommendations, one for equipped and the other for resource poor settings. This is ethically wrong, and places such children at an unacceptable disadvantage.

Completing guidelines are totally pointless if they are not circulated, read, and widely available. Many doctors are unaware of published guidelines (Wilmshurst et al., 2013). Most health care workers in RPCs, where most people with epilepsy reside, have no access to guidelines, or do not believe they are of relevance to them (Wilmshurst et al., 2013). As a result, however, good the guideline, it is pointless unless it is read and understood by the health care worker.

Effective strategies to promote the use of recommendations by decision-makers (clinicians, public health officers, policymakers) are important (Fretheim et al., 2006) Use of educational materials, educational meetings, consensus processes, educational outreach, opinion leaders, patient-directed interventions, audit and feedback, reminders, recruitment of other professionals (mass media and marketing), financial interventions, organizational interventions, structural interventions and regulatory interventions should be part of the on-going process (Grimshaw et al., 2004).

Effective guidelines require local adaptation, implementation, impact assessment, and program revision (Katchanov and Birbeck, 2012). Sociocultural and financial barriers that impede the implementation of the guidelines should be identified and ameliorated. Strong advocacy for guideline adoption by health authorities at the national, provincial, district, and institutional levels are required. Collaborations with local stake-holders, i.e., traditional healers, are essential in developing programs and program-evaluation processes. Barriers at the patient, healthcare worker and macro level threaten the implementation of guidelines.

For better results from the integration of guidelines it would be more effective to look at the best standard management for the specific clinical setting, to make recommendations approachable, viable and relevant and to highlight where this is based on expert opinion and common practice. The simpler a guideline can be the better. Once in place the outcomes must be measured through audit of practice and an assessment of consistent practice in different settings. There should be caution of fixed guidelines, as these can have disastrous effects for lobbying capacity if they do not allow for capacity building.

The need to be more flexible with guidelines, especially in resource poor settings, where incorporation of lower quality evidence, adapting existing guidelines to be in-line with local capacity and building on these approaches to improve care has been proposed (English and Opiyo, 2011). Most guidelines are carefully formulated at an expert level by highly qualified specialists, skilled in performing meta-analyses of relevant data. Whilst this generates the "pure" form of the literature assessment, these guides must be adapted at each local level to be truly relevant and useful, and to be actually used by the working practitioner.

References

- Alam S, Lux AL. Epilepsies in infancy. *Arch Dis Child* 2012; 97: 985-92.
- Atkins D, Best D, Briss PA, et al. Grading quality of evidence and strength of recommendations. *BMJ* 2004a; 328: 1490.
- Bahi-Buisson N, Mention K, Leger PL, et al. Neonatal epilepsy and inborn errors of metabolism. *Arch Pediatrie* 2006; 13: 284-92.
- Baumann RJ, Duffner PK. Treatment of children with simple febrile seizures: the AAP practice parameter. American Academy of Pediatrics. *Pediatr Neurol* 2000; 23: 11-7.
- Berg AT, Shinnar S. Complex febrile seizures. *Epilepsia* 1996; 37: 126-33.
- Bittigau P, Sifringer M, Genz K, et al. Antiepileptic drugs and apoptotic neurodegeneration in the developing brain. *Proc Natl Acad Sci USA* 2002; 99: 15089-94.
- Brunklaus A, Ellis R, Reavey E, Forbes GH, Zuberi SM. Prognostic, clinical and demographic features in SCN1A mutation-positive Dravet syndrome. *Brain* 2012; 135: 2329-36.

- Camfield CS, Camfield PR, Gordon K, Wirrell E, Dooley JM. Incidence of epilepsy in childhood and adolescence: a population-based study in Nova Scotia from 1977 to 1985. *Epilepsia* 1996; 37: 19-23.
- Capovilla G. Shaking body attacks: a new type of benign non-epileptic attack in infancy. *Epileptic Disord* 2011; 13: 140-4.
- Capovilla G, Mastrangelo M, Romeo A, Vigevano F. Recommendations for the management of "febrile seizures": Ad Hoc Task Force of LICE Guidelines Commission. *Epilepsia* 2009; 50 (suppl 1): 2-6.
- Chugani HAT, Conti JR. Etiologic classification of infantile spasms in 140 cases: role of positron emission tomography. *J Child Neurol* 1996; 11: 44-8.
- Chugani HT, Shields WD, Shewmon DA, Olson DM, Phelps ME, Peacock WJ. Infantile spasms: I. PET identifies focal cortical dysgenesis in cryptogenic cases for surgical treatment. *Ann Neurol* 1990; 27: 406-13.
- Co JP, Elia M, Engel J Jr, *et al.* Proposal of an algorithm for diagnosis and treatment of neonatal seizures in developing countries. *Epilepsia* 2007; 48: 1158-64.
- Cross JH, Jayakar P, Nordli D, *et al.* Proposed criteria for referral and evaluation of children for epilepsy surgery: recommendations of the Subcommission for Pediatric Epilepsy Surgery. *Epilepsia* 2006; 47: 952-9.
- Doose H, Sitepu B. Childhood epilepsy in a German city. *Neuropediatrics* 1983; 14: 220-4.
- Dunkley C, Cross JH. NICE guidelines and the epilepsies: how should practice change? *Arch Dis Child* 2006; 91: 525-8.
- Dura-Trave T, Yoldi-Petri ME, Gallinas-Victoriano F. Incidence of epilepsies and epileptic syndromes among children in Navarre, Spain: 2002 through 2005. *J Child Neurol* 2008; 23: 878-82.
- Edlund W, Gronseth G, So Y, Franklin G (eds). *Clinical Practice Guideline Process Manual.* St Paul: American Academy of Neurology, 2004.
- Eisermann M, Kaminska A, Moutard ML, Soufflet C, Plouin P. Normal EEG in childhood: from neonates to adolescents. *Clin Neurophysiol* 2013; 43: 35-65.
- Eltze CM, Chong WK, Cox T, *et al.* A population-based study of newly diagnosed epilepsy in infants. *Epilepsia* 2013; 54: 437-45.
- English M, Opiyo N. Getting to grips with GRADE-perspective from a low-income setting. *J Clin Epidemiol* 2011; 64: 708-10.
- Flink R, Pedersen B, Guekht AB, *et al.* Guidelines for the use of EEG methodology in the diagnosis of epilepsy. International League Against Epilepsy: commission report. Commission on European Affairs: Subcommission on European Guidelines. *Acta Neurol Scand* 2002; 106: 1-7.
- Forcelli PA, Janssen MJ, Vicini S, Gale K. Neonatal exposure to antiepileptic drugs disrupts striatal synaptic development. *Ann Neurol* 2012; 72: 363-72.
- Freeman JM, Vining EP, Pillas DJ, *et al.* The efficacy of the ketogenic diet-1998: a prospective evaluation of intervention in 150 children. *Pediatrics* 1998; 102: 1358-63.
- Freitag CM, May TW, Pfafflin M, Konig S, Rating D. Incidence of epilepsies and epileptic syndromes in children and adolescents: a population-based prospective study in Germany. *Epilepsia* 2001; 42: 979-85.
- Fretheim A, Schunemann HJ, Oxman AD. Improving the use of research evidence in guideline development: 15. Disseminating and implementing guidelines. *BioMed Central* 2006; 4: 27.
- Gaillard WD, Chiron C, Cross JH, *et al.* and ILAE, Committee for Neuroimaging, Subcommittee for Pediatric. Guidelines for imaging infants and children with recent-onset epilepsy. *Epilepsia* 2009; 50: 2147-53.
- Glass HC, Wusthoff CJ, Shellhaas RA, *et al.* Risk factors for EEG seizures in neonates treated with hypothermia: A multicenter cohort study. *Neurology* 2014 [Epub ahead of print].

- Glauser T, Ben-Menachem E, Bourgeois B, *et al*. Updated ILAE evidence review of antiepileptic drug efficacy and effectiveness as initial monotherapy for epileptic seizures and syndromes. *Epilepsia* 2013; 54: 551-63.
- Go CY, Mackay MT, Weiss SK, Child Neurology Society, *et al*. Evidence-based guideline update: medical treatment of infantile spasms. Report of the Guideline Development Subcommittee of the American Academy of Neurology and the Practice Committee of the Child Neurology Society. *Neurology* 2012; 78: 1974-80.
- Granieri E, Rosati G, Tola R, *et al*. A descriptive study of epilepsy in the district of Copparo, Italy, 1964-1978. *Epilepsia* 1983; 24: 502-14.
- Grimshaw J, Eccles M, Tetroe J.Implementing clinical guidelines: current evidence and future implications. *J Contin Educ Health Prof* 2004; 24 (suppl 1): S31-7.
- Gronseth G, French J. Practice parameters and technology assessments: what they are, what they are not, and why you should care. *Neurology* 2008; 71: 1639-43.
- Hancock EC, Osborne JP, Edwards SW. Treatment of infantile spasms. *Cochrane Database Syst Rev* 2013; 6: CD001770.
- Hattori J, Ouchida M, Ono J, *et al*. A screening test for the prediction of Dravet syndrome before one year of age. *Epilepsia* 2008; 49: 626-33.
- Hesdorffer DC, Shinnar S, Lewis DV, *et al*. Risk Factors for Febrile Status Epilepticus: A Case-Control Study. *J Pediatr* 2013; 163: 1147-51.
- Hirtz DG, Ellenberg JH, Nelson KB. The risk of recurrence of nonfebrile seizures in children. *Neurology* 1984; 34: 637-41.
- Hsieh DT, Chang T, Tsuchida TN, *et al*. New-onset afebrile seizures in infants: role of neuroimaging. *Neurology* 2010; 74: 150-6.
- Johnson CP, Myers SM, American Academy of Pediatrics Council on Children With Disabilities. Identification and evaluation of children with autism spectrum disorders. *Pediatrics* 2007; 120: 1183-215.
- Katchanov J, Birbeck GL. Epilepsy care guidelines for low- and middle- income countries: From WHO mental health GAP to national programs. *BMC medicine* 2012; 10.
- Kontio T, Toet MC, Hellstrom-Westas L, *et al*. Early neurophysiology and MRI in predicting neurological outcome at 9-10 years after birth asphyxia. *Clin Neurophysiol* 2013; 124: 1089-94.
- Korff CM, Nordli DR, Jr. The clinical-electrographic expression of infantile seizures. *Epilepsy Res* 2006; 70 (suppl 1): S116-31.
- Kurtz Z, Tookey P, Ross E. Epilepsy in young people: 23 year follow up of the British national child development study. *BMJ* 1998; 316: 339-42.
- Low E, Boylan GB, Mathieson SR, *et al*. Cooling and seizure burden in term neonates: an observational study. *Arch Dis Child Fetal Neonatal Ed*. 2012; 97 (suppl 4): F267-72.
- Lux AL, Edwards SW, Hancock E, *et al*. The United Kingdom Infantile Spasms Study (UKISS) comparing hormone treatment with vigabatrin on developmental and epilepsy outcomes to age 14 months: a multicentre randomised trial. *Lancet Neurol* 2005; 4: 712-7.
- Mbuba CK, Ngugi AK, Newton CR, Carter JA. The epilepsy treatment gap in developing countries: a systematic review of the magnitude, causes, and intervention strategies. *Epilepsia* 2008; 49: 1491-503.
- Mung'ala-Odera V, White S, Meehan R, *et al*. Prevalence, incidence and risk factors of epilepsy in older children in rural Kenya. *Seizure* 2008; 17: 396-404.
- National Society of Genetic Counselors' Definition Task Force. A new definition of Genetic Counseling: National Society of Genetic Counselors' Task Force report. *J Genet Counsel* 2006; 15: 77-83.
- O'Callaghan FJ, Lux AL, Darke K, *et al*. The effect of lead time to treatment and of age of onset on developmental outcome at 4 years in infantile spasms: evidence from the United Kingdom Infantile Spasms Study. *Epilepsia* 2011; 52: 1359-64.

- Offringa M, Newton R. Prophylactic drug management for febrile seizures in children. *Cochrane Database System Reviews* 2011; 4: CD003031.
- Olafsson E, Ludvigsson P, Gudmundsson G, *et al*. Incidence of unprovoked seizures and epilepsy in Iceland and assessment of the epilepsy syndrome classification: a prospective study. *Lancet Neurol* 2005; 4: 627-34.
- Orbach SA, Bonifacio SL, Kuzniewicz MW, Glass HC. Lower incidence of seizure among neonates treated with therapeutic hypothermia. *J Child Neurol* 2014; 29: 1502-7.
- Orosz I, McCormick D, Zamponi N, *et al*. Vagus nerve stimulation for drug-resistant epilepsy: a European long-term study up to 24 months in 347 children. *Epilepsia* 2014; 55(10): 1576-84.
- Ottman R, Hirose S, Jain S, *et al*. Genetic testing in the epilepsies--report of the ILAE Genetics Commission. *Epilepsia* 2010; 51: 655-70.
- Shinnar S, Berg AT, Moshe SL, *et al*. The risk of seizure recurrence after a first unprovoked afebrile seizure in childhood: an extended follow-up. *Pediatrics* 1996; 98 (2 Pt 1): 216-25.
- Surtees R, Wolf N. Treatable neonatal epilepsy. *Arch Disease Child* 2007; 92: 659-61.
- van Rooij LG, Toet MC, van Huffelen AC, *et al*. Effect of treatment of subclinical neonatal seizures detected with aEEG: randomized, controlled trial. *Pediatrics* 2010; 125: e358-66.
- Verity CM, Ross EM, Golding J. Epilepsy in the first 10 years of life: findings of the child health and education study. *BMJ* 1992; 305: 857-61.
- Wilmshurst JM, Badoe E, Wammanda RD, *et al*. Child neurology services in Africa. *J Child Neurol* 2011; 26: 1555-63.
- Wilmshurst JM, Cross JH, Newton C, *et al*. Children with epilepsy in Africa: recommendations from the international child neurology association/african child neurology association workshop. *J Child Neurol* 2013; 28: 633-44.
- Wolf NI, Bast T, Surtees R. Epilepsy in inborn errors of metabolism. *Epileptic Disord* 2005; 7: 67-81.
- Yu HJ, Lee CG, Nam SH, Lee J, Lee M. Clinical and ictal characteristics of infantile seizures: EEG correlation *via* long-term video EEG monitoring. *Brain Dev* 2013; 35:771-7.

IMPRIM'VERT®

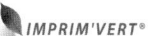

Achevé d'imprimer par　　Corlet, Imprimeur, S.A.
14110 Condé-sur-Noireau
N° d'Imprimeur : 169039 - Dépôt légal : mars 2015

Imprimé en France